FREE Study Skills Videos/DVD Offer

Dear Customer,

Thank you for your purchase from Mometrix! We consider it an honor and a privilege that you have purchased our product and we want to ensure your satisfaction.

As a way of showing our appreciation and to help us better serve you, we have developed Study Skills Videos that we would like to give you for FREE. These videos cover our *best practices* for getting ready for your exam, from how to use our study materials to how to best prepare for the day of the test.

All that we ask is that you email us with feedback that would describe your experience so far with our product. Good, bad, or indifferent, we want to know what you think!

To get your FREE Study Skills Videos, you can use the **QR code** below, or send us an **email** at studyvideos@mometrix.com with *FREE VIDEOS* in the subject line and the following information in the body of the email:

- The name of the product you purchased.
- Your product rating on a scale of 1-5, with 5 being the highest rating.
- Your feedback. It can be long, short, or anything in between. We just want to know your impressions and experience so far with our product. (Good feedback might include how our study material met your needs and ways we might be able to make it even better. You could highlight features that you found helpful or features that you think we should add.)

If you have any questions or concerns, please don't hesitate to contact me directly.

Thanks again!

Sincerely,

Jay Willis
Vice President
jay.willis@mometrix.com
1-800-673-8175

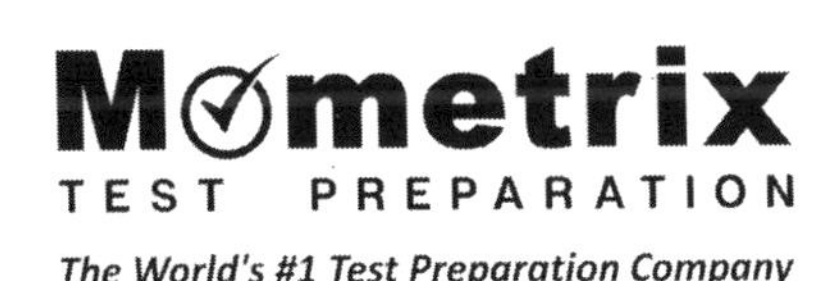

Adult-Gerontology CNS Exam

SECRETS

Study Guide

Your Key to Exam Success

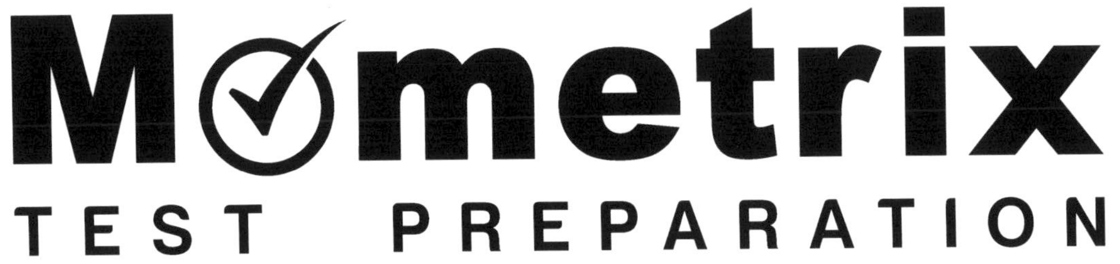

Written and edited by the Mometrix Nurse Specialist Certification Test Team

Printed in the United States of America

This paper meets the requirements of ANSI/NISO Z39.48-1992 (Permanence of Paper).

Paperback
ISBN 13: 978-1-63094-286-1
ISBN 10: 1-63094-286-3

Ebook
ISBN 13: 978-1-5167-0234-3
ISBN 10: 1-5167-0234-4

Hardback
ISBN 13: 978-1-5167-1148-2
ISBN 10: 1-5167-1148-3

DEAR FUTURE EXAM SUCCESS STORY

First of all, **THANK YOU** for purchasing Mometrix study materials!

Second, congratulations! You are one of the few determined test-takers who are committed to doing whatever it takes to excel on your exam. **You have come to the right place.** We developed these study materials with one goal in mind: to deliver you the information you need in a format that's concise and easy to use.

In addition to optimizing your guide for the content of the test, we've outlined our recommended steps for breaking down the preparation process into small, attainable goals so you can make sure you stay on track.

We've also analyzed the entire test-taking process, identifying the most common pitfalls and showing how you can overcome them and be ready for any curveball the test throws you.

Standardized testing is one of the biggest obstacles on your road to success, which only increases the importance of doing well in the high-pressure, high-stakes environment of test day. Your results on this test could have a significant impact on your future, and this guide provides the information and practical advice to help you achieve your full potential on test day.

Your success is our success

We would love to hear from you! If you would like to share the story of your exam success or if you have any questions or comments in regard to our products, please contact us at **800-673-8175** or **support@mometrix.com**.

Thanks again for your business and we wish you continued success!

Sincerely,
The Mometrix Test Preparation Team

Need more help? Check out our flashcards at:
http://mometrixflashcards.com/CNS

TABLE OF CONTENTS

Introduction

Thank you for purchasing this resource! You have made the choice to prepare yourself for a test that could have a huge impact on your future, and this guide is designed to help you be fully ready for test day. Obviously, it's important to have a solid understanding of the test material, but you also need to be prepared for the unique environment and stressors of the test, so that you can perform to the best of your abilities.

For this purpose, the first section that appears in this guide is the **Secret Keys**. We've devoted countless hours to meticulously researching what works and what doesn't, and we've boiled down our findings to the five most impactful steps you can take to improve your performance on the test. We start at the beginning with study planning and move through the preparation process, all the way to the testing strategies that will help you get the most out of what you know when you're finally sitting in front of the test.

We recommend that you start preparing for your test as far in advance as possible. However, if you've bought this guide as a last-minute study resource and only have a few days before your test, we recommend that you skip over the first two Secret Keys since they address a long-term study plan.

If you struggle with **test anxiety**, we strongly encourage you to check out our recommendations for how you can overcome it. Test anxiety is a formidable foe, but it can be beaten, and we want to make sure you have the tools you need to defeat it.

Secret Key #1 – Plan Big, Study Small

There's a lot riding on your performance. If you want to ace this test, you're going to need to keep your skills sharp and the material fresh in your mind. You need a plan that lets you review everything you need to know while still fitting in your schedule. We'll break this strategy down into three categories.

Information Organization

Start with the information you already have: the official test outline. From this, you can make a complete list of all the concepts you need to cover before the test. Organize these concepts into groups that can be studied together, and create a list of any related vocabulary you need to learn so you can brush up on any difficult terms. You'll want to keep this vocabulary list handy once you actually start studying since you may need to add to it along the way.

Time Management

Once you have your set of study concepts, decide how to spread them out over the time you have left before the test. Break your study plan into small, clear goals so you have a manageable task for each day and know exactly what you're doing. Then just focus on one small step at a time. When you manage your time this way, you don't need to spend hours at a time studying. Studying a small block of content for a short period each day helps you retain information better and avoid stressing over how much you have left to do. You can relax knowing that you have a plan to cover everything in time. In order for this strategy to be effective though, you have to start studying early and stick to your schedule. Avoid the exhaustion and futility that comes from last-minute cramming!

Study Environment

The environment you study in has a big impact on your learning. Studying in a coffee shop, while probably more enjoyable, is not likely to be as fruitful as studying in a quiet room. It's important to keep distractions to a minimum. You're only planning to study for a short block of time, so make the most of it. Don't pause to check your phone or get up to find a snack. It's also important to **avoid multitasking**. Research has consistently shown that multitasking will make your studying dramatically less effective. Your study area should also be comfortable and well-lit so you don't have the distraction of straining your eyes or sitting on an uncomfortable chair.

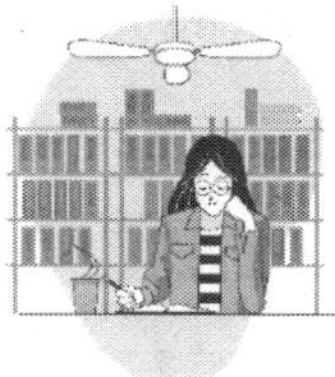

The time of day you study is also important. You want to be rested and alert. Don't wait until just before bedtime. Study when you'll be most likely to comprehend and remember. Even better, if you know what time of day your test will be, set that time aside for study. That way your brain will be used to working on that subject at that specific time and you'll have a better chance of recalling information.

Finally, it can be helpful to team up with others who are studying for the same test. Your actual studying should be done in as isolated an environment as possible, but the work of organizing the information and setting up the study plan can be divided up. In between study sessions, you can discuss with your teammates the concepts that you're all studying and quiz each other on the details. Just be sure that your teammates are as serious about the test as you are. If you find that your study time is being replaced with social time, you might need to find a new team.

Secret Key #2 – Make Your Studying Count

You're devoting a lot of time and effort to preparing for this test, so you want to be absolutely certain it will pay off. This means doing more than just reading the content and hoping you can remember it on test day. It's important to make every minute of study count. There are two main areas you can focus on to make your studying count.

Retention

It doesn't matter how much time you study if you can't remember the material. You need to make sure you are retaining the concepts. To check your retention of the information you're learning, try recalling it at later times with minimal prompting. Try carrying around flashcards and glance at one or two from time to time or ask a friend who's also studying for the test to quiz you.

To enhance your retention, look for ways to put the information into practice so that you can apply it rather than simply recalling it. If you're using the information in practical ways, it will be much easier to remember. Similarly, it helps to solidify a concept in your mind if you're not only reading it to yourself but also explaining it to someone else. Ask a friend to let you teach them about a concept you're a little shaky on (or speak aloud to an imaginary audience if necessary). As you try to summarize, define, give examples, and answer your friend's questions, you'll understand the concepts better and they will stay with you longer. Finally, step back for a big picture view and ask yourself how each piece of information fits with the whole subject. When you link the different concepts together and see them working together as a whole, it's easier to remember the individual components.

Finally, practice showing your work on any multi-step problems, even if you're just studying. Writing out each step you take to solve a problem will help solidify the process in your mind, and you'll be more likely to remember it during the test.

Modality

Modality simply refers to the means or method by which you study. Choosing a study modality that fits your own individual learning style is crucial. No two people learn best in exactly the same way, so it's important to know your strengths and use them to your advantage.

For example, if you learn best by visualization, focus on visualizing a concept in your mind and draw an image or a diagram. Try color-coding your notes, illustrating them, or creating symbols that will trigger your mind to recall a learned concept. If you learn best by hearing or discussing information, find a study partner who learns the same way or read aloud to yourself. Think about how to put the information in your own words. Imagine that you are giving a lecture on the topic and record yourself so you can listen to it later.

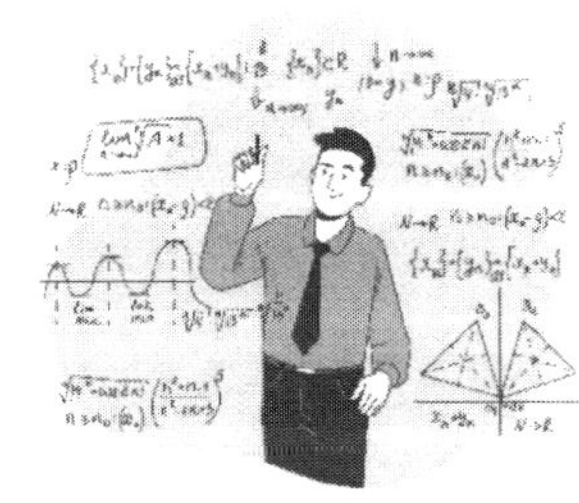

For any learning style, flashcards can be helpful. Organize the information so you can take advantage of spare moments to review. Underline key words or phrases. Use different colors for different categories. Mnemonic devices (such as creating a short list in which every item starts with the same letter) can also help with retention. Find what works best for you and use it to store the information in your mind most effectively and easily.

Secret Key #3 – Practice the Right Way

Your success on test day depends not only on how many hours you put into preparing, but also on whether you prepared the right way. It's good to check along the way to see if your studying is paying off. One of the most effective ways to do this is by taking practice tests to evaluate your progress. Practice tests are useful because they show exactly where you need to improve. Every time you take a practice test, pay special attention to these three groups of questions:

- The questions you got wrong
- The questions you had to guess on, even if you guessed right
- The questions you found difficult or slow to work through

This will show you exactly what your weak areas are, and where you need to devote more study time. Ask yourself why each of these questions gave you trouble. Was it because you didn't understand the material? Was it because you didn't remember the vocabulary? Do you need more repetitions on this type of question to build speed and confidence? Dig into those questions and figure out how you can strengthen your weak areas as you go back to review the material.

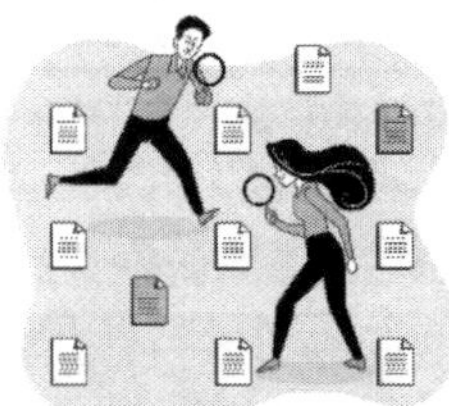

Additionally, many practice tests have a section explaining the answer choices. It can be tempting to read the explanation and think that you now have a good understanding of the concept. However, an explanation likely only covers part of the question's broader context. Even if the explanation makes perfect sense, **go back and investigate** every concept related to the question until you're positive you have a thorough understanding.

As you go along, keep in mind that the practice test is just that: practice. Memorizing these questions and answers will not be very helpful on the actual test because it is unlikely to have any of the same exact questions. If you only know the right answers to the sample questions, you won't be prepared for the real thing. **Study the concepts** until you understand them fully, and then you'll be able to answer any question that shows up on the test.

It's important to wait on the practice tests until you're ready. If you take a test on your first day of study, you may be overwhelmed by the amount of material covered and how much you need to learn. Work up to it gradually.

On test day, you'll need to be prepared for answering questions, managing your time, and using the test-taking strategies you've learned. It's a lot to balance, like a mental marathon that will have a big impact on your future. Like training for a marathon, you'll need to start slowly and work your way up. When test day arrives, you'll be ready.

Start with the strategies you've read in the first two Secret Keys—plan your course and study in the way that works best for you. If you have time, consider using multiple study resources to get different approaches to the same concepts. It can be helpful to see difficult concepts from more than one angle. Then find a good source for practice tests. Many times, the test website will suggest potential study resources or provide sample tests.

Practice Test Strategy

If you're able to find at least three practice tests, we recommend this strategy:

Untimed and Open-Book Practice

Take the first test with no time constraints and with your notes and study guide handy. Take your time and focus on applying the strategies you've learned.

Timed and Open-Book Practice

Take the second practice test open-book as well, but set a timer and practice pacing yourself to finish in time.

Timed and Closed-Book Practice

Take any other practice tests as if it were test day. Set a timer and put away your study materials. Sit at a table or desk in a quiet room, imagine yourself at the testing center, and answer questions as quickly and accurately as possible.

Keep repeating timed and closed-book tests on a regular basis until you run out of practice tests or it's time for the actual test. Your mind will be ready for the schedule and stress of test day, and you'll be able to focus on recalling the material you've learned.

Secret Key #4 – Pace Yourself

Once you're fully prepared for the material on the test, your biggest challenge on test day will be managing your time. Just knowing that the clock is ticking can make you panic even if you have plenty of time left. Work on pacing yourself so you can build confidence against the time constraints of the exam. Pacing is a difficult skill to master, especially in a high-pressure environment, so **practice is vital**.

Set time expectations for your pace based on how much time is available. For example, if a section has 60 questions and the time limit is 30 minutes, you know you have to average 30 seconds or less per question in order to answer them all. Although 30 seconds is the hard limit, set 25 seconds per question as your goal, so you reserve extra time to spend on harder questions. When you budget extra time for the harder questions, you no longer have any reason to stress when those questions take longer to answer.

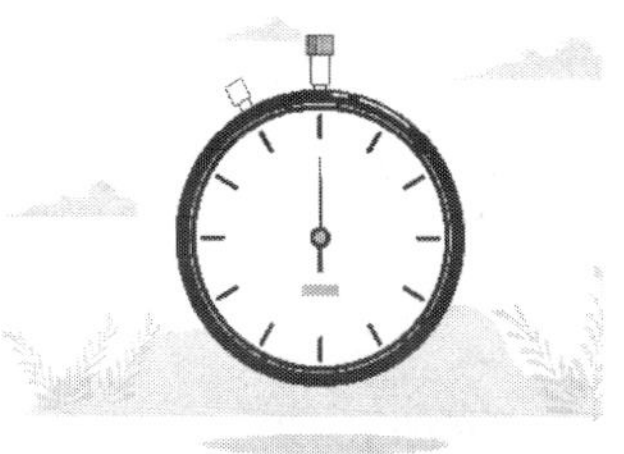

Don't let this time expectation distract you from working through the test at a calm, steady pace, but keep it in mind so you don't spend too much time on any one question. Recognize that taking extra time on one question you don't understand may keep you from answering two that you do understand later in the test. If your time limit for a question is up and you're still not sure of the answer, mark it and move on, and come back to it later if the time and the test format allow. If the testing format doesn't allow you to return to earlier questions, just make an educated guess; then put it out of your mind and move on.

On the easier questions, be careful not to rush. It may seem wise to hurry through them so you have more time for the challenging ones, but it's not worth missing one if you know the concept and just didn't take the time to read the question fully. Work efficiently but make sure you understand the question and have looked at all of the answer choices, since more than one may seem right at first.

Even if you're paying attention to the time, you may find yourself a little behind at some point. You should speed up to get back on track, but do so wisely. Don't panic; just take a few seconds less on each question until you're caught up. Don't guess without thinking, but do look through the answer choices and eliminate any you know are wrong. If you can get down to two choices, it is often worthwhile to guess from those. Once you've chosen an answer, move on and don't dwell on any that you skipped or had to hurry through. If a question was taking too long, chances are it was one of the harder ones, so you weren't as likely to get it right anyway.

On the other hand, if you find yourself getting ahead of schedule, it may be beneficial to slow down a little. The more quickly you work, the more likely you are to make a careless mistake that will affect your score. You've budgeted time for each question, so don't be afraid to spend that time. Practice an efficient but careful pace to get the most out of the time you have.

Secret Key #5 – Have a Plan for Guessing

When you're taking the test, you may find yourself stuck on a question. Some of the answer choices seem better than others, but you don't see the one answer choice that is obviously correct. What do you do?

The scenario described above is very common, yet most test takers have not effectively prepared for it. Developing and practicing a plan for guessing may be one of the single most effective uses of your time as you get ready for the exam.

In developing your plan for guessing, there are three questions to address:

- When should you start the guessing process?
- How should you narrow down the choices?
- Which answer should you choose?

When to Start the Guessing Process

Unless your plan for guessing is to select C every time (which, despite its merits, is not what we recommend), you need to leave yourself enough time to apply your answer elimination strategies. Since you have a limited amount of time for each question, that means that if you're going to give yourself the best shot at guessing correctly, you have to decide quickly whether or not you will guess.

Of course, the best-case scenario is that you don't have to guess at all, so first, see if you can answer the question based on your knowledge of the subject and basic reasoning skills. Focus on the key words in the question and try to jog your memory of related topics. Give yourself a chance to bring the knowledge to mind, but once you realize that you don't have (or you can't access) the knowledge you need to answer the question, it's time to start the guessing process.

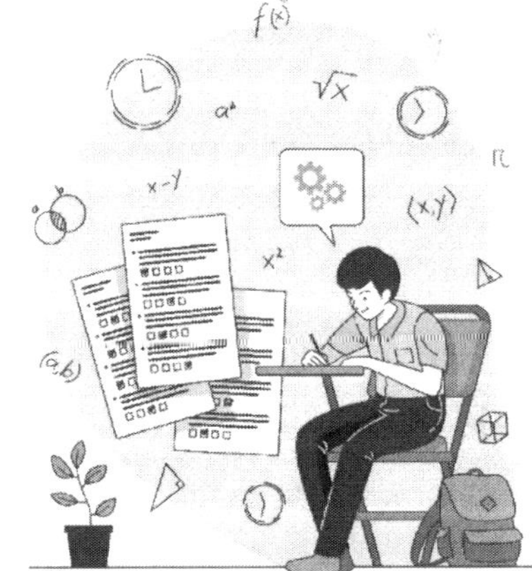

It's almost always better to start the guessing process too early than too late. It only takes a few seconds to remember something and answer the question from knowledge. Carefully eliminating wrong answer choices takes longer. Plus, going through the process of eliminating answer choices can actually help jog your memory.

Summary: Start the guessing process as soon as you decide that you can't answer the question based on your knowledge.

How to Narrow Down the Choices

The next chapter in this book (**Test-Taking Strategies**) includes a wide range of strategies for how to approach questions and how to look for answer choices to eliminate. You will definitely want to read those carefully, practice them, and figure out which ones work best for you. Here though, we're going to address a mindset rather than a particular strategy.

Your odds of guessing an answer correctly depend on how many options you are choosing from.

Number of options left	5	4	3	2	1
Odds of guessing correctly	20%	25%	33%	50%	100%

You can see from this chart just how valuable it is to be able to eliminate incorrect answers and make an educated guess, but there are two things that many test takers do that cause them to miss out on the benefits of guessing:

- Accidentally eliminating the correct answer
- Selecting an answer based on an impression

We'll look at the first one here, and the second one in the next section.

To avoid accidentally eliminating the correct answer, we recommend a thought exercise called **the $5 challenge**. In this challenge, you only eliminate an answer choice from contention if you are willing to bet $5 on it being wrong. Why $5? Five dollars is a small but not insignificant amount of money. It's an amount you could afford to lose but wouldn't want to throw away. And while losing $5 once might not hurt too much, doing it twenty times will set you back $100. In the same way, each small decision you make—eliminating a choice here, guessing on a question there—won't by itself impact your score very much, but when you put them all together, they can make a big difference. By holding each answer choice elimination decision to a higher standard, you can reduce the risk of accidentally eliminating the correct answer.

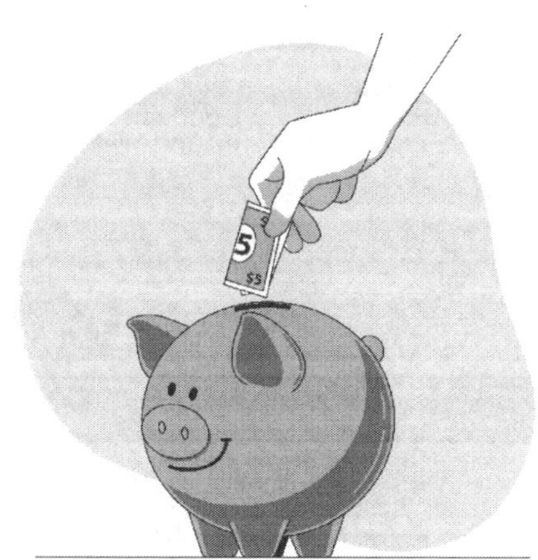

The $5 challenge can also be applied in a positive sense: If you are willing to bet $5 that an answer choice *is* correct, go ahead and mark it as correct.

Summary: Only eliminate an answer choice if you are willing to bet $5 that it is wrong.

Which Answer to Choose

You're taking the test. You've run into a hard question and decided you'll have to guess. You've eliminated all the answer choices you're willing to bet $5 on. Now you have to pick an answer. Why do we even need to talk about this? Why can't you just pick whichever one you feel like when the time comes?

The answer to these questions is that if you don't come into the test with a plan, you'll rely on your impression to select an answer choice, and if you do that, you risk falling into a trap. The test writers know that everyone who takes their test will be guessing on some of the questions, so they intentionally write wrong answer choices to seem plausible. You still have to pick an answer though, and if the wrong answer choices are designed to look right, how can you ever be sure that you're not falling for their trap? The best solution we've found to this dilemma is to take the decision out of your hands entirely. Here is the process we recommend:

Once you've eliminated any choices that you are confident (willing to bet $5) are wrong, select the first remaining choice as your answer.

Whether you choose to select the first remaining choice, the second, or the last, the important thing is that you use some preselected standard. Using this approach guarantees that you will not be enticed into selecting an answer choice that looks right, because you are not basing your decision on how the answer choices look.

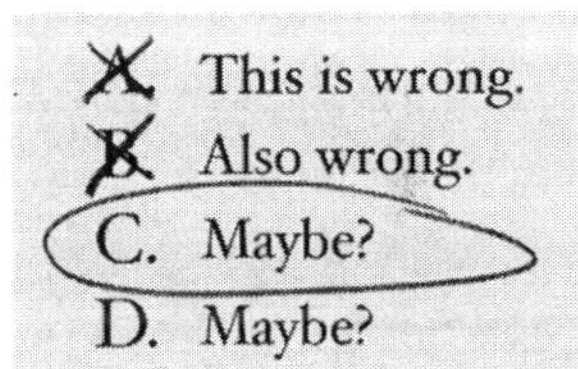

This is not meant to make you question your knowledge. Instead, it is to help you recognize the difference between your knowledge and your impressions. There's a huge difference between thinking an answer is right because of what you know, and thinking an answer is right because it looks or sounds like it should be right.

Summary: To ensure that your selection is appropriately random, make a predetermined selection from among all answer choices you have not eliminated.

Test-Taking Strategies

This section contains a list of test-taking strategies that you may find helpful as you work through the test. By taking what you know and applying logical thought, you can maximize your chances of answering any question correctly!

It is very important to realize that every question is different and every person is different: no single strategy will work on every question, and no single strategy will work for every person. That's why we've included all of them here, so you can try them out and determine which ones work best for different types of questions and which ones work best for you.

Question Strategies

✓ Read Carefully

Read the question and the answer choices carefully. Don't miss the question because you misread the terms. You have plenty of time to read each question thoroughly and make sure you understand what is being asked. Yet a happy medium must be attained, so don't waste too much time. You must read carefully and efficiently.

✓ Contextual Clues

Look for contextual clues. If the question includes a word you are not familiar with, look at the immediate context for some indication of what the word might mean. Contextual clues can often give you all the information you need to decipher the meaning of an unfamiliar word. Even if you can't determine the meaning, you may be able to narrow down the possibilities enough to make a solid guess at the answer to the question.

✓ Prefixes

If you're having trouble with a word in the question or answer choices, try dissecting it. Take advantage of every clue that the word might include. Prefixes and suffixes can be a huge help. Usually, they allow you to determine a basic meaning. *Pre-* means before, *post-* means after, *pro-* is positive, *de-* is negative. From prefixes and suffixes, you can get an idea of the general meaning of the word and try to put it into context.

✓ Hedge Words

Watch out for critical hedge words, such as *likely, may, can, sometimes, often, almost, mostly, usually, generally, rarely*, and *sometimes*. Question writers insert these hedge phrases to cover every possibility. Often an answer choice will be wrong simply because it leaves no room for exception. Be on guard for answer choices that have definitive words such as *exactly* and *always*.

✓ Switchback Words

Stay alert for *switchbacks*. These are the words and phrases frequently used to alert you to shifts in thought. The most common switchback words are *but, although*, and *however*. Others include *nevertheless, on the other hand, even though, while, in spite of, despite*, and *regardless of*. Switchback words are important to catch because they can change the direction of the question or an answer choice.

✅ Face Value

When in doubt, use common sense. Accept the situation in the problem at face value. Don't read too much into it. These problems will not require you to make wild assumptions. If you have to go beyond creativity and warp time or space in order to have an answer choice fit the question, then you should move on and consider the other answer choices. These are normal problems rooted in reality. The applicable relationship or explanation may not be readily apparent, but it is there for you to figure out. Use your common sense to interpret anything that isn't clear.

Answer Choice Strategies

✅ Answer Selection

The most thorough way to pick an answer choice is to identify and eliminate wrong answers until only one is left, then confirm it is the correct answer. Sometimes an answer choice may immediately seem right, but be careful. The test writers will usually put more than one reasonable answer choice on each question, so take a second to read all of them and make sure that the other choices are not equally obvious. As long as you have time left, it is better to read every answer choice than to pick the first one that looks right without checking the others.

✅ Answer Choice Families

An answer choice family consists of two (in rare cases, three) answer choices that are very similar in construction and cannot all be true at the same time. If you see two answer choices that are direct opposites or parallels, one of them is usually the correct answer. For instance, if one answer choice says that quantity x increases and another either says that quantity x decreases (opposite) or says that quantity y increases (parallel), then those answer choices would fall into the same family. An answer choice that doesn't match the construction of the answer choice family is more likely to be incorrect. Most questions will not have answer choice families, but when they do appear, you should be prepared to recognize them.

✅ Eliminate Answers

Eliminate answer choices as soon as you realize they are wrong, but make sure you consider all possibilities. If you are eliminating answer choices and realize that the last one you are left with is also wrong, don't panic. Start over and consider each choice again. There may be something you missed the first time that you will realize on the second pass.

✅ Avoid Fact Traps

Don't be distracted by an answer choice that is factually true but doesn't answer the question. You are looking for the choice that answers the question. Stay focused on what the question is asking for so you don't accidentally pick an answer that is true but incorrect. Always go back to the question and make sure the answer choice you've selected actually answers the question and is not merely a true statement.

✅ Extreme Statements

In general, you should avoid answers that put forth extreme actions as standard practice or proclaim controversial ideas as established fact. An answer choice that states the "process should be used in certain situations, if..." is much more likely to be correct than one that states the "process should be discontinued completely." The first is a calm rational statement and doesn't even make a definitive, uncompromising stance, using a hedge word *if* to provide wiggle room, whereas the second choice is far more extreme.

⊘ Benchmark

As you read through the answer choices and you come across one that seems to answer the question well, mentally select that answer choice. This is not your final answer, but it's the one that will help you evaluate the other answer choices. The one that you selected is your benchmark or standard for judging each of the other answer choices. Every other answer choice must be compared to your benchmark. That choice is correct until proven otherwise by another answer choice beating it. If you find a better answer, then that one becomes your new benchmark. Once you've decided that no other choice answers the question as well as your benchmark, you have your final answer.

⊘ Predict the Answer

Before you even start looking at the answer choices, it is often best to try to predict the answer. When you come up with the answer on your own, it is easier to avoid distractions and traps because you will know exactly what to look for. The right answer choice is unlikely to be word-for-word what you came up with, but it should be a close match. Even if you are confident that you have the right answer, you should still take the time to read each option before moving on.

General Strategies

⊘ Tough Questions

If you are stumped on a problem or it appears too hard or too difficult, don't waste time. Move on! Remember though, if you can quickly check for obviously incorrect answer choices, your chances of guessing correctly are greatly improved. Before you completely give up, at least try to knock out a couple of possible answers. Eliminate what you can and then guess at the remaining answer choices before moving on.

⊘ Check Your Work

Since you will probably not know every term listed and the answer to every question, it is important that you get credit for the ones that you do know. Don't miss any questions through careless mistakes. If at all possible, try to take a second to look back over your answer selection and make sure you've selected the correct answer choice and haven't made a costly careless mistake (such as marking an answer choice that you didn't mean to mark). This quick double check should more than pay for itself in caught mistakes for the time it costs.

⊘ Pace Yourself

It's easy to be overwhelmed when you're looking at a page full of questions; your mind is confused and full of random thoughts, and the clock is ticking down faster than you would like. Calm down and maintain the pace that you have set for yourself. Especially as you get down to the last few minutes of the test, don't let the small numbers on the clock make you panic. As long as you are on track by monitoring your pace, you are guaranteed to have time for each question.

⊘ Don't Rush

It is very easy to make errors when you are in a hurry. Maintaining a fast pace in answering questions is pointless if it makes you miss questions that you would have gotten right otherwise. Test writers like to include distracting information and wrong answers that seem right. Taking a little extra time to avoid careless mistakes can make all the difference in your test score. Find a pace that allows you to be confident in the answers that you select.

⊘ Keep Moving

Panicking will not help you pass the test, so do your best to stay calm and keep moving. Taking deep breaths and going through the answer elimination steps you practiced can help to break through a stress barrier and keep your pace.

Final Notes

The combination of a solid foundation of content knowledge and the confidence that comes from practicing your plan for applying that knowledge is the key to maximizing your performance on test day. As your foundation of content knowledge is built up and strengthened, you'll find that the strategies included in this chapter become more and more effective in helping you quickly sift through the distractions and traps of the test to isolate the correct answer.

Now that you're preparing to move forward into the test content chapters of this book, be sure to keep your goal in mind. As you read, think about how you will be able to apply this information on the test. If you've already seen sample questions for the test and you have an idea of the question format and style, try to come up with questions of your own that you can answer based on what you're reading. This will give you valuable practice applying your knowledge in the same ways you can expect to on test day.

Good luck and good studying!

Assessment and Diagnosis

Normal Age-Related Changes

Growth and Development in Late Adolescence/Young Adulthood

Late adolescence/young adulthood, **18-21,** is the time when adolescents begin to take on more adult roles and responsibilities, entering the world of work or going to college. Most have come to terms with their sexuality and have a more mature understanding of people's motivations. Some young people will continue to engage in high-risk behaviors. Many of the problems associated with middle adolescence may continue if unresolved, interfering with the transition to adulthood. **Developmental concerns** include the following:

- Failure to take on adult roles, no life goals or future plans.
- Low self-esteem.
- Lack of intimate relationships, sexual identification concerns.
- Gang association.
- Continued identification with peer group or dependence on parents.
- High-risk sexual behavior, multiple partners and unprotected sex.
- Poor academic progress or ability.
- Psychosomatic complaints, depression.
- Lack of impulse control.
- Poor nutrition.
- Poor dental health.
- Chronic disease.
- Obesity.
- Lack of exercise.

Additional Age-Related Changes

Age-related changes are as follows:

- **Heart** - The heart muscle thickens and arteries thicken, so the heart must work harder to pump blood, but the maximum pumping rate decreases. The body is less able to extract oxygen from blood, and blood oxygenation levels begin to decline.
- **Lungs** - Between 40 and 70, the maximum breathing capacity decreases by about 40%.
- **Brain** - The brain begins to lose some axons and neurons. Mild short-term memory loss is common.
- **Eyes** - Clouding of the lens occurs with aging as cells die and accumulate. A cataract, opacity of the lens that interferes with vision, can occur in one eye or bilaterally and usually progresses slowly. Incidence is >50% by age 80. People may have difficulty focusing, decreased night vision, and increased photophobia. People tend to become farsighted with age.
- **Kidney/Bladder** - Kidneys are less efficient at removing wastes from blood, and bladder capacity declines, often resulting in frequency and urgency.

- **Skin** - As people age, Langerhans cells in the skin decrease in number, making the skin more prone to cancer, and the inflammatory reactions decrease. The sweat glands, vascularity, and subcutaneous fat all decrease, interfering with thermoregulation and contributing to dryness and irritation of the skin. The epidermal-dermal junction flattens, resulting in skin prone to tearing. The elastin in the skin degrades with age and solar exposure. The thinning of the hypodermis can lead to pressure ulcers.
- **Fat** - Body fat increases until middle age, stabilizes, and decreases in older age. Fat is redistributed from skin to deeper organs, usually to the abdomen rather than the hips.
- **Muscles** - Between ages 30 and 70, males lose 23% of muscle mass and females 22% without compensatory exercise.
- **Bones** - Bone mineral loss exceeds replacement in women >35, accelerating after menopause, and in males >65, resulting in osteoporosis if preventive measures, such as exercise and calcium supplements, are not taken.

Cognitive Changes Associated with Aging

There are large individual differences in the **effect of age on cognition**. Age-related changes in *cognition* do not usually occur before age 70. Research indicates that approximately 65 percent of individuals exhibit a slight decline in cognitive abilities by age 81. While fluid intelligence (the ability to process information) decreases somewhat, crystallized intelligence (the ability to solve practical problems) is usually unaffected by aging and may actually improve. Acquired knowledge often remains intact. Older adults may find it difficult to apply new information to the solution of complex problems. Even if their intellect is unaffected, older adults may have trouble paying attention for any significant length of time. Individuals older than 60 may take longer to react to situations and may take longer to complete cognitive tasks. Working memory is affected by age. While implicit memory (skills) is unaffected by increasing age, explicit memory (information) may decline.

Cardiovascular Changes Associated with Aging

Cardiovascular changes that are associated with aging include the following:

- There is an age-related reduction in the ability of the cardiovascular system to pump blood. This results in a decrease in oxygen delivery.
- Reduced cardiac output causes circulation time to increase.
- Arteries lose elasticity with age, leading to an increase in blood pressure at rest and during exercise.
- The left ventricle may enlarge (hypertrophy).
- The baroreceptor response may decrease.
- Diastolic dysfunction may be evident.
- An age-related reduction in the resting and maximal heart rates results in a slower response to situations that call for increased oxygen.
- The atria may enlarge: This is correlated with atrial fibrillation, atrial flutter, and congestive heart failure (CHF).

It should be remembered that there are distinct individual differences in the response of the heart to aging. Some individuals experience much more serious age-related changes than others.

Neurological Changes Associated with Aging

Neurological changes associated with aging include the following:

- The number of nerve cells in the brain and spinal cord decreases with increasing age.
- There is a slight reduction in brain mass.
- The loss of neurons occurs particularly in the frontal lobes.
- There is also a decrease in cerebral blood flow.
- Short-term memory loss may occur with increasing age. Cognitive processes are not usually affected unless there is an underlying brain disease or disorder. For example, Alzheimer's disease and stroke may affect mentation.
- Some neurofibrillary tangles may be present in the normally aging brain.
- Skeletal muscles may atrophy with age as a result of peripheral nerve cell degeneration. The ability of peripheral nerves to repair themselves is reduced.
- The speed of conduction of peripheral nerves may decrease, resulting in a loss of sensation and slower reflexes.
- There may be changes in the autonomic nervous system, resulting in reduced perspiration.

Pulmonary Changes Associated with Aging

Pulmonary changes that occur with normal aging include the following:

- There is a decrease in the elasticity of the lungs.
- The alveoli flatten and the alveolar ducts enlarge. As a result, the air tends to stay in the alveolar ducts rather than in the alveoli. This decreases the efficiency of oxygen exchange.
- There is an increase in the residual volume of the lungs.
- There is a reduction in forced expiratory volume (FEV) and forced vital capacity (FVC) in older adults.
- Because older adults experience a decrease in overall strength, they are less able to breathe deeply.
- The cough reflex is reduced. Ciliary action decreases with age.
- Protective laryngeal reflexes may be lost.
- Total lung capacity does not change with age.

Sensory Changes Associated with Aging

A number of **sensory changes** occur in older adults:

- Older adults frequently experience deteriorating *vision* (such as presbyopia and cataracts), which prevents them from reading and navigating safely. Most people older than 60 years of age require glasses.
- Adults may become *less sensitive to color differences* (particularly blues and greens) as they age.
- Night vision decreases.
- *Hearing impairment* may necessitate periodic cleaning of the ears or hearing aids.
- *Taste and smell*, which are both required to taste, are not usually significantly affected by normal aging. Most changes in taste and smell are caused by disease and/or drugs rather than aging.

- The *sense of touch*, including the ability to sense vibration, temperature, and pain, is usually somewhat reduced in older adults. However, it is unclear if this is a normal change or related to morbidity or drugs.
- A reduction in *sensitivity to temperature* (hot and cold) may put older adults at risk for burns, hyperthermia, and hypothermia.

Skin Changes Associated with Aging

The characteristics of the **skin** change throughout life. The skin of an infant is thinner than that of an adult. The epidermis is fully developed at birth, but the dermis is not and continues to become thicker after birth. During adolescence, the hair follicles in the skin become active, and the dermis becomes thinner. It also takes longer for the cells of the epidermis to regenerate, increasing the time needed for healing. With increasing age, there is a reduction in the number of Langerhans cells. This increases the risk of skin cancer. As the aging process continues, the sweat glands and blood vessels decrease in number, and the amount of subcutaneous fat decreases. This makes the skin drier and more likely to become irritated. The junction between the epidermis and dermis flattens, increasing the risk of tearing. Age and exposure to the sun break down elastin, which gives skin strength and resilience.

Postmenopausal Changes

The female reproduction system undergoes a number of **postmenopausal changes.** The ovaries still produce some hormones, but by late postmenopause, the production of estrogen has dropped by 80 percent and progesterone by 60 percent. Mental functioning may be affected. The decrease in estrogen levels may result in cognitive decline, insomnia, and depression. The skin becomes thinner and loses collagen. Hair follicles become dry. Bones lose calcium and become more porous. As connective tissue is lost, breasts begin to droop. The bladder starts to function less efficiently. The ovaries atrophy. The uterus shrinks to about 50 percent of its original size and may not be palpable in women older than age 75. The cervix may retract. The vagina becomes shorter. The walls of the vagina become thinner and lose elasticity and lubrication; this may result in painful sexual intercourse. The vaginal fluid becomes more alkaline. The labia majora shrink and separate. This exposes the inner structures and increases the risk of infection.

Pathophysiology Across the Lifespan: Elderly

Gait and Mobility Issues

Approximately 20 percent of noninstitutionalized adults and 54 percent of institutionalized adults older than age 85 have **gait and mobility issues** that limit their independence and predispose them to falls. Risk factors include arthritis, peripheral neuropathy, hypothyroidism, Parkinson's disease, orthostatic hypotension, deformities, stroke and heart attack, medication effects, and orthopedic problems. Weakness, loss of muscle mass and tone, and confusion may contribute to gait disorders. An older patient should be observed for gait abnormalities, including unsteadiness, uneven weight distribution, and abnormal positioning of limbs. A slow gait, covering five meters in less than 0.6 m/second, is predictive of functional limitations. In the Timed Up and Go (TUG) test, the patient stands from a sitting position in a chair with armrests, walks three meters and turns, walks back to the chair, and sits down again. Those requiring 14 seconds or more are at risk for falls. The Performance Oriented Mobility Assessment (POMA) tests mobility and gait under different conditions. Treatment for mobility issues includes identifying and treating the underlying cause, gait and strength training, environmental modifications, assistive devices, and orthotics.

Osteoporosis

Osteoporosis is a condition involving low bone mass and structural deterioration. More bone is lost than gained. The condition leads to thin, porous bones that break easily. Osteoporosis occurs most commonly in postmenopausal women, although men older than age 65 experience bone loss at the same rate as women. Primary osteoporosis occurs as part of normal aging. Bone mass density (BMD) can be tested to determine the extent of osteoporosis. The *risk factors* for osteoporosis can be arranged to spell the word **FRACTURED** and are as follows:

F = ***f***ractures
R = ***r***ace
A = ***a***ge and gender
C = ***c***hronic disease/medication
T = ***t***hin bones and low weight
U = ***u***nderactive/inadequate exercise
R = ***r***educed estrogen
E = ***e***xcessive alcohol intake and smoking
D = ***d***iet

Cancer survivors and individuals with chronic disease are at increased risk for osteoporosis. Treatments include the following medications: bisphosphonates, hormones (not recommended), selective estrogen receptor modulator, calcitonin, and recombinant human parathyroid hormone. A diet high in calcium and vitamin D may be recommended. Balance training, strength training, and regular weight-bearing exercise will often improve symptoms of osteoporosis.

Hip Fracture

Falls occur in 30 percent of those older than age 65, and 50 percent of those older than age 80. About five percent of these falls result in fractures. **Hip fractures** pose the greatest risk to the older adult. Osteoporosis increases risk of fracture. Bone deterioration may cause pain in the hip, and the patient may have difficulty bearing weight prior to a fall. The most common fracture sites are the femoral neck and the intertrochanteric region. Patients may have comorbidities and may present with dehydration and blood loss. The mortality rate is 10 percent during initial treatment and 25 percent or more over the next year. Various types of repair are performed, including cannulated screw fixation, internal fixation, total hip replacement, extramedullary implant (sliding screw and plate), intramedullary implant (Gamma nail), or hip compression screw and side plate. Yearly infusion of Reclast started within three months of a fracture has been shown to reduce the incidence of new fractures and to increase survival rate.

Cataracts

As cells die and accumulate in the eye, the lens of the eye clouds. A **cataract** (opacity of the lens that interferes with vision) can occur in one eye or in both eyes. The condition usually progresses slowly. By the age of 80, the incidence of cataracts is 50 percent. The most frequent complaint in individuals with cataracts is blurred vision without pain. Other symptoms include astigmatism, diplopia, color shift, and reduction in light transmission. A patient with cataracts should be referred to an ophthalmologist for evaluation. The condition may be surgically repaired. There are three primary types of age-related cataracts: nuclear, cortical, and posterior subcapsular.

- *Nuclear cataracts* are associated with myopia and tend to worsen myopia and blur vision.
- *Cortical cataracts* involve the anterior, posterior, or equatorial lens cortex. This condition causes vision to worsen in bright light.

- *Posterior subcapsular cataracts* are anterior to the posterior capsule and tend to develop in younger people or those taking corticosteroids over a long period of time. An affected eye becomes increasingly photophobic and near vision diminishes.

Hearing Deficits in Older Adults

Conductive hearing deficits result from abnormalities in the structures of the outer and/or middle ear that interfere with function. Cerumen is a common cause of conductive hearing loss. Cerumen can result in significant hearing deficit when 95 percent occlusion occurs. Cerumen becomes hard and dry because of the atrophy of the modified apocrine glands, which thin cerumen. Removing the cerumen restores hearing. Benign growths, tympanic membrane perforation, and middle ear effusions may also impair hearing.

Sensory hearing deficits result from damage to the auditory or cochlear nerves in the inner ear. Damage may occur suddenly or progress over an extended period of time. The nerves of the ears may be damaged by Ménière's disease, viral infections, perilymph fistula, vascular occlusive disorders, and autoimmune disorders. Exposure to high-intensity sounds over an extended period of time can result in noise-induced hearing loss. Presbycusis is the most common hearing disorder. It is caused by physiological changes related to aging. Presbycusis causes bilateral high-frequency hearing loss.

Macular Degeneration

Macular degeneration is the most common cause of blindness in the Caucasian population. The condition rarely occurs in other groups. There are two types of macular degeneration: dry and wet.

- *Dry macular degeneration* is more common and occurs when hyaline bodies, called drusen, are deposited near the retina. Dry macular degeneration begins in middle age. The condition progresses slowly and causes a loss of vision in the central part of the eye. It does not usually result in legal blindness. However, it can develop into wet macular degeneration.
- *Wet macular degeneration* occurs when capillaries invade the retina and grow behind the macula of the eye. Wet macular degeneration can result in legal blindness. There is no cure for macular degeneration. Vitamins A, D, and E slow the progression of dry macular degeneration. Some medications (such as Lucentis, Macugen, and Visudyne) and surgery may improve vision in individuals with wet macular degeneration. The disease appears to be heritable, and prevention is important. Eating food high in carotenoids, quitting smoking, and protecting the eyes from ultraviolet light can reduce risk.

Glaucoma

Glaucoma is a group of eye conditions characterized by damage to the optic nerve and vision impairment. Risk factors include being older than 40 years of age, a family history of the disease, cardiovascular disease, myopia, migraine syndromes, corticosteroid use, diabetes, and being of African American descent. Glaucoma involves an increase in intraocular pressure (normally 10-21 mm Hg) resulting from inadequate drainage of aqueous fluid. Fluid may fail to drain properly due to blockages in the drainage system and/or a decreased angle (< 45°) between the iris and cornea. There are different types of glaucoma, but the symptoms for each are similar: blurred vision, halos around lights, lack of focus, eye discomfort, headache, and difficulty seeing in low light. Referral should be made to an ophthalmologist for evaluation. Treatment may include topical beta-blockers, miotics, adrenergic agonists, carbonic anhydrase inhibitors, and prostaglandins. Surgical management includes laser trabeculoplasty, laser iridotomy, filtering procedures, trabeculectomy, and drainage implants/shunts.

Dental Conditions

Approximately 28 percent of individuals younger than age 75 are **edentulous**, while 43 percent of individuals older than age 75 are edentulous. Some edentulous individuals wear dentures, but others eventually stop wearing dentures due to poor fit or because the dentures have caused oral lesions (30%). If patients have had the same dentures for a number of years, the dentures may need to be refitted or replaced. Approximately one-third of older adults have untreated **caries**. Frequently, these are root caries, which occur because of the recession of gum tissue**. Gum-tissue recession** occurs in about 86 percent of those older than age 65. Gum-tissue recession leaves the roots exposed and increases the risk of developing periodontal disease. **Periodontal disease** affects about 85 percent of older adults with 25 percent exhibiting loss of supporting structures. Periodontal disease is characterized by pockets of swollen, bleeding, erythematous gingiva around the teeth. Effective oral hygiene, including brushing and flossing, use of mouthwashes, and cleaning, is important in combating periodontal disease. Surgical treatment may be required.

Effects of Dentition Problems and Functional Impairment on Eating

Older patients should be assessed for dentition and functional impairment. **Dentition** relates directly to the ability to chew food and eat, so ill-fitting dentures, caries, or an edentulous condition may require intervention or adjustment of diet. **Functional impairment** may adversely affect the ability to prepare foods, eat an adequate diet, and drink an adequate amount of fluid. A functional assessment evaluates ability to participate in activities of daily living (ADLs) and instrumental activities of daily living (IADL). ADLs are those activities necessary for self-care. They include dressing, bathing, and preparing food. Inability to carry out ADLs may relate to physical impairment (paralysis, paresis, and frailty) or cognitive impairment (dementia and confusion). IADLs include such activities as managing affairs (including finances), arranging transportation, using prosthetic devices, shopping, and telephoning. The inability to carry out IADLs may relate to cognitive impairment, poverty, or inaccessibility and can prevent people from shopping for or ordering food.

Dysarthria

Dysarthria (unclear speech, slurring) in older adults may be related to lack of teeth, neurological disorders (Parkinson's, Huntington's, MS), stroke, Bell's palsy, alcohol intoxication, brain injury, and excessive use of drugs such as narcotics and phenytoin. Dysarthria is unrelated to intelligence or hearing, so the nurse should use age-appropriate vocabulary and materials. The nurse should speak in a normal tone of voice, facing the patient, so the nurse can observe gestures and facial expressions that the patient may use as augmentative and assistive communication (AAC). If the patient uses assistive materials (flip-charts, letter boards, computer programs, or speech-generating devices) these should be available and the nurse knowledgeable about the use of the equipment. If the patient is not able to speak at all (oral surgery, tracheotomy), then the patient's ability to indicate yes/no by blinking or nodding should be assessed. In general, yes/no questions are easiest for patients with dysarthria. It's important not to rush patients or try to complete their statements for them.

Diet Deficiencies in Older Adults

Diet deficiencies are common in many patient populations, especially older adults. The diets of older adults are frequently nutritionally inadequate and often contain excessive amounts of fat (especially saturated fat), cholesterol, and sodium. The diets of older adults are often deficient in protein, vitamins, and minerals. In addition, older adults are often not sufficiently hydrated. Poor diet may be related to chronic disease, lack of dentition, inability to prepare meals, or poverty. Individuals who are frail and require assistance with activities of daily living tend to have the most deficient diets, and those older than age 85 frequently have inadequate caloric intake. The diets of older adults are often deficient in calcium, vitamin D, vitamin C, vitamin B_6, thiamine, riboflavin, and all minerals, especially magnesium and zinc. Older adults may benefit from food programs (Meals on Wheels, for example) and dietary counseling. In addition, older adults should be advised to take a daily multivitamin to ensure that they receive adequate amounts of vitamins and trace minerals.

Risk Factors and Indicators of Malnutrition

There are a number of risk factors for **malnutrition**. Hypermetabolism can result from various diseases (acquired immunodeficiency syndrome [AIDS], for example) and other conditions (such as stress). It can also result from trauma. Weight loss is a risk factor for malnutrition, especially a sudden weight loss or the loss of 10 percent of normal weight over a three-month period. Low body weight (less than 90 percent of the ideal body weight for age) is a risk factor for malnutrition. Low body mass index (BMI) (less than 18.5) is associated with malnutrition. Immunosuppressive drugs can interfere with the absorption of nutrients. Malabsorption of nutrients may be caused by diseases such as chronic kidney or liver failure. Changes in appetite may decrease intake of nutrients. Food intolerances may result from lack of enzymes necessary to digest certain foods. Dietary restrictions, such as the need to limit protein intake with kidney failure, can result in malnutrition. Functional limitations may impair the ability to take in nutrients. The lack of teeth or functioning dentures may limit food intake. Alterations in taste and smell may render food unpalatable.

Asthma

Asthma in seniors may be a continuing condition from childhood, but it may also develop in older people. Asthma may be diagnosed as a new disorder in seniors. The symptoms of asthma include wheezing, tightness of the chest, shortness of breath, and coughing. The symptoms are episodic and do not appear continually through the day. The symptoms usually worsen at night and while exercising. Airborne allergens can exacerbate or trigger the symptoms. The patient may exhibit allergic rhinitis and/or atopic dermatitis. Physical examination may show hyperextension of the patient's thorax. The condition tends to be hereditary; the patient may have relatives with the disorder. The symptoms of asthma are not always present. A diagnosis of asthma cannot be excluded because symptoms are absent at the time of examination. Episodic airflow obstruction that is partly reversible is diagnosed by spirometry. Further tests include pulmonary function studies, bronchoprovocation, allergy tests, and chest x-rays. In seniors, asthma is often complicated by age and comorbid conditions.

Care of Skin

The skin of older adults is often friable and bruises easily. Therefore, it should be treated with care. Excessive palpitation and pulling should be avoided. The skin should be examined for lesions or indications of pressure ulcers. Older adults often have benign skins lesions, including, acrochordons (skin tags), actinic keratoses, cherry hemangiomas, dermatofibromas, lentigines (liver spots), nevi (moles), sebaceous hyperplasia, and seborrheic keratoses. Some of these types of lesions, such as actinic keratoses, are precancerous and should be examined carefully as they may become squamous cell or basal cell carcinoma. Malignant melanoma can occur in individuals of any age. These lesions occur most frequently on the torso, head, and neck of males and the legs of females.

Delirium

Delirium is an acute, sudden change in consciousness. It is characterized by reduced ability to focus or sustain attention, language and memory impairment, disorientation, confusion, audiovisual hallucinations, sleep disturbance, and psychomotor activity disorder. The symptoms of delirium fluctuate. Delirium occurs in 10 to 40 percent of hospitalized older adults and in about 80 percent of terminally ill patients. Delirium may result from the use of certain drugs (such as anticholinergics) and from numerous conditions including infection, hypoxia, trauma, dementia, depression, vision and hearing loss, surgery, alcoholism, untreated pain, fluid/electrolyte imbalance, and malnutrition. Delirium increases the risk of morbidity and death, especially if untreated. Diagnosis is based on patient interview and history and chart review. Asking the patient to count backward from 20 to 1 and spell his or her first name backward can identify an attention deficit. Treatment includes decreasing the dosage of hypnotics and psychotropics. Medications administered to reduce symptoms include trazodone, lorazepam, and haloperidol.

Loneliness and Social Isolation

Social isolation is pervasive especially among older adults and is correlated with feelings of loneliness. The social activity of individuals decreases as they age. Family and friends die, move to nursing homes, or relocate. **Loneliness** is especially common among adults who are widowed. Surprisingly, loneliness is common among older adults living with their grown children. Social isolation and loneliness are exacerbated by disease and anxiety. Older adults often have very little social interaction and many are neglected by family and friends. Loneliness can lead to stress-related disorders (hypertension, cardiovascular disease, and diabetes mellitus, for example). Research has demonstrated that although older women tend to be more isolated than men, men suffer more acutely from loneliness than women. Loneliness appears to increase the risk of dementia associated with Alzheimer's disease. Loneliness may have a negative effect on the nervous system. Effective interventions include involving older adults in group activities that promote social interaction.

Confusion, Dependence, and Passivity

Older adults coping with loss may exhibit **confusion, dependence, and passivity.** The frequency and speed of changes and loss may overwhelm the older adult, resulting in increasing confusion. This is especially true if the person has even a mild degree of cognitive impairment. However, even those without dementia may exhibit the same symptoms, such as forgetting to take medications, missing appointments, and confusing directions. The person may appear disoriented. In response to stress, some older adults become very dependent on others often to the point of being clingy and demanding of attention. They may call family members constantly or demand attention to receive reassurance. They may become very distressed if asked to make independent decisions. Some older adults begin to believe that they have no control and become very passive, allowing others to make decisions in matters concerning them. These patients are not engaged in their life or health concerns, deferring to doctors, nurses, and family members.

Loss of Independence and Autonomy

The **loss of independence and autonomy** associated with aging is profoundly disturbing to many older adults. Losing the ability to live independently increases overall dependency on others, especially if older adults must live with family members or in a long-term care facility. Losing the ability to drive can prevent older adults from shopping and engaging in social activities. This loss may be devastating to some individuals and may increase symptoms of depression. Many people, especially males, do not willingly give up driving and are forced to do so because of safety concerns by family or physicians. These individuals may become very angry and resentful. Role reversal may occur as older adults' children become their care providers and increasingly make decisions for them. This may cause conflicts that are draining to both parties, and some older adults become increasingly dependent and demanding. Assistance with instrumental activities of daily living (IADLs) and activities of daily living (ADLs) is often necessary, but older adults who want to remain autonomous may resist the help.

SEXUALITY

Human **sexuality** is important to adults of all ages. Older adults need and often crave intimacy with others, including sexual intimacy. Health-care providers should address this issue directly with their older patients as patients may be embarrassed or reluctant to ask questions. Although the issue of sexual intimacy in older adults may be uncomfortable, nurses should not avoid the topic because of personal anxiety. Further, the nurse should respect different attitudes and behavior. Assessment should be done in private, ensuring confidentiality. Questioning should progress from general topics ("Do you have a good relationship with your partner?") to more specific questions related to sexual issues ("Is intercourse uncomfortable for you?"). Older adults may need to know how to deal with physical or environmental limitations. Some older adults engage in sexual behavior that puts them at increased risk of human immunodeficiency virus (HIV) or sexually transmitted diseases (STDs). Discussing sexual issues provides an opportunity for education and counseling.

HUMAN SEXUALITY AND CARDIOVASCULAR CONSIDERATIONS

Older adults with **cardiovascular disease** (such as myocardial infarction and angina) may be very anxious and fearful about sexual activity, but the risks associated with sexual activity are very low, and most heart recovery programs encourage exercise. There are a number of things to keep in mind. The participants should be well rested, so morning or after a nap may be the best time for sexual activity. The participants should wait one to three hours after eating before engaging in sexual activity. The couple should use whatever position is comfortable for them. If pressure on the chest is an issue, the couple may feel less anxious in side-lying positions. The couple should engage in foreplay so that the heart rate increases and strengthens in preparation for sexual intercourse. If one of the participants is taking nitroglycerin for angina, he or she should take the medication prior to sexual activity to prevent angina.

HUMAN SEXUALITY AND CHRONIC HEALTH PROBLEMS

Chronic health problems that affect stamina and mobility may pose challenges for older adults engaging in sexual activity. There are several actions that can make things easier. The participant with the health problem should be well rested and engage in sexual activities at the time of day when he or she has the most energy. This is usually in the morning. A person with chronic pain should engage in sexual activity when pain medication is at peak effectiveness. It should be noted that orgasm releases endorphins that may relieve pain for hours after sexual activity. Taking a warm bath prior to sexual activity may relax the muscles and relieve stiffness. It may take some experimentation for the couple to find a position that is comfortable for both. Males with Foley catheters can fold the catheter up against the shaft of the penis and apply a condom to secure it. Females with Foley catheters can position the catheter upward and away from the vagina. The couple may engage in manual and/or oral stimulation.

INAPPROPRIATE SEXUAL BEHAVIOR

The sexual feelings of older adults with dementia or cognitive impairment may be expressed inappropriately. These individuals may undress, masturbate, request sexual favors, use obscene language, or behave aggressively. Such inappropriate behavior may be out of character for the individual. **Inappropriate sexual behavior** may be prompted by lack of inhibition and decreased reasoning ability. This behavior may be of brief duration during a phase or may persist for a prolonged period of time (months or years). In some cases, such as disrobing publicly, the person may simply be hot or need to urinate or defecate. People may relieve themselves in inappropriate places, such as a wastebasket, in response to physical need. If the individual exhibits violent sexual behavior, medication may be prescribed to try to manage it. However, in general, medication does little to prevent or lessen inappropriate behavior. Inappropriate sexual behavior is best managed by supervision. The patient may exhibit certain patterns of behavior (such as pulling at clothes) before engaging in inappropriate sexual behavior. The behavior may be prevented if the patient is distracted.

Sexually Transmitted Diseases

Older adults are more active and healthier than ever before, and the incidence of **sexually transmitted diseases** among older adults is increasing. However, older adults often practice unsafe sex and fail to use condoms. The **Centers for Disease Control has developed six steps to prevent and control the spread of sexually transmitted diseases:**

1. Identify symptomatic and asymptomatic infected persons.
2. Diagnose and treat all infected individuals.
3. Prevent the infected individual from infecting sex partners through evaluation, treatment, and counseling.
4. Provide preexposure vaccination to individuals at risk.
5. Educate individuals at risk about ways to prevent infection.
6. Obtain sexual histories of patients and assess their risk.

The **4-P approach** (omitting pregnancy) to questioning is advocated: ***p***artners, gender and number; ***p***rotection, methods used; ***p***ractices, type of sexual practices (oral, anal, vaginal) and use of condoms; and ***p***ast history of sexually transmitted diseases.

Pathophysiology Across the Lifespan: Cardiac

Cardiac Metabolic Requirements

Cardiac metabolic requirements are high because the heart has a central role in metabolism for the entire body; increased demands result in increased heart rate, cardiac output, and stroke volume. The heart depends on adequate oxygenation, provided through the coronary arteries, which branch from the aorta, so the heart muscle is nourished first. Energy in the normal heart is derived primarily from glucose uptake. Glucose is metabolized into pyruvate and adenosine triphosphate (ATP), which releases energy. Fatty acids are also important and supply 60 to 70% of cardiac energy needs, but fatty acids require 10% more oxygen than glucose to provide an equivalent amount of ATP. During times of stress or with some diseases, such as diabetes, glucose uptake is depressed, and fatty acid uptake increases to 90 to 100% of energy needs. This decreases the contractility of the cardiac muscle. Interference with glucose metabolism may result in ischemia.

Hypertension

Hypertension is commonly called high blood pressure. Blood pressure is defined as the pressure of the blood exerted against the walls of the arteries. An individual's blood pressure results from a combination of cardiac output and peripheral resistance. Hypertension can occur from a change in either one of these factors. Blood pressure is expressed as systolic over diastolic. Normal blood pressure is a systolic pressure less than 120 and a diastolic pressure less than 80. Hypertension is defined as a systolic pressure greater than 140 and a diastolic pressure greater than 90. Primary hypertension is idiopathic, meaning no cause can be identified. Secondary hypertension is defined as hypertension with a known cause (for example, renal disease or thyroid disease). In essential hypertension, cardiac output is within normal limits and peripheral resistance is increased. Hypertension may be caused by an insufficient number of nephrons to adequately clear fluids, stress, genetic anomalies, and obesity.

Hypotension

Hypotension is abnormally low blood pressure. The condition can be life threatening. Low blood pressure is defined as a systolic pressure of 90 mm Hg (millimeters of mercury) or lower and a diastolic pressure of 60 mm Hg or lower. Hypotension can be caused by reduced blood volume (hypovolemia), decreased cardiac output in the presence of normal blood volume, and excessive vasodilation. There are a number of hypotensive syndromes, including orthostatic hypotension, neurocardiogenic syncope, and postprandial hypotension. Orthostatic hypotension is also called postural hypotension. This type of hypotension occurs after following a change the position of the body. Neurocardiogenic syncope occurs as a result of an increase in the activity of the vagus nerve. Postprandial hypotension occurs 30 to 75 minutes after a heavy meal. Orthostatic hypotension and postprandial hypotension occur most commonly in those older than age 65.

Heart Failure

Classes of Heart Failure

The term **heart failure** encompasses contraction disorders and/or filling disorders. Contraction disorders involve systolic dysfunction, and filling disorders involve diastolic dysfunction. Heart failure may include pulmonary edema, peripheral edema, or systemic edema. Heart failure has several causes. The most common of these include coronary artery disease, systemic or pulmonary hypertension, cardiomyopathy, abnormal heart valves, and congenital heart disease. Heart failure is classified according to the symptoms involved and the prognosis.

- **Class I:** Symptoms are not evident during normal activities, and pulmonary congestion and peripheral hypotension are absent. The patient's activities are not restricted. Prognosis is good.
- **Class II:** Symptoms are usually absent at rest but become evident with physical exertion. Slight pulmonary edema may be present as evidenced by basilar rales. Prognosis is good.
- **Class III**: Activities of daily living are affected, and the patient experiences discomfort on exertion. Prognosis is fair.
- **Class IV:** The patient exhibits symptoms at rest. Prognosis is poor.

Review Video: Coronary Artery Disease
Visit mometrix.com/academy and enter code: 950720

Acute and Chronic Heart Failure

Acute heart failure can develop within hours or days. It occurs when a functional or structural problem impairs the ability of the heart to pump sufficient blood for the body's needs. The ability of the myocardium to contract decreases. The peripheral blood vessels narrow. Fluid and sodium are retained in an attempt to control hypotension. Heart rate increases. The lack of sufficient oxygen leads to events such as tissue necrosis, cardiotoxicity, pulmonary edema, and organ failure.

Chronic heart failure has a slower development than acute heart failure. The myocardium becomes damaged by insufficient oxygenation and nutrition. Myocardial cells die, and areas of the heart become necrotic. Fibroblasts are produced in response, and dead myocardial cells are replaced with collagen. This process results in a fibrotic heart muscle. Existing myocardial cells enlarge and become weaker. Cardiac dilation and vascular resistance are the end results.

Diastolic Heart Failure

The clinical symptoms of diastolic heart failure and systolic heart failure are similar. In **diastolic heart failure**, the heart muscle cannot relax sufficiently to allow the ventricles to fill. This is similar to what occurs in systolic heart failure, when myocardial hypertrophy causes stiffening of the muscle. Diastolic heart failure occurs more commonly in women older than 75 years of age. In diastolic heart failure, the intracardiac pressure is usually within the normal range. However, the pressure increases substantially on exertion. The ventricles of the heart do not expand adequately for the fill volume, and the heart is unable to increase stroke volume during exercise because of the delay in muscle relaxation. Dyspnea, fatigue, and pulmonary edema are evident on exercise as a result. Ejection fractions are generally greater than 40 or 50 percent. There is a rise in left ventricular end-diastolic pressure (LVEDP). Left ventricular end-diastolic volume (LVEDV) decreases.

Systolic Heart Failure

Systolic heart failure is left-sided heart failure. This type of heart failure decreases the volume of blood pumped from the ventricles during each contraction. The sympathetic nervous system produces epinephrine and norepinephrine to support the heart muscle. Down-regulation eventually results, and the beta and adrenergic receptors are destroyed. This causes further damage to the heart muscle. The reduced perfusion stimulates the kidneys to produce renin. This promotes the release of angiotensin I, which is converted to angiotensin II. Angiotensin II is a vasoconstrictor. This stimulates the production of aldosterone, which causes sodium and fluid to be retained. Preload and afterload are increased as a result of these processes, adding to the workload of the heart. The myocardium loses its ability to contract, and blood accumulates in the ventricles. The myocardium is stretched, and the ventricles enlarge. The heart muscle thickens, and ischemia results due to an insufficient blood supply.

Myocardial Infarction

Myocardial infarction (MI) results when the supply of oxygen to the heart is not sufficient to meet its requirements. MI is on the acute coronary syndrome (ACS) continuum. An MI may result after any of the following events: an episode of unstable angina resulting from rupture of an atherosclerotic plaque, thrombosis associated with coronary artery spasm, vasoconstriction, acute blood loss, a reduction in the oxygen supply, and cocaine ingestion. Myocardial damage usually occurs in the following stages:

1. Ischemia develops with decreasing oxygen levels, resulting in an ischemic zone.
2. Cellular damage occurs to the cells surrounding the site of infarction.
3. Tissue becomes necrotic at the site of infarction, and the cells are replaced with scar tissue.

A myocardial infarction (MI) is categorized according to the extent of the damage and necrosis, the location of the damage, and the muscle layers affected.

Clinical Manifestations

The **clinical manifestations of MI** vary considerably among individuals. Males usually exhibit the more classical symptoms of MI. Females often do not exhibit these symptoms. Patients with diabetes may have reduced pain sensation because of neuropathy. A diabetic patient with MI may complain primarily of weakness. Elderly patients may also have a reduced sensation of pain and complain of weakness during MI. Older individuals with MI are more likely to exhibit pulmonary edema, left ventricular wall rupture, or papillary muscle rupture. Signs and symptoms of MI include chest pain (66%), dyspnea (20-59%), neurological symptoms (15-33%), and gastrointestinal tract disorders (20%). Other signs and symptoms may include hypertension and hypotension. Electrocardiogram (ECG) changes may be evident (arrhythmia, tachycardia, bradycardia, or dysrhythmia).

CAD

Coronary (arteriosclerotic) artery disease (CAD) is the most frequently occurring cardiovascular disorder. Increased high-density lipoprotein (HDL) cholesterol levels initiate an inflammatory process, which damages the arterial lining. Low-density lipoprotein (LDL) cholesterol and monocytes then enter the tissue. A percentage of the monocytes turn into macrophages. The macrophages in combination with LDL cholesterol form foam cells. Foam cells are an indicator of atherosclerosis. HDL aids in clearing cholesterol from the lining of the artery. Plaques with a procoagulant lipid center and fibrous cap develop. If the cap ruptures, the lipids are released and may block the lumen. This can result in a thrombosis and lead to myocardial infarction if there is insufficient collateral circulation. Plaques may decrease in size with a decrease in serum cholesterol level. In this case, the lipid core shrinks and inflammation decreases. However, the fibrous cap of the plaque remains intact. HDL may be raised and LDL lowered by medications and changes in diet.

PAD

Peripheral vascular insufficiency is inadequate peripheral blood flow. It can involve both veins and arteries. Peripheral venous insufficiency is a chronic disorder and does not usually cause crises requiring acute care. Peripheral arterial disease (PAD) affects the aorta, arteries, and arterioles. In PAD, the arteries of the legs are often occluded. This causes extreme pain and ischemia. The distal aorta and femoral, popliteal, and iliac arteries are the vessels most commonly affected by peripheral arterial disease. Atherosclerosis is the most frequent cause of peripheral disease. Symptoms of PAD include intermittent claudication (cramping pain while walking), rest pain, and tissue changes (thickening of the nails, hair loss, dry skin, and ulcerations). These symptoms require treatment to remove the blockage (catheter or surgery). Acute occlusion may present with pain, lack of pulses, reduced skin temperature, reduced sensation, and loss of function. Acute occlusion requires immediate surgical intervention.

Cardiac Dysrhythmias

Cardiac dysrhythmias are abnormal heart rhythms. They often occur as a result of damage to the conduction system. Damage may occur during major cardiac surgery or after a myocardial infarction.

Bradydysrhythmias involve abnormally slow pulse rates.

- Complete atrioventricular (AV) block may be congenital or occur as a response to surgical trauma.
- Sinus bradycardia may be caused by the autonomic nervous system or occur because of hypotension and a decrease in available oxygen.
- Junctional/nodal rhythms occur frequently in postsurgical patients when the P wave is absent. Heart rate and output generally remain stable. Unless there is compromise, no treatment is necessary.

Tachydysrhythmias are abnormally fast pulse rates.

- Sinus tachycardia is often caused by illness.
- Supraventricular tachycardia (200-300 beat per minute) often has a sudden onset and if untreated leads to congestive heart failure.
- Conduction irregularities are irregular heart rhythms that occur postoperatively. They are usually of no significance.
- Premature contractions originate in the atria or ventricles.

Sinus Bradycardia

Sinus bradycardia (SB) results from a decreased impulse rate from the sinus node. The pulse and electrocardiogram (ECG) are abnormally slow but otherwise normal. SB is characterized by a regular heart rhythm with a pulse rate of fewer than 60 beats per minute (bpm). P waves are in front of QRS waves, which are generally normal in shape and duration. The PR interval is 0.12-0.20 seconds, and the P:QRS ratio is 1:1. There are a number of factors that can cause SB:

- Conditions that reduce the body's metabolic requirements (for example, hypothermia or sleep).
- Some medications (such as calcium channel blockers and beta-blockers).
- Vagal stimulation resulting from vomiting, suctioning, or defecating.
- Increased intracranial pressure.
- Myocardial infarction.

SB is treated by eliminating the cause of the disorder (for example, changing medications). Atropine 0.5-1.0 mg may be administered intravenously to block vagal stimulation.

Sinus Node Dysrhythmia

Sinus Arrhythmia

Sinus arrhythmia (SA) originates in the sinus node. The arrhythmia is often paradoxical, which means it increases with inspiration and decreases with expiration. This occurs because the vagal nerve is stimulated during inspiration. A negative hemodynamic effect rarely occurs as a result of sinus arrhythmia. Cyclical changes often occur in the pulse during respiration in both children and young adults. These changes often decrease with age. In some adults, they may persist. In some cases, sinus arrhythmia is associated with heart or valvular disease. Vagal stimulation that occurs during suctioning, vomiting, or defecating may increase sinus arrhythmia.

Sinus Tachycardia

Sinus tachycardia (ST) occurs as a result of an increase in the frequency of the sinus node impulse. ST is characterized by a regular pulse greater than 100 bpm. P waves occur before the QRS waves but are sometimes part of the preceding T wave. The shape and duration of the QRS waves are usually normal, but they may be consistently irregular. The PR interval is 0.12-0.20 seconds, and the P:QRS ratio is 1:1. The rapid pulse results in a decrease in the diastolic filling time and a reduction in cardiac output, resulting in hypotension. Decreased ventricular filling may lead to acute pulmonary edema. A number of factors may cause ST:

- Acute blood loss
- Shock
- Anemia
- Hypovolemia
- Sinus arrhythmia
- Heart failure (hypovolemic)
- Hypermetabolic conditions
- Fever
- Anxiety
- Exertion
- Medications (such as sympathomimetic drugs).

Treatment for ST includes eliminating the precipitating factors and reducing heart rate by means of calcium channel blockers and beta-blockers.

Atrial Dysrhythmia

Premature Atrial Contractions

A **premature atrial contraction (PAC)** is an extra beat caused by an electrical impulse to the atrium occurring before the sinus node impulse. This occurrence may be the result of alcohol, caffeine, or nicotine intake. PACs may also occur as a result of hypervolemia, hypokalemia, hypermetabolic conditions, atrial ischemia, or infarction. There is an irregular pulse because of extra P waves. Although the shape and duration of the QRS wave is usually normal, it may be abnormal. The PR interval is between 0.12-0.20 seconds. The P:QRS ratio is 1:1. PACs can occur in healthy hearts and are not cause for concern unless they occur at a rate of more than six per hour and cause severe palpitations. In severe cases, atrial fibrillation may be the cause and antidysrhythmic drugs may be required. Eliminating the cause usually helps to control the PACs.

Atrial Flutter

Atrial flutter (AF) results from an atrial rate that is faster (250-400 beats per minute [bpm]) than the conduction rate of the atrioventricular (AV) node. Not all of the impulses continue through into the ventricles. The impulses are blocked at the AV node. AF is caused by coronary artery disease, valvular disease, pulmonary disease, heavy alcohol ingestion, and cardiac surgery. Atrial rates reach 250-400, while ventricular rates reach 75-150; the ventricular rate is generally regular. The P waves are saw-toothed. These are referred to as fibrillatory (F) waves. The shape and duration of QRS waves are usually normal. It is difficult to calculate the PR interval because of F waves. The P:QRS ratio is 2:1-4:1. Symptoms include chest pain, dyspnea, and hypotension. There are a number of treatments for atrial fibrillation. Cardioversion is performed if the condition is unstable. Medications may be administered to control the heart rate. Medications may also be given to cause conversion to sinus rhythm.

Atrial Fibrillation

Atrial fibrillation (A Fib) involves rapid, disorganized atrial beats. A Fib can cause the formation of thrombus and emboli. The ventricular rate increases, while the stroke volume decreases. Cardiac output decreases, and myocardial ischemia increases. There are a number of causes for A Fib, including coronary artery disease, valvular disease, pulmonary disease, heavy alcohol ingestion, and cardiac surgery. In A Fib, the pulse is very irregular; the atrial rate is 300-600 bpm, and the ventricular rate is 120-200 bpm. Generally, the shape and duration of QRS waves are normal. Instead of P waves, fibrillatory (F) waves are seen. It is impossible to measure the PR interval. The P:QRS ratio varies. Cardioversion may be required if A Fib lasts longer than 48 hours. However, the condition frequently converts to normal sinus rhythm within 24 hours. There are a number of medications administered to treat A Fib. Ibutilide, procainamide, and digoxin are used to treat acute A Fib. Quinidine and amiodarone are administered to maintain rhythm. Ventricular rate is controlled by means of beta-blockers, calcium channel blockers, and verapamil. Heparin and Coumadin are given to prevent clotting.

Ventricular Dysrhythmia

Premature Ventricular Contractions

In a **premature ventricular contraction (PVC)** the electrical impulse starts in the ventricles and continues through the ventricles before the next sinus impulse. There may be one site (unifocal) or multiple sites (multifocal) stimulating the ectopic beats. For this reason, QRS complexes vary in shape. Unless there is an underlying heart condition or an acute myocardial infarction (MI), PVCs do not usually cause death. Characteristics of PVCs include an irregular heartbeat, an oddly shaped QRS wave that is greater than or equal to 0.12 seconds, an absent P wave or a P wave that precedes or follows the QRS wave, a PR interval of less than 0.12 seconds in cases in which a P wave is present, and a P:QRS ratio of 0:1-1:1. PVCs are often left untreated in healthy individuals, but lidocaine may be administered as a short-term treatment. PVCs may be triggered by caffeine, nicotine, or alcohol. PVCs may occur in conjunction with any type of supraventricular dysrhythmia, so the underlying rhythm must be determined as well.

Ventricular Fibrillation

Ventricular fibrillation (VF) is a rapid and very irregular ventricular rate. The ventricles beat at more than 300 beats per minute (bpm), but no atrial activity is observable on the electrocardiogram (ECG). The condition results from disorganized electrical activity in the ventricles. The QRS complex is not discernable; the ECG shows irregular undulations. The causes of ventricular fibrillation are the same as for ventricular tachycardia (VT). These include alcohol, caffeine, and nicotine intake and underlying coronary disease. If VT is left untreated, VF may result. Electrical shock can induce VF. Congenital disorders, such as Brugada syndrome, can also cause VF. Individuals with VF do not have a palpable pulse or audible pulse and lack respirations. VF is a life-threatening condition, and emergency defibrillation is necessary. The cause of the condition should be determined after normal rhythm is established. Antiarrhythmic agents (such as amiodarone) may be alternated with defibrillation to convert the heart rhythm to normal rhythm. If VF occurs as a result of MI, the mortality rate is high.

Ventricular Tachycardia

Ventricular tachycardia (VT) is defined as three or more PVCs in sequence with a ventricular rate of 100-200 bpm. Ventricular tachycardia and PVCs may have the same triggers, and both may be related to underlying coronary artery disease. However, the rapid rate of contractions during VT makes the condition dangerous. The heart does not pump blood efficiently during VT, and the ineffective beats may cause unconsciousness. If a rate is detectable, it is usually regular. The oddly shaped QRS complex is greater than or equal to 0.12 seconds. The P wave may or may not be present. If the P wave is present, the PR interval is irregular. The P:QRS ratio may be difficult to detect because of the absence of P waves. Treatment varies, depending on the severity of the condition. It may be necessary to use cardioversion to restore a normal sinus rhythm, but ventricular tachycardia (VT) may convert spontaneously. If the patient is unconscious and no pulse can be felt, defibrillation is usually administered as an emergency measure.

First-Degree AV Block

First-degree atrioventricular (AV) block describes a situation in which the atrial impulses are conducted through the AV node to the ventricles at a slower-than-normal rate. The P waves and QRS complex are usually normal. The PR interval is greater than 0.20 seconds, and the P:QRS ration is 1:1. If the QRS complex is narrow, it indicates that the conduction abnormality is only in the AV node. A widened QRS complex indicates that the bundle branches are also damaged. Chronic first-degree AV block may result from the fibrosis/sclerosis associated with coronary artery disease, valvular disease, and cardiac myopathies. This type of block is not usually associated with morbidity. Acute first-degree block is potentially much more serious and may occur as a result of digoxin toxicity, beta-blockers, amiodarone, myocardial infarction, hyperkalemia, or edema resulting from valvular surgery. The condition is correlated with increasing age. The incidence of first-degree AV block is low in young adults. However, elderly individuals have a lower rate of first-degree AV block (at 5%) than do athletes (8.7%).

SECOND-DEGREE AV BLOCK

Second-degree AV block describes a situation in which some of the atrial beats are blocked at the AV node. Second-degree AV block is divided into two types based on the pattern of blockage:

- **Mobitz type I block (Wenckebach):** In type I block, the interval between the atrial impulses in a group of beats increases until one fails to conduct (the PR interval progressively increases). This results in more P waves than QRS waves. However, the shape and duration of the QRS complex is usually normal. The sinus node conducts impulses at a regular rate, so the P-P interval is regular. However, the R-R interval usually becomes shorter with each impulse. The P:QRS ratio varies (for example, 3:2, 4:3, or 5:4). This type of block does not usually cause significant morbidity unless it is associated with inferior-wall myocardial infarction. If this occurs, a temporary pacemaker may be needed.
- In **Mobitz type II block,** some of the atrial impulses are conducted unpredictably through the AV node to the ventricles. The block always occurs below the AV node in the bundle of His, the bundle branches, or the Purkinje fibers. If the impulses are conducted, the PR intervals do not vary. In most cases, the QRS complex is widened. The P:QRS ratio varies (for example, 2:1, 3:1, and 4:1). Type II block is more serious than type l block. Type II block progress to complete AV block and may cause Stokes-Adams syncope. In addition, if the block occurs at the Purkinje fibers, there is no escape impulse. In the case of type II block, a transcutaneous cardiac pacemaker and defibrillator should be kept at the patient's bedside. If the heart block is caused by myocarditis or myocardial ischemia, chest pain may be experienced.

In a **2:1 block,** every other atrial impulse (P:QRS ratio of 2.1) is conducted through the AV node. A 2:1 block may be referred to as advanced second-degree AV block.

THIRD-DEGREE AV BLOCK

In **third-degree AV block,** the P waves outnumber the QRS waves and there is no clear relationship between the two. The atrial rate is 2-3 times the speed of the pulse rate. Because of this, the PR interval is irregular. In the case of sinoatrial (SA) node malfunction, the AV node fires at a lower rate. In the case of AV node malfunction, the pacemaker site in the ventricles takes over, resulting in a bradycardic rate. If there is a complete AV block, the heart still contracts. However, the contractions are often ineffectual. Atrioventricular dissociation occurs because the atrial P wave (sinus rhythm or atrial fibrillation) and the ventricular QRS wave (ventricular escape rhythm) are stimulated by different impulses. While the heart may be able to compensate at rest, it cannot compensate when placed under stress (exertion). Bradycardia results and may lead to congestive heart failure, syncope (fainting), or sudden death. Conduction abnormalities usually worsen gradually over time. Symptoms include dyspnea (shortness of breath), chest pain, and hypotension. Atropine is administered intravenously for these symptoms. The use of a transcutaneous pacemaker may be required. Complete persistent atrioventricular (AV) block normally requires an implanted pacemaker, usually dual chamber.

Pathophysiology Across the Lifespan: Respiratory

CHRONIC BRONCHITIS

Chronic bronchitis is a pulmonary airway disease defined by severe cough with sputum production lasting at least two years. Irritation of the airways causes an inflammatory response that increases the number of mucus-secreting glands and goblet cells. Ciliary function also decreases, allowing the extra mucus to plug the airways. In addition, the bronchial walls become thicker, and alveoli near the inflamed bronchioles become fibrotic. These changes prevent the alveolar macrophages from functioning properly. As a result, susceptibility to infection is increased. Chronic bronchitis occurs most frequently in individuals older than age 45. It occurs twice as often in females than in males. Symptoms include persistent cough with increasing amounts of sputum, dyspnea, and frequent respiratory tract infections. Treatment for chronic bronchitis includes bronchodilators, long-term continuous oxygen therapy, supplemental oxygen during exercise as required, pulmonary rehabilitation to improve exercise and breathing, antibiotics for infection, and corticosteroids for acute episodes.

EMPHYSEMA

Emphysema involves abnormal enlargement of air spaces at the ends of terminal bronchioles and destruction of the alveolar walls. As a result, gas exchange decreases and dead space increases. These changes lead to hypoxemia, hypercapnia, and respiratory acidosis. The capillary bed is damaged, resulting in an increased pulmonary blood flow and raised pressure in the right atrium (cor pulmonale) and pulmonary artery. Cardiac failure results from these changes. Complications of emphysema include respiratory insufficiency and failure. The two primary types of emphysema are centrilobular and panlobular. These may occur together.

- *Centrilobular* is the most common type. It affects the central portion of the respiratory lobule, sparing distal alveoli and usually the upper lobes. Symptoms include abnormal ventilation-perfusion ratios, hypoxemia, hypercapnia, and polycythemia with right-sided heart failure.
- *Panlobular* emphysema is an enlargement of all air spaces, including the bronchiole, alveolar duct, and alveoli. However, there is minimal inflammatory disease. Symptoms include hyperextended, rigid, barrel chest; marked dyspnea; weight loss; and active expiration.

COPD

Chronic obstructive lung disease (COPD) includes emphysema and chronic bronchitis. These disorders may occur separately or in combination. COPD causes a progressive limitation in airflow. The disease process includes an inflammatory response that results in a narrowing of the peripheral airways and thickening of the pulmonary blood vessel walls. Symptoms include chronic cough, dyspnea, and orthopnea. Acute episodes can result in decompensation with hypoxemia (arterial oxygen saturation [SAO_2] less than 90 with tachycardia, tachypnea, cyanosis, and change in mental status) and hypercapnia (mental status change and hypopnea). Assessment for severity includes pulmonary function tests, arterial blood gas (ABG) level, chest x-ray (to rule out pneumonia or other complications), and echocardiogram. Treatments include oxygen with nasal cannula, face mask, Venturi mask, or nonrebreathing mask to elevate partial pressure of oxygen in arterial blood (PAO_2) to greater than 60 mm Hg or SAO_2 to greater than 90 percent; beta-2 adrenergic agonists by nebulizer for bronchodilation; anticholinergics (ipratropium bromide by metered inhaler); corticosteroids (60-180 mg/day for 7-14 days in decreasing doses); antibiotics for infection; and assisted ventilation for muscle fatigue and respiratory acidosis.

PNEUMONIA

Pneumonia is an inflammation of the lung parenchyma; the alveoli fill with exudate. Pneumonia is a common disease, occurring in children and adults. Pneumonia may be a primary or secondary disease. It may occur as a result of another infection or disease. Pneumonia may be caused by bacteria, viruses, parasites, or fungi. There are a number of common causes for community-acquired pneumonia: *Streptococcus pneumoniae*, legionella species, *Haemophilus influenzae*, *Staphylococcus aureus*, *Mycoplasma pneumoniae*, and viruses.

Chemical damage may also cause pneumonia. Pneumonia is categorized according to site of infection. Lobar pneumonia involves one or more lobes of the lungs. If the pneumonia involves lobes in both lungs, it is referred to as bilateral or double pneumonia. Bronchial/lobular pneumonia involves the terminal bronchioles, and exudate pneumonia can involve the adjacent lobules. The pneumonia usually occurs in scattered patches throughout the lungs. Interstitial pneumonia primarily affects the interstitium and alveoli. White blood cells and plasma fill the alveoli, causing inflammation and creating fibrotic tissue as the alveoli are destroyed.

Aspiration Pneumonitis and Pneumonia

Aspiration pneumonitis and pneumonia result from the inhalation of toxic substances (for example, stomach contents). The inhaled substance damages the lungs. The risk factors for aspiration pneumonitis and pneumonia include an altered level of consciousness related to illness or sedation, certain diseases (such as Alzheimer's and Parkinson's), depression of the gag or swallowing reflex, intubation or feeding tubes, ileus or gastric distention, and gastrointestinal disorders (for example, gastroesophageal reflux disorders). Diagnosis is based on clinical findings, arterial blood gases showing hypoxemia, infiltrates observed on x-ray and an increased white blood cell count if infection is present. Symptoms are similar to other pneumonias and include cough (often with copious sputum), dyspnea, respiratory distress, cyanosis, tachycardia, and hypotension. Treatment includes suctioning as needed to clear the upper airway, supplemental oxygen, antibiotic therapy as indicated, and symptomatic respiratory support.

Asthma

An **acute asthma attack** occurs as a result of a precipitating stimulus, such as a substance that triggers an allergic response. An inflammatory cascade results that causes edema of the mucous membranes (swollen airway), contraction of smooth muscles (bronchospasm), increased mucus production (cough and obstruction), and hyperinflation of the airways (decreased ventilation and shunting). Mast cells and T lymphocytes produce cytokines. The cytokines cause increased blood flow, vasoconstriction, and bronchoconstriction. This causes fluid to leak from the blood vessels. Epithelial cells and cilia are destroyed, exposing nerves and causing hypersensitivity. Bronchodilation is stimulated by sympathetic nervous system receptors in the bronchi. The three main symptoms of asthma are cough, wheezing, and dyspnea. In cough-variant asthma, a severe cough may be the only symptom at the onset of the condition.

Reducing Exposure to Allergens

It is difficult if not impossible to control **asthma** without reducing or at best eliminating exposure to allergens. When this accomplished, asthma severity drastically decreases and quality of life increases for the patient:

- To control animal dander, it may be necessary to remove the pet from the home or at least from the patient's bedroom.
- Air filters placed over bedroom vents help to control air circulation.
- Dust mites can be controlled by encasing mattresses and pillowcases in allergen proof covers.
- Removing carpet is helpful to keep dust mites down.
- Humidity in the home should be less than 50%. Insect infestation should be controlled as well as mold and fungi.
- In extreme cases, one should limit exposure to the outside environment, especially during times of high pollen count or increased smog.

Lung Cancer

Lung cancer is the leading cause of cancer-related death in adults older than age 65. Approximately 80 to 90 percent of lung cancer is related to a history of smoking. Four types of lung cancer occur commonly in older adults: 1) Squamous cell cancer (40-50%) affects the central airway and is slow growing. 2) Adenocarcinoma (30-35%) affects the bronchial/mucosal glands and is more lethal than squamous cell cancer. 3) Large-cell cancer (15%) affects the bronchial/mucosal glands. 4) Small-cell (oat-cell) cancer (25%) affects the submucosal tissue, grows rapidly, and metastasizes rapidly (often by the time of diagnosis).

Symptoms depend on whether the cancer is localized or has spread. Symptoms can include cough, respiratory obstruction, pain, dyspnea, hoarseness, superior vena cava syndrome pneumonitis, pleural effusion, dysphagia, bronchoesophageal fistula, arrhythmia, and heart failure. Initial diagnosis is based on x-ray and computed tomography (CT). However, false negatives can occur. Cytologic screening may not detect cancer in the early stages. Treatment depends on the stage of the cancer and may include chemotherapy, surgery, or palliative care.

Tuberculosis

Tuberculosis (TB) is caused by *Mycobacterium tuberculosis. M. tuberculosis* is an extracellular agent and needs oxygen. It is attracted to the upper respiratory tract. It is also a facultative intracellular invader and is able to evade the immune system. The immune system of the host attempts to control the spread of the bacterium by walling it off with macrophages. This causes a positive skin reaction (cell-mediated immune response) but no infection. TB is particularly dangerous to immunocompromised individuals. Symptoms of TB may include weight loss, general debility, night sweats, and fever. A progressive cough with dyspnea and bloody sputum is common in pulmonary involvement. The disease is transmitted through airborne particles. These particles suspend in the air and are inhaled. The following steps can be taken to prevent the spread of the disease: prompt diagnosis; administration of antituberculosis drugs; airborne infection isolation, skin testing, and x-rays for exposed individuals; and preventive isoniazid therapy for those with latent infection or those newly converted to positive on TB testing.

Pathophysiology Across the Lifespan: GI/GU

Risk Factors for Fecal Incontinence

Common risk factors for **fecal incontinence** include the following:

- *Age*: Fecal incontinence is most common among elderly people with health problems, such as urinary incontinence.
- *Sex*: Women are more likely than men to experience fecal incontinence because women often suffer damage to the sphincter during childbirth. For example, scar tissue that forms after episiotomy may cause fecal incontinence. In addition, muscles weaken after multiple childbirths.
- *Neurological damage*: Congenital or acquired neurological defects are highly associated with fecal incontinence. In addition, progressive neuropathy (such as diabetes mellitus or multiple sclerosis) may result in the inability to control defecation.
- *Dementia/Alzheimer's disease*: Both fecal and urinary incontinence occur in late-stage Alzheimer's disease.

- *Physical disability*: Physical disability, either congenital or acquired, may lead to fecal incontinence. Accessing a toilet may be difficult for individuals with a disability. Some individuals may be unable to express the need to defecate. Others may not be able to physically manage toileting without assistance.

Constipation and Fecal Impaction

Constipation is a condition in which bowel movements are abnormally infrequent for an individual or in which hard, small stools are evacuated from the bowels fewer than three times per week. Food travels from the small intestine to the colon in semiliquid form. Fluid is absorbed in the colon, which is responsible for the consistency of the stool. If too much fluid is absorbed, the stool can become too dry. An individual with constipation may have abdominal distention and cramps and need to strain for defecation.

Fecal impaction occurs when hard stool in the rectum becomes a large, dense, immovable mass that cannot be expelled even with straining. Fecal impaction usually occurs as a result of chronic constipation. A person with fecal impaction may experience abdominal cramps and distention and intense rectal pressure and pain. The individual may feel a sense of urgency to defecate. Symptoms may include nausea and vomiting. In a case of fecal impaction, hemorrhoids will often become engorged. Fecal incontinence, with liquid stool leaking out around the impaction, may occur.

Factors Contributing to Bowel Dysfunction

Bowel dysfunction can be caused by factors that can be corrected and factors that require compensation. Bowel dysfunction includes diarrhea, constipation, and gas. Dietary factors that can contribute to bowel dysfunction include insufficient fiber and fluids and ingestion of certain foods. Some clinical conditions (such as hemorrhoids) may cause pain that delays defecation. Surgical treatment of hemorrhoids, fistulas, or the rectum may cause injury to the sphincters. Chronic diseases (such as irritable bowel syndrome and multiple sclerosis) may be associated with bowel dysfunction. Dementia may be associated with the inability to manage toileting. Delay of defecation is the most common cause of constipation, impaction, and fecal incontinence. Delay of defecation may result from functional disability or dementia. Medications frequently cause constipation. Some medications (antacids and antibiotics, for example) can cause diarrhea. Laxative abuse results in the development of laxative tolerance. Physical inactivity reduces bowel motility and increases constipation.

Bowel Obstruction and Infarction

Bowel obstruction can occur for the following reasons: an obstruction of the passage of intestinal contents because of constriction of the lumen, occlusion of the lumen, or lack of muscular contractions (paralytic ileus). Obstruction may be caused by congenital or acquired abnormality. Symptoms of bowel obstruction include abdominal pain and distention, abdominal rigidity, vomiting and dehydration, diminished or absent bowel sounds, severe constipation (obstipation), respiratory distress (resulting from pressure exerted by the diaphragm), shock (resulting from diminishing plasma volume and the movement of electrolytes from the bloodstream into the intestines), and sepsis (resulting from bacteria proliferation in the bowel and invasion of the bloodstream by bacteria).

Bowel infarction is ischemia of the intestines resulting from a severely restricted blood supply. It can be the result of a number of different conditions, such as strangulated bowel or occlusion of arteries of the mesentery. It may occur subsequent to untreated bowel obstruction. Patients present with acute abdomen and shock. The mortality rate is very high even with resection of the infarcted section of bowel.

Diarrhea

Diarrhea is a condition in which an individual passes liquid or semiliquid stool more frequently than is normal. Diarrhea is often accompanied by abdominal cramping, distention, and sense of urgency to defecate. Individuals with severe diarrhea may need to defecate hourly. Diarrhea is characterized according to color, odor, consistency, and frequency of defecation. Diarrhea may be acute or chronic. Acute diarrhea usually has a sudden onset and may be caused by chemotherapy, irritating foods, gastrointestinal organisms, and stress. Diarrhea may be watery or bloody. It may be accompanied by flatus. Acute diarrhea usually resolves without treatment within a few days or responds to antidiarrheals. Chronic diarrhea persists more than three days and is usually the result of a long-term disease process (such as Crohn's disease) or trauma (such as radiation therapy). Certain foods may irritate the gastrointestinal tract and cause chronic diarrhea. Chronic diarrhea may also result from laxative overuse, in which there may be a cycle of constipation followed by diarrhea.

Urinary Incontinence

Causes

There are many potential causes of **urinary incontinence**:

- *Pregnancy/childbirth*: Childbirth weakens the muscles of the pelvic floor and urethral sphincter. Nerve damage and bladder prolapse are also possible complications of pregnancy that can contribute to incontinence.
- *Postmenopausal changes*: Menopause involves a loss of estrogen. This can cause bladder and urethral tissues to weaken.
- *Hysterectomy*: This surgery can damage the muscles and nerves in the urinary tract because of the proximity of the urinary tract and the uterus.
- *Interstitial cystitis*: This is an inflammation that sometimes causes incontinence.
- *Prostate enlargement*: The enlarging prostate constricts the urethra and leads to urgency or overflow incontinence.
- *Prostate cancer*: Incontinence may be caused directly by the cancer or may occur in response to radiation or the surgical removal of the prostate.
- *Bladder cancer*: Dysuria and incontinence are common symptoms.
- *Neurological deficits*: Neurological deficits present at birth or caused by injury or disease can result in the inability to control urination.
- *Urinary tract obstruction*: An obstruction anywhere in the urinary tract can cause overflow incontinence.

Types

The different types of **urinary incontinence** are as follows: urge, stress, overflow, functional, reflex, mixed, and induced. An individual may have more than one type of incontinence.

- An individual with *urge incontinence* feels a pressing need to urinate as soon as the bladder feels full. As a result, the individual may urinate on the way to the toilet or in bed during the night. Diuretics may worsen urge incontinence.
- *Stress incontinence* involves a sudden increase in bladder pressure resulting from such actions as coughing, laughing, or bending. Stress incontinence causes small amount of urine to leak from the bladder. It is common in people who are obese.
- *Overflow incontinence* usually occurs when the bladder is overfull. Small amounts of urine dribble from the urinary tract, and the leakage can be almost constant.

- *Functional incontinence* results from physical or mental impairment or environmental barriers to urination, such as the lack of an accessible bathroom.
- *Reflex urination* involves the loss of urine without the individual's awareness. It occurs as a result of a fistula or bladder leak.

Overactive Bladder

Overactive bladder is a condition involving urgency, frequency, and nocturia but not incontinence. The urge to urinate may be as frequent as every 20 to 30 minutes in extreme cases. If nocturia is present, people may become sleep deprived. If overactive bladder includes incontinence, it is known as urge incontinence. The treatments are similar for overactive bladder and urge incontinence. Treatment includes drug therapy, specific exercises, behavioral modification, fluid management, and dietary changes. Anticholinergics (antimuscarinics) such as Detrol and Ditropan relax the bladder muscle and relieve symptoms. Pelvic-floor muscle exercises include Kegel exercises and vaginal weight training as well as biofeedback or pelvic-floor electrical stimulation conducted in conjunction with the Kegel exercise program. Behavioral modification involves bladder training, including scheduled voiding with increasing time between urinations, and strategies to delay urination. Prompted urination may be needed for some people, especially those with dementia. Fluid management involves decreasing fluids in the evening while still maintaining adequate fluid intake. Reducing caffeine and other ingested bladder irritants may reduce contractions.

Urinary Tract Infections

Urinary infections develop in the urinary tract (kidneys, ureters, bladder, and urethra). These are common and often recurring low-grade infections. The prompt treatment of urinary infections is very important. Some symptoms of urinary tract infection appear as changes in the character of the urine. The urine may become cloudy from mucus or purulent material. Blood may be evident in the urine. The urine may take on a dark yellow, orange, or brown color as it becomes more concentrated. The urine may have a very strong or foul odor. Urinary output may decrease markedly. A urinary tract infection may cause pain in the lower back or flank, resulting from inflammation of the kidneys. Systemic symptoms include fever, chills, headache, and general malaise. Some people suffer lack of appetite, nausea, and vomiting. Fever usually indicates that the infection has affected the kidneys. The treatment for urinary tract infection includes increased fluid intake and antibiotics.

Bladder Cancer

Bladder cancer originates in the lining of the urinary organs and then invades the deeper layers. The bladder wall and lining of the urinary tract are composed of several layers, listed here from the inner to the outer layer: the urothelium (mucosa), urothelial (transitional) cells lining the inside layer of the urinary tract; the lamina propria (submucosa), a thin layer of connective tissue; the muscularis propria, a thicker layer of muscle; the serosa, fatty connective tissue covering the superior surfaces; and the adventitia, covering areas with no serosa.

There are several *symptoms* of bladder cancer. Gross hematuria is the presence of blood in the urine. Bright red blood may be evident. The urine may be brown or rust colored. Blood in the urine may appear intermittently. The patient may exhibit microscopic hematuria; in this case, the blood is visible only under a microscope. The patient may experience dysuria. Bladder cancer may cause burning or pain on urination and a feeling that the bladder does not empty completely. Urination may be frequent.

Renal Metabolic Requirements

The kidneys comprise approximately 0.5% of the total body mass of an adult but consume approximately 7% of the total body oxygen, so **renal metabolic requirements** are high relative to size. Approximately 1200 mL of blood flows through the kidneys each minute, or 25% of the cardiac output at rest. The kidneys consume twice as much oxygen as the brain while receiving 7 times more blood; the flow of oxygen through the kidneys far exceeds metabolic needs and is directly related to the need for a high glomerular filtration rate, required to regulate body fluids and electrolytes. The kidneys' relatively high consumption of oxygen is directly related to sodium reabsorption. The more sodium reabsorbed, the higher the consumption of oxygen. Thus, if the kidneys are not functioning, the GFR stops, and sodium is not being reabsorbed, and the kidneys' need for oxygen drops to 25% of the normal, indicating the basal metabolic requirements to nourish the kidney and remove cellular waste products.

Renal Failure

Renal failure is the inability of the kidneys to filter waste products, excrete waste products, concentrate urine, and maintain electrolyte balance. Renal failure may occur because of hypoxia, kidney disease, or obstruction of the urinary tract. It leads to azotemia (accumulation of nitrogenous waste in the blood) followed by uremia (toxic symptoms caused by accumulation of nitrogenous wastes). The kidneys cannot perform necessary functions after 50 percent of functional renal capacity is lost. Loss of renal function leads to progressive deterioration and eventually end-stage renal disease. Initial symptoms are often nonspecific and include loss of appetite, loss of energy, weight loss, muscle cramping, fatigue, bruising of the skin, dry or itching skin, increase in blood urea nitrogen (BUN) and serum creatinine, fluid retention (leading to edema), hyperkalemia, metabolic acidosis, calcium and phosphorus depletion (leading to altered bone structure and metabolism), and uremic syndrome. Treatment for renal failure includes dialysis and transplantation. The patient receives supportive care and symptomatic therapy.

Pyelonephritis

Pyelonephritis is a bacterial infection of the parenchyma of the kidney. The infection has the potential to permanently damage the kidneys. Pyelonephritis can lead to abscess formation, sepsis, and kidney failure. Pyelonephritis is especially dangerous to individuals who have compromised immune systems, are pregnant, or have diabetes. Most infections are caused by *Escherichia coli*. Symptoms vary widely but can include dysuria, frequent urination, hematuria, flank and/or low-back pain, fever and chills, costovertebral angle tenderness, and changes in mental status (geriatric). Patients may need to be hospitalized and require careful follow-up. Diagnosis is based on urinalysis and blood and urine cultures. Treatments include analgesia, antipyretics, intravenous fluids, and antibiotics. Antibiotics used to treat pyelonephritis include ceftriaxone and fluoroquinolone.

Dehydration

Older adults do not conserve water efficiently, have a less pronounced sense of thirst, and may have impaired sodium balance. For many older adults, lean body mass decreases from 65 percent to 40 percent; fat increases and total body water decreases. **Dehydration** results when total body water decreases but total body sodium does not decrease. This can result from inadequate fluid intake, excess water loss, disease, nasogastric suctioning, drugs, diarrhea, vomiting, and fever. Dehydration can be mild, moderate, or severe. Diagnostic criteria include increased hematocrit, blood urea nitrogen (BUN)/creatinine ratio, and urine sodium (less than 20 mEq/L). Treatment includes estimating fluid loss and replacing 50 percent of the loss within the first 12 hours.

- **Mild dehydration** involves a *five percent loss* of total body water. Symptoms include dizziness, lethargy, altered mentation, decreased skin turgor, dry mucous membranes, dysrhythmia, and orthostatic hypotension. Treatment includes increasing oral fluids or the administration of intravenous fluids.
- **Moderate dehydration** involves a *10 percent loss* of total body water. Symptoms include confusion, resting hypotension, tachycardia, and oliguria/anuria.
- **Severe dehydration** involves a *greater than 15 percent loss* of total body water. Marked hypotension and anuria occur at this stage.

Gastrointestinal Hemorrhage

A **gastrointestinal (GI) hemorrhage** may occur in either the upper or lower GI tract. The main cause of GI hemorrhage (50 to 70% of cases) is peptic ulcer disease (gastric and duodenal ulcers). Peptic ulcer disease causes the gastromucosal lining to break down, which compromises the glycoprotein mucous barrier and the gastroduodenal epithelial cells that provide protection from gastric secretions. The gastric secretions erode the mucosal and submucosal layers, damaging blood vessels and causing hemorrhage. The primary causes are nonsteroidal anti-inflammatory drugs (NSAIDs) and infection by the *Helicobacter pylori* bacterium. Symptoms include abdominal pain and distention, bloody or tarry stools, hypotension, and tachycardia. Treatment includes fluid replacement; antibiotic therapy for *H. pylori* infection; endoscopic thermal therapy to cauterize; injection therapy (hypertonic saline, epinephrine, and ethanol) to cause vasoconstriction; and arteriography with intra-arterial infusion of vasopressin and/or embolizing agents (such as stainless-steel coils, platinum microcoils, or Gelfoam pledgets). A vagotomy and pyloroplasty are performed if bleeding persists.

GERD

Gastroesophageal reflux disease (GERD) is the regurgitation of the stomach contents into the esophagus. It usually results from decreased tone in the gastroesophageal valve and hiatal hernia. The stomach contents damage the mucosal lining of the esophagus. A number of conditions may develop from GERD. These include chronic esophagitis, strictures, Barrett's esophagus (abnormal changes in the cells of the distal esophagus), and esophageal cancer. GERD symptoms include epigastric pain, heartburn, dysphagia, chronic cough (particularly at night), hoarseness, earache, and sinusitis. There are a number of treatments. Patients are advised to avoid eating large meals and snacking after dinner. Eating at least three hours before bedtime is recommended.

Certain foods, such as coffee, alcohol, fatty foods, spicy foods, and cruciferous vegetables, should be avoided. The patient is advised to sleep on the left side with the head of the bed elevated. The condition is also treated with medications, including histamine-2 receptor blockers (famotidine and ranitidine), proton pump inhibitors, alginic acid (Gaviscon), and antacids (without aluminum). Surgical repair, called fundoplication, may be necessary.

Hiatal Hernias

The esophagus exits the pleural cavity and enters the abdominal cavity through an opening in the diaphragm. The diaphragm should surround the esophagus tightly to prevent the stomach from entering the pleural cavity. A **hiatal hernia** results when a defect in the diaphragm causes it to loosen and permits a portion of the stomach to swell into the chest cavity. Hiatal hernias occur more often in women than in men. There are two main types of hiatal hernia: sliding and paraesophageal (rolling). Some individuals may have a combined form.

- A *sliding hiatal hernia* occurs when the gastroesophageal junction and the proximal stomach slide in and out of the chest cavity. This is the most common form (about 90%) of hiatal hernia. A sliding hiatal hernia occurs because of a laxity in the gastroesophageal junction, and the condition often involves reflux, regurgitation, and heartburn.
- A *paraesophageal hiatal hernia* is one in which all or part of the stomach swells up into the chest cavity while the gastroesophageal junction remains in place. This does not cause symptoms of reflux.

Types of Colorectal Cancers

Types of **colorectal cancers** include the following:

- *Adenocarcinomas,* which account for 90 to 95 percent of colorectal cancers, originate in epithelial tissue in adenomatous polyps. There are two subtypes. *Signet ring* is a very aggressive form of adenocarcinoma. It is hard to treat but accounts for only 0.1 percent of adenocarcinomas. *Mucinous* is also an aggressive form of adenocarcinoma. This form is composed of about 60 percent mucus, which allows the cells to spread faster and makes the cancer difficult to treat. Mucinous adenocarcinoma accounts for 10 to 15 percent of adenocarcinomas.
- *Sarcomas* (leiomyosarcomas) develop in smooth muscle. Sarcomas account for less than two percent of colorectal cancers; however, over 50 percent of sarcomas metastasize.
- *Carcinoids* are slow-growing tumors that rarely spread and are most frequently found in the rectum. Carcinoids account for less than one percent of colorectal cancers.
- *Lymphoma* is a rare type of colorectal cancer. Lymphomas are primary tumors that usually occur in the rectum, while secondary metastatic tumors usually occur in the colon.
- *Melanomas* are tumors that have usually metastasized from other parts of body. They account for less than two percent of colorectal cancers.

Types of Primary Cancer of the Small Intestine

The small intestine does not develop cancerous lesions as frequently as other parts of the gastrointestinal tract. The four main types of **primary small intestine cancer** are named according to the type of cells from which they develop.

- *Adenocarcinomas* are the most commonly occurring type of primary small intestine cancer. Adenocarcinomas originate in the lining of intestine and usually occur in the duodenum.
- *Carcinoids* originate in hormone-producing cells in the small bowel. Carcinoids occur most frequently in the ileum and sometimes in the appendix.
- *Lymphomas* originate in the lymph tissue. They are generally of the non-Hodgkin's type and occur most frequently in the jejunum or ileum.
- *Sarcomas* originate in the supportive tissues, such as fat and muscle. *Leiomyosarcomas* generally develop in the muscle wall of the ileum. Gastrointestinal stromal tumors may originate in any section of the small intestine.

Right-Sided (Ascending) Colon Cancer

Stool enters the cecum and ascending colon in liquid form; therefore, cancers arising in these areas may grow to a large size before they cause obstruction and obvious symptoms. Lesions frequently ulcerate the intestine and cause chronic bleeding that may not change the character or the appearance of the stool. Liquid stool is able to pass through a very narrow opening. Twenty-two percent of colorectal tumors originate in the ascending colon. Symptoms of **ascending colon cancer** include the following:

- Fatigue
- Generalized weakness
- Pallor
- Dull abdominal pain
- Loss of appetite
- Weight loss
- Occult blood or melena (tarry stools)
- Hypochromic microcytic anemia
- Chronic iron deficiency anemia
- Palpitations (related to anemia)
- Congestive heart failure (related to anemia)
- Palpable abdominal mass (may be evident with large tumors)
- Chronic diarrhea (may result with some large right-sided lesions)
- Bowel obstruction (in the late stages).

Transverse, Descending, Sigmoid, and Rectal Cancers

Fluid in the intestines is absorbed in the ascending colon, so stool in the transverse and descending colon is more solid. Lesions originating in the transverse and descending colon are usually annular constrictive lesions. These encircle the intestine and cause to obstruction. Tumors of the sigmoid colon and rectum may exert pressure on adjacent structures (such as the vagina, prostate, and bladder).

Characteristics of **transverse and descending colon cancers** include changes in bowel habits; abdominal cramping, especially in the left-lower quadrant; pencil-thin stools from narrowing of the lumen; constipation; abdominal distention; intestinal obstruction; perforation of the bowel; and peritonitis.

Characteristics of **sigmoid colon and rectal cancers** include tenesmus (painful, ineffective straining to pass stool); pain in rectal or perianal area; feeling of fullness and incomplete evacuation of stool; alternating constipation and diarrhea; frank blood in stool; blood clots; pencil-thin stools from narrowing of the lumen; abdominal pain and cramping; urinary symptoms; and vaginal fistulae.

Compensated Cirrhosis and Decompensated Cirrhosis

Cirrhosis of the liver is a condition in which the liver is scarred. The two types of cirrhosis are compensated and decompensated. The term compensated means that the liver is still capable of coping with the damage. In this case, there is no sign of liver failure.

- *Compensated cirrhosis* is usually indicated by nonspecific symptoms, such as intermittent fever, epistaxis, edema, indigestion, abdominal pain, and palmar erythema. Hepatomegaly and splenomegaly may also be present. Many people with compensated cirrhosis are stable for years before the liver starts to fail. Liver failure does not occur suddenly, but slowly. Signs that the liver is starting to fail are evident for some time before failure occurs.
- *Decompensated cirrhosis* occurs when the liver is no longer capable of synthesizing proteins, clotting factors, and other necessary substances. It is indicated by the development of one or more of the following symptoms: jaundice (yellow discoloration of the skin and eyes), variceal hemorrhage, fluid in the peritoneal cavity (ascites), and encephalopathy.

Liver Failure and Portal Hypertension

The right and left hepatic arteries supply the liver with oxygenated blood. The liver also receives nutrient-rich blood from the intestinal tract via the portal vein. Blood from the portal vein is filtered in the liver. Pathogens and nutrients from the blood are absorbed and metabolized in the liver by the hepatocytes. The liver stores nutrients and excretes unwanted substances into the hepatic veins and inferior vena cava. In **liver failure,** portal hypertension impairs this process.

In **portal hypertension**, the portal vein becomes blocked, and blood flow is reduced. This increases blood pressure in the portal venous system, which is already compressed by cirrhotic changes. Because the liver cannot adequately filter the blood, increased pressure creates collateral blood vessels that bypass the obstruction. Unfiltered blood returns to the systemic circulation via the collateral vessels. Varices form in the esophagus and other areas as a result of the collateral vessels. Increased aldosterone causes sodium and fluid to be retained. Plasma albumin decreases, causing fluid to leak from the vascular system. Ascites results from this process.

Hepatorenal Syndrome and Hepatic Encephalopathy

Hepatorenal syndrome and hepatic encephalopathy are part of the syndrome of **hepatic failure.**

- *Hepatorenal syndrome* involves a marked decrease in renal blood flow resulting in azotemia (abnormal levels of nitrogenous substances). Sodium level falls and potassium level increases. The syndrome involves abnormalities in blood chemistry and clotting time. Hepatorenal syndrome is related to hepatic encephalopathy.
- *Hepatic encephalopathy* occurs when ammonia crosses the blood-brain barrier and is absorbed by brain tissue. Under normal circumstances, protein is digested in the intestines and the ammonia that is produced as a waste product is filtered by the liver and broken down to form urea. Restricted blood flow from the portal system causes the level of ammonia in the blood to increase. Ammonia causes mental confusion, stupor, and finally, coma. Marked changes are observable on an electroencephalogram (EEG).

Prostatitis and Benign Prostatic Hypertrophy

Prostatitis is an acute infection of the prostate gland. It is caused by bacteria such as *Escherichia coli, Pseudomonas*, or *Staphylococcus*. Symptoms include fever and chills lower back pain, frequent urination, dysuria, painful ejaculation, and perineal discomfort. Diagnosis is based on physical assessment showing perineal tenderness and spasm of the rectal sphincter. Treatment includes 500 mg of ciprofloxacin taken orally twice a day for one month (treatment of choice) and trimethoprim/sulfamethoxazole double-strength (TMP/SMX DS) twice daily for one month. A urethral culture is taken to check for sexually transmitted diseases (STDs).

Benign prostatic hypertrophy/hyperplasia usually develops in men after the age of 40. The prostate enlarges gradually, but the surrounding tissue limits outward growth, so the gland compresses the urethra. The bladder wall also exhibits changes. It becomes thicker and irritated and begins to spasm, causing frequent urination. With time, the bladder muscle weakens and the bladder does not empty completely on urination. Symptoms include urgency, dribbling, frequent urination, nocturia, incontinence, urine retention, and bladder distention. Diagnostic methods include intravenous pyelogram (IVP), cystogram, and prostate-specific antigen (PSA). Treatment methods include catheterization for urine retention and surgical excision.

Sexual Dysfunction

Sexual activity lessens with age. However, approximately 50 percent of individuals older than age 60 engage in sexual activity. Typically, sexual desire decreases with age. Women have more difficulty reaching orgasm as they age. Vaginal lubrication decreases, and **vaginal atrophy** may be present. Men require more stimulation to achieve an erection, which may not be as firm. The amount of ejaculate may be decreased. **Dyspareunia** (painful intercourse) may be treated with vaginal estrogen preparations in the form of creams and tablets. Water-based products may be used to provide lubrication. **Erectile dysfunction** may result from vascular disease, diabetes, smoking, urinary tract infections (UTIs), alcohol use, obesity, and lack of testosterone. Various medications may also cause erectile dysfunction. Treatment may include oral medications (such as Viagra, Cialis), intracorporeal injections (injections into the corpus cavernosa), or intraurethral medications (pellets inserted into the urethra with an applicator). Mechanical devices to treat erectile dysfunction include external vacuum tumescence devices (an elastic ring at the base of the penis inhibits venous drainage to maintain erection) and the penile prosthesis (a surgical procedure used if other means fail).

Vulvovaginitis

Vulvovaginitis is a condition in which the vulva and vaginal tissues are inflamed. There are a number of different causes: bacterial (*Gardnerella vaginalis*), fungal (usually *Candida albicans*), or parasitic (*Trichomonas vaginalis*). Vulvovaginitis can be caused by an allergy to soaps or other irritants (allergic-contact vaginitis). In addition, atrophic vaginitis occurs in women who are postmenopausal. Symptoms of the condition include vaginal odor, swelling, discharge, bleeding, pain, and itching. Diagnosis is based on physical examination, culture (discharge), and pH testing. Treatment depends on the cause of the condition. Bacterial infections are treated with all of the following medications simultaneously: metronidazole orally, metronidazole gel intravaginally, and clindamycin cream. Fungal infections are treated with Diflucan or vaginal creams, tablets, or suppositories (such as Femstat or Vagistat). Parasitic (*Trichomonas*) infections are treated with metronidazole orally.

Pathophysiology Across the Lifespan: Musculoskeletal

Osteoarthritis and Rheumatoid Arthritis

Osteoarthritis often occurs following injury, but it may be idiopathic. The disease is progressive, with symptoms occurring after age 60. Osteoarthritis involves deterioration of the cartilage. Signs and symptoms of the disease include increasing pain with use and/or weight bearing and stiffness. The involvement is local and unilateral. Treatment includes nonsteroidal anti-inflammatory drugs (NSAIDs), heat, weight reduction, joint rest, orthotic devices, postural exercises, osteotomy, and arthroplasty (with joint replacement).

Rheumatoid arthritis is a systemic autoimmune inflammatory disorder. Its cause is unknown. It has an acute onset, and is first evident in the hands, wrists, and feet. The disease usually develops between the ages of 25 to 50 years. Rheumatoid arthritis causes joint inflammation and deformity. Signs and symptoms include pain, stiffness, swelling, erythema, nodules, generalized weakness, fatigue, weight loss, and fever. The involvement is systemic, bilateral, and symmetric. Treatment includes light exercise to prevent contractures. Medications used to treat the disease include salicylates (e.g., ASA), NSAIDs, cyclo-oxygenase-2 (COX-2) inhibitors (e.g., Celebrex), disease-modifying antirheumatic drugs (gold-containing compounds, methotrexate, azathioprine, and adalimumab), immunomodulators (e.g., abatacept), interleukin 1 receptor inhibitors (e.g., anakinra), and glucocorticoids (e.g., prednisone) and topical analgesics.

Musculoskeletal Deformities

Musculoskeletal deformities may interfere with mobility and independence or cause serious health problems. As a person ages, bones become more porous, muscle mass reduces, and ligaments and tendons lose strength and elasticity. Foot deformities (such as bunions, hammertoes, corns, calluses, and bone spurs) may cause pain and inflammation and limit mobility. Hand deformities (such as those caused by arthritis or carpal tunnel syndrome) may increase dependence. Overuse syndromes and decreased sensation of touch are common. The hands may feel cold due to vascular insufficiency. Spinal deformities include kyphosis, lordosis, and scoliosis.

- *Kyphosis* is a convex angulation of the thoracic spine. It may occur as a consequence of arthritis or compression fractures. Kyphosis may cause compression of thoracic and abdominal structures and lead to decreased ventilation and perfusion.
- *Lordosis* is a frequently painful concave angulation of the lumbar spine. It is often associated with obesity, flexion hip contracture, and slipped femoral capital epiphysis.
- *Scoliosis* is a lateral and rotational curvature of the spine. It can cause alterations in the structure of the pelvis and chest.

Pathophysiology Across the Lifespan: Endocrine

Type 1 Diabetes

The most commonly occurring metabolic disorder is diabetes mellitus. **Type 1 diabetes** is an autoimmune disease. Insufficient insulin production occurs as a result of the destruction of pancreatic beta cells. This results in a lack of insulin. The lack of insulin first leads to an increase in fasting blood glucose and then to an increase in urine glucose. Individuals with the disorder exhibit pronounced polyuria and polydipsia. The disease has a fast onset. Individuals with the disorder may be overweight or have experienced a recent weight loss. Ketoacidosis may be present. Insulin is needed to control blood sugar. This type of diabetes is fatal without treatment using exogenous insulin. Glucose monitoring is necessary one to four times each day. The patient's intake of carbohydrates is controlled. Exercise is prescribed.

Type 2 Diabetes

Type 2 diabetes is more common, and the incidence increases with age. The disease used to be called adult-onset diabetes; however, the incidence of type 2 diabetes is increasing in children due increasing rates of obesity. In type 2 diabetes, the pancreas does not produce sufficient insulin or the body cannot efficiently use the insulin produced by the pancreas. This is called insulin resistance. The disease has a slow onset. It is associated with obesity. Nonketotic hyperglycemia may occur in individuals with the disease. Ketoacidosis is not common. The development of type 2 diabetes may be prevented or slowed by eating a proper diet and exercising. Type 2 diabetes is a chronic disease, and there is no known cure. Treatment is aimed at reducing mortality and morbidity and preserving quality of life. The disease is treated by diet and exercise. Oral medications are available.

Risk Factors for Neuropathic/Diabetic Ulcers

There are a number of **risk factors** for the development of neuropathic/ diabetic ulcers:

- *Sensory loss* can cause sores and ulcers to go undetected in the early stages.
- *Vascular insufficiency,* especially peripheral artery disease, occurs 4 times more frequently in diabetics.
- *Autonomic neuropathy* decreases sweating, leaving feet dry and more prone to cracks and sores.
- Long-term diabetes mellitus with poor glucose control causes severe damage to the circulatory system.

- *Smoking* increases vascular damage and arterial insufficiency.
- *Deformities or lack of mobility* may increase risk of developing ulcers or having ulcers remain undetected.
- *Obesity* decreases circulation and interferes with control of diabetes. Between 80-90% of diabetics are overweight.
- *Male gender* increases risk.
- *Poor vision* may cause people to overlook dangers or prevent them from examining the feet and skin.
- *Age* is associated with increased danger of ulcers.
- *Ethnic background* can determine genetic risks: Native Americans, Hispanic Americans, African Americans and Pacific Islanders are more prone to these ulcers.
- Improperly fitted and non-supportive footwear can cause ulcerations.

Hyperglycemia

Hyperglycemia is a condition in which the serum glucose is elevated to 180 mg/dL or higher. However, symptoms may not be evident until serum glucose reaches 270 mg/dL or higher. The most common cause of hyperglycemia is diabetes mellitus, but the condition may also result from chronic pancreatitis, acromegaly, Cushing's syndrome, and adverse reactions to certain drugs (furosemide, glucocorticoids, growth hormone, oral contraceptives, and thiazides). Symptoms of hyperglycemia are similar to those that occur with chronic diabetes. Symptoms include ketoacidosis, polyuria, polydipsia, polyphagia, weight loss, and encephalopathy. Stress-related hyperglycemia may occur after stroke and myocardial infarction and increases the risk of mortality. Physiological stress associated with infection may also increase glucose levels. Hyperglycemia can be treated with insulin and by addressing the underlying cause.

Ketoacidosis

Ketoacidosis is a complication of diabetes mellitus. Because of an insufficient production of insulin, glucose is unavailable for metabolism. As a result, fat is broken down as an alternate fuel source. Glycerol in both fat cells and the liver is converted to ketone bodies (beta-hydroxybutyrate, acetoacetic, and acetone), which are then used for cellular metabolism. Fat is a less efficient fuel than glucose. The excess ketone bodies are excreted in the urine (ketonuria) or in exhalations. The ketone bodies lower serum pH, leading to ketoacidosis. Symptoms include Kussmaul respirations (hyperventilation to eliminate buildup of carbon dioxide), fluid imbalance (resulting in dehydration and diuresis with excess thirst), cardiac arrhythmias (sometimes resulting in cardiac arrest), and hyperglycemia (blood glucose 300-800 mg/dL). Treatment includes insulin therapy by continuous infusion, rehydration, and electrolyte replacement.

Hypoglycemia

Acute hypoglycemia (hyperinsulinism) may result from a number of conditions. Pancreatic islet tumors and hyperplasia increase insulin production, which decreases blood sugar. The use of insulin to control diabetes mellitus may cause a decrease in blood sugar. Hyperinsulinism can cause damage to the central nervous system and cardiopulmonary system. Causes of acute hypoglycemia include genetic defects in chromosome 11 (short arm); severe infections (gram-negative sepsis and endotoxic shock, for example); toxic ingestion of alcohol or drugs (such as salicylates); too much insulin for body needs; and too little food or excessive exercise. Symptoms include blood glucose level less than 50 to 60 mg/dL, seizures, altered consciousness, lethargy, loss of appetite, vomiting, myoclonus, respiratory distress, diaphoresis, hypothermia, cyanosis, diaphoresis, tremor, tachycardia, palpitation, hunger, and anxiety.

Treatment depends on underlying cause and includes glucose or glucagon administration to elevate blood glucose levels, diazoxide (Hyperstat) to inhibit release of insulin, and somatostatin (Sandostatin) to suppress insulin production.

Hypothyroidism

Hypothyroidism is a condition in which the thyroid produces inadequate amounts of thyroid hormones. The condition may range from mild to severe. There are a number of causes: chronic lymphocytic thyroiditis (Hashimoto's thyroiditis); excessive treatment for hyperthyroidism; atrophy of the thyroid gland; medications, such as lithium and iodine compounds; radiation to the area of the thyroid; diseases that affect the thyroid, such as scleroderma; and iodine imbalances. Signs and symptoms include chronic fatigue, menstrual disturbances, hoarseness, subnormal temperature, low pulse rate, weight gain, thinning hair, and thickening skin. Some dementia may occur in advanced cases. Clinical findings may include increased cholesterol levels with associated atherosclerosis and coronary artery disease. Myxedema may occur. Signs and symptoms include changes in respiration with hypoventilation and CO_2 retention resulting in coma. Treatment involves hormone replacement with synthetic levothyroxine (Synthroid) based on thyroid-stimulating hormone (TSH) levels. However, this increases the oxygen requirements of the body, necessitating careful monitoring of cardiac status to avoid myocardial infarction while establishing the normal hormone levels.

Hyperthyroidism

Hyperthyroidism (thyrotoxicosis) is a condition in which excessive amounts of thyroid hormones are produced by the thyroid gland. This occurs as a result of abnormal stimulation of the thyroid gland by immunoglobulins. Other causes include thyroiditis (inflammation of the thyroid) and excessive amounts of thyroid medication. Symptoms vary and may be nonspecific, especially in the elderly. Symptoms include hyperexcitability, tachycardia, atrial fibrillation, increased systolic (but not diastolic) blood pressure, poor heat tolerance, flushed skin, diaphoresis, dry skin, pruritis (especially in the elderly), hand tremor, progressive muscular weakness, exophthalmos (bulging eyes), and increased appetite and food intake with weight loss. Treatment involves a series of actions. Radioactive iodine is administered to destroy the thyroid gland. Propranolol may be used to prevent thyroid storm. Thyroid hormones are given for resultant hypothyroidism. Antithyroid medications, such as Propacil or Tapazole, are administered to block the conversion of thyroxine (T4) to triiodothyronine (T3). The thyroid is surgically removed if the patient cannot tolerate other treatments or if there is a large goiter involved. One-sixth of the thyroid is usually left in place.

Thyrotoxic Storm

A **thyrotoxic storm** is a severe form of hyperthyroidism. A toxic storm is precipitated by stress. Toxic storms occur in individuals with untreated or inadequately treated hyperthyroidism. If not treated promptly, the condition is fatal. The incidence of the condition has decreased with the advent of antithyroid medications, but it may still occur in medical emergencies or during pregnancy. Signs and symptoms include temperature increase to 38.5 degrees Celsius or more; tachycardia; atrial fibrillation; heart failure; gastrointestinal disorders (such as nausea, vomiting, diarrhea, and abdominal discomfort); and altered mental status (delirium progressing to coma). Diagnostic findings include increased T3 uptake and decreased thyroid-stimulating hormone (TSH). Treatment includes controlling the production of thyroid hormone through the use of antithyroid medications (such as propylthiouracil and methimazole), inhibiting the release of thyroid hormone with iodine therapy (or lithium), and controlling peripheral activity of thyroid hormone with propranolol. In addition, treatment may include fluid and electrolyte replacement, administration of glucocorticoids (such as dexamethasone), the use of cooling blankets, and the administration of antiarrhythmics and anticoagulants.

Pathophysiology Across the Lifespan: Electrolyte Imbalances

Sodium Electrolyte Imbalances

The normal sodium level is 135 to 145 mEq/L. Hyponatremia and hypernatremia are **sodium electrolyte imbalances.**

Hyponatremia is defined as a sodium level of less than 135 mEq/L. The condition may result from an insufficient intake of sodium or an abnormal loss of sodium through diarrhea, vomiting, and nasogastric suctioning. It can occur following severe burns and as a result of fever and illnesses such as syndrome of inappropriate antidiuretic hormone secretion (SIADH) and ketoacidosis. Symptoms vary and may include irritability, lethargy, and alterations in consciousness. Cerebral edema can lead to seizures and coma. Dyspnea can lead to respiratory failure. Treatment involves identifying and treating the underlying cause and providing sodium replacement.

Hypernatremia is defined as a sodium level of greater than 145 mEq/L. Hypernatremia may occur as a result of renal disease, diabetes insipidus, or fluid depletion. Signs and symptoms of hypernatremia include irritability, lethargy, confusion, coma, seizures, flushing, muscle weakness and spasms, and thirst. Treatment includes identification and treatment of the underlying cause and intravenous fluid replacement.

Hyperkalemia

Hyperkalemia is an abnormally high level of potassium (greater than 5.5 mEq/L). Hyperkalemia may be caused by renal disease, adrenal insufficiency, metabolic acidosis, severe dehydration, burns, hemolysis, and trauma. The disorder rarely occurs without renal disease but may be induced by treatment (such as nonsteroidal anti-inflammatory drugs [NSAIDs] and potassium-sparing diuretics). Untreated renal disease results in reduced excretion of potassium. Individuals with Addison's disease and a deficiency of adrenal hormones may suffer a sodium loss that results in potassium retention. The primary symptoms relate to the effect on the cardiac muscle. Signs and symptoms are as follows: ventricular arrhythmias leading to cardiac and respiratory arrest, weakness with ascending paralysis and hyperreflexia, diarrhea, and increasing mental confusion. Treatment includes identification of the underlying cause, discontinuation of sources of excess potassium, administration of calcium gluconate to decrease cardiac effects, administration of sodium bicarbonate (to shift potassium into the cells temporarily), administration of insulin and hypertonic dextrose (to shift potassium into the cells temporarily), use of cation exchange resin (Kayexalate) (to decrease potassium), and peritoneal dialysis or hemodialysis.

Hypokalemia

Hypokalemia is an abnormally low potassium level. Potassium is the primary electrolyte in intracellular fluid. Approximately 98 percent of the potassium in the body is found inside cells, and only 2 percent is found in the extracellular fluid. Potassium affects the activity of the skeletal and cardiac muscles. Potassium level is dependent on renal functioning, because 80 percent is excreted in urine and 20 percent in feces and sweat. The normal potassium level is 3.5 to 5.5 mEq/L. In hypokalemia, the level of potassium is less than 3.5 mEq/L. Hypokalemia may be caused by loss of potassium through diarrhea, vomiting, gastric suction, diuresis, alkalosis, decreased potassium intake with starvation, and nephritis. Signs and symptoms of hypokalemia include lethargy, weakness, nausea, vomiting, paresthesia, dysrhythmia, premature ventricular contractions (PVCs), flattened T waves, muscle cramps with hyporeflexia, hypotension, and tetany. Treatment includes the identification of the underlying cause of the disorder and potassium replacement.

Hypophosphatemia and Hyperphosphatemia

Phosphorus, or phosphate (PO_4), is necessary for neuromuscular and red blood cell function and for the maintenance of acid-base balance. Phosphorus provides structure for teeth and bones. About 85 percent is in the bones, 14 percent in soft tissue, and less than 1 percent in extracellular fluid. The normal level of phosphorus is 2.4 to 4.5 mEq/L. In hypophosphatemia, the phosphorus level is less than 2.4 mEq/L. In hyperphosphatemia, the level is greater than 4.5 mEq/L.

Hypophosphatemia occurs in the following situations: severe protein-calorie malnutrition; excessive use of antacids containing magnesium, calcium, or aluminum; hyperventilation; severe burn injuries; and diabetic ketoacidosis. Signs and symptoms include irritability, tremors, seizures, coma, hemolytic anemia, decreased myocardial function, and respiratory failure. Treatment involves identification of the underlying cause and phosphorus replacement.

Hyperphosphatemia occurs in the following situations: renal failure, hypoparathyroidism, excessive intake of phosphate, neoplastic disease, diabetic ketoacidosis, muscle necrosis, and chemotherapy. Signs and symptoms include tachycardia, muscle cramping, hyperreflexia, tetany, nausea, and diarrhea. Treatment involves identification of the underlying cause, correction of hypocalcemia, and provision of antacids and dialysis.

Hypocalcemia and Hypercalcemia

One percent of the **calcium** in the body is in the serum. Serum calcium is important for transmitting nerve impulses and regulating muscle contraction and relaxation. Calcium activates enzymes that stimulate chemical reactions, and it plays a role in blood clotting. The normal calcium level is 8.8 to 10.7 mg/dL. In hypocalcemia, the level is less than 8.8 mg/dL. In hypercalcemia, the level is greater than 10.7 mg/dL.

Hypocalcemia may be caused by hypoparathyroidism. It also occurs after thyroid and parathyroid surgery and as a result of pancreatitis, renal failure, inadequate vitamin D intake, alkalosis, magnesium deficiency and low serum albumin. Signs and symptoms include tetany, tingling, seizures, altered mental status, and ventricular tachycardia. Treatment includes calcium replacement and vitamin D supplementation.

Hypercalcemia may be caused by acidosis, kidney disease, hyperparathyroidism, prolonged immobilization, and malignancies. A hypercalcemic crisis carries a 50 percent mortality rate. Signs and symptoms include muscle weakness with hypotonicity, anorexia, nausea, vomiting, constipation, bradycardia, and cardiac arrest. Treatment includes identification and treatment of the underlying cause and administration of loop diuretics and IV fluids.

Hypomagnesemia and Hypermagnesemia

Magnesium (Mg) is the second most common intracellular electrolyte (after potassium). Magnesium activates many intracellular enzyme systems. It is important for carbohydrate and protein metabolism, neuromuscular function, and cardiovascular function. Magnesium produces vasodilation and directly affects the peripheral arterial system. The normal level of magnesium is 1.4 mEq/L. In hypomagnesemia, magnesium level is less than 1.4 mEq/L. In hypermagnesemia, magnesium level is greater than 1.4 mEq/L.

Hypomagnesemia occurs in the following situations: chronic diarrhea, chronic renal disease, chronic pancreatitis, excessive diuretic or laxative use, hyperthyroidism, hypoparathyroidism, severe burn injuries, and diaphoresis. Signs and symptoms include neuromuscular excitability/tetany, mental confusion, headaches, dizziness, seizure, coma, tachycardia with ventricular arrhythmia, and respiratory depression. Treatment involves identification of the underlying cause and magnesium replacement.

Hypermagnesemia occurs in the following situations: renal failure or inadequate renal function, diabetic ketoacidosis, hypothyroidism, and Addison's disease. Signs and symptoms include muscle weakness, seizures, dysphagia with decreased gag reflex, and tachycardia with hypotension. Treatment includes identification of the underlying cause, intravenous hydration with calcium, and dialysis.

Pathophysiology Across the Lifespan: Acidosis/Alkalosis

Metabolic Acidosis

Metabolic acidosis is an increase in the acidity of the plasma. It involves a disruption of the body's acid-base balance. A number of different disorders can lead to metabolic acidosis. These include kidney failure, diabetic ketoacidosis, starvation, and shock. In addition, the disorder can be caused by ingesting certain toxic substances (such as antifreeze and large amounts of aspirin). Metabolic acidosis may result in shock or death. Signs and symptoms of this disorder include rapid breathing, mental confusion, lethargy, arrhythmia, nausea, vomiting, and abdominal pain. The condition can be a mild, chronic disorder in some cases. Diagnostic tests include arterial blood gas, metabolic panel, and blood count. Treatment includes addressing the underlying cause. Bicarbonate may be administered. This treatment can decrease the blood's acidity.

Metabolic Alkalosis

Metabolic alkalosis is a disorder involving an abnormally elevated blood pH. The disorder can be caused by excessive vomiting over a prolonged period of time, severe dehydration, the ingestion of alkali substances, and the administration of diuretics. Endocrine disorders (such as Cushing's syndrome) can also cause metabolic alkalosis. Hypokalemia and hypocalcemia may accompany metabolic alkalosis. Metabolic alkalosis may indicate dysfunction of a major organ. Symptoms include slow breathing, cyanosis, dizziness, mental confusion, tremors, muscle cramping, tetany, tachycardia, arrhythmia, nausea, vomiting, loss of appetite, and compensatory hypoventilation. Metabolic alkalosis is diagnosed based on the patient's symptoms. The disorder is confirmed with laboratory tests. A blood pH of more than 7.45 is confirmative. The levels of other components of the blood (potassium, chloride, and sodium, for example) are below normal. Serum bicarbonate level is elevated. The aim of treatment is to restore the acid-base balance. Treatment includes the administration of normal saline and potassium chloride. Medication may be administered to regulate blood pressure and heart rate. The underlying condition must be treated.

Respiratory Acidosis

Respiratory acidosis is an abnormal drop in the pH level of the blood. This condition occurs because of reduced ventilation of the alveoli. This leads to a rapid increase in the concentration of carbon dioxide in the arteries. The body fluids become increasingly acidic. The condition can be acute or chronic. In the acute form, the carbon dioxide increases too rapidly for the kidneys to compensate. In the chronic form, respiratory acidosis takes place over a longer period, allowing the kidneys time to compensate. In chronic respiratory acidosis, the kidneys produce chemicals to control the acid-base balance. Causes of respiratory acidosis include asthma and chronic obstructive pulmonary disease, skeletal disorders that prevent the lungs from filling efficiently, nerve disorders that interfere with lung inflation or deflation, obesity, and ingestion of certain drugs (such as narcotics and benzodiazepines). Signs and symptoms include mental confusion, lethargy, and shortness of breath. Diagnostic techniques include tests of pulmonary function, chest x-ray, computed tomography (CT) scan, and arterial blood gas. Treatment includes bronchodilator medications, noninvasive positive-pressure ventilation, mechanical ventilation, and oxygen administration.

RESPIRATORY ALKALOSIS

Respiratory alkalosis is a disorder in which the blood contains abnormally low levels of carbon dioxide. Respiratory alkalosis occurs as a result of alveolar hyperventilation. Respiratory alkalosis may be acute or chronic. In the chronic state, the body compensates and reduces the effect of alkalosis. Respiratory alkalosis has a number of causes, including hyperventilation, anxiety, hysteria, fever, stroke, and use of certain drugs (such as doxapram). Caffeine and aspirin overdose can also cause this disorder. Signs and symptoms include dizziness, light-headedness, and numbness in the extremities. Seizures may occur in severe cases, but this is extremely uncommon. Diagnosis is based on arterial blood gas, chest x-ray, and pulmonary function tests. Treatment for respiratory alkalosis depends on the cause of the disorder. The underlying condition must be addressed. A rebreathing mask may be used.

Pathophysiology Across the Lifespan: Infectious Disease

HIV

Human immunodeficiency virus, commonly referred to as **HIV**, is a slow-acting retrovirus of the genus lentivirus. The virus is spread through contact with infected body fluids. HIV attacks the body by binding with cells that have CD4 receptors. These are primarily CD4+ T cells and other cells of the immune system. The virus enters the cells and starts replicating. The virus destroys the host cells in a number of ways: The virus disrupts the cell membrane when large numbers of viral cells push through the cell membrane. Cell function is disrupted when large numbers of viral cells accumulate within a host cell. Syncytia are formed when HIV-infected host cells fuse with nearby cells. This process creates giant cells and facilitates the spread of the virus. The virus also signals uninfected cells to self-destruct. The binding of HIV cells to host cell membranes causes the host cell to be targeted by killer T cells as part of the immune response.

AIDS

Acquired immunodeficiency syndrome (AIDS) is caused by HIV. Individuals older than age 50 comprise the fastest growing group of AIDS patients. As people age and acquire other diseases in addition to AIDS, management becomes complicated. The diagnostic criteria for AIDS include HIV infection; a CD4 count of less than 200 cells/mm^3; and AIDS-defining conditions, such as opportunistic infections (cytomegalovirus, tuberculosis), wasting syndrome, neoplasms (Kaposi's sarcoma), or AIDS dementia complex. Because of the wide range of AIDS-defining conditions, the patient may present with many types of symptoms. However, more than half of patients exhibit fever, lymphadenopathy, pharyngitis, rash, and myalgia/arthralgia. It is important to review the following when making a diagnosis: CD4 counts (to determine immune status), white blood cell count and differential (for signs of infection), cultures (to help identify any infective agents), and complete blood count (to evaluate for signs of bleeding or thrombocytopenia). Treatment is designed to cure or manage opportunistic conditions and control the underlying HIV infection. Highly active antiretroviral therapy (HAART) is administered. Three or more drugs are used concurrently.

Pathophysiology Across the Lifespan: Neurological

THERMOREGULATION

Thermoregulation is the ability of an organism to maintain an optimum temperature in the presence of a variety of external conditions. The body maintains its core temperature by balancing heat gains and losses. The feedback system of the human body regulates the temperature so that it remains at a nearly constant 98.6 degrees Fahrenheit (F). Thermoregulation is controlled by the central nervous system. Generally, thermoregulation is possible when the environmental temperature is between 68 degrees F and 130 degrees F. When thermoregulation breaks down and body temperature increases significantly above normal, hyperthermia occurs. When the temperature drops significantly below normal, hypothermia occurs. Older adults do not thermoregulate as efficiently as younger individuals. Older adults are less tolerant of changes in ambient temperature. Older adults should be kept warm and comfortable during physical examinations.

APHASIA

Aphasia is the loss of ability to use and/or understand written and spoken language because of damage to the speech center of the brain caused by brain tumors, brain injury, and stroke. The speech pathologist should assess the patient and provide guidance in communicating with the patient. There are different types of aphasia:

- *Global*: This involves difficulty understanding and producing language in speaking, reading, and writing although patients may understand gestures. Use pictures, diagrams, and gestures to convey meaning. Picture charts are useful.
- *Broca's*: Individuals with this form of aphasia can understand but have difficulty producing language to varying degrees. Speak slowly and clearly, facing the person and be patient. Picture charts may be useful to help the patient communicate.
- *Wernicke's*: Patients with Wernicke's aphasia have difficulty understanding language but can understand gestures and are able to produce language, although with some impairment. For example, these individuals may use incorrect words or sounds. Patients may be able to write or use letter boards to assist communication.

DYSPHAGIA

Dysphagia is exhibited as difficulty swallowing solids and thin liquids. It occurs in approximately 10 percent of noninstitutionalized older adults. Symptoms of the disorder include tightness or pain in the chest, regurgitation, choking, esophageal reflux, and aspiration pneumonia. Dysphagia may result in weight loss and dehydration. Diagnosis of the disorder is based on symptoms, barium swallow, and endoscopy. The patient is instructed to eat sitting upright, avoid eating before lying down, chew foods slowly, sip water after swallowing, thicken thin liquids, and limit bite size. The variety of *underlying causes* must be treated:

- *Stroke*: Approximately 30 percent of stroke patients have dysphagia.
- *Neuromuscular diseases*: Individuals with Parkinson's disease, myasthenia gravis, multiple sclerosis, and amyotrophic lateral sclerosis (ALS) may have dysphagia.
- *Drugs*: Phenothiazines may cause dysphagia.
- *Dementia*: Individuals with dementia may not chew food sufficiently or may neglect to swallow.
- *Achalasia*: If the esophagus does not contract effectively and the sphincter does not relax, then dysphagia can result.

- *Esophageal stricture, diverticulum, or web* (from iron deficiency) may lead to dysphagia.
- *Esophageal cancer* causes dysphagia.

Oropharyngeal Dysphagia

Dysphagia is a complex problem that can be related to a number of different abnormalities. Food is masticated and then moved to the back of the throat, triggering the pharyngeal swallow reflex. At the same time, the larynx closes and the epiglottis prevents aspiration. In **oropharyngeal dysphagia**, this process can be impaired. Neuromuscular disorders (stroke, multiple sclerosis, and Parkinson's disease) and masses that affect the tongue, pharynx, and upper sphincter of the esophagus can cause oropharyngeal dysphagia. Affected individuals may have difficulty swallowing and may cough early in the swallow or regurgitate food into the nose. People may also exhibit dysphonia, dysarthria, and hyposalivation.

Esophageal Dysphagia

Food enters the esophagus, and peristalsis moves the food to the lower esophageal sphincter, which opens so the food can pass into the stomach. In **esophageal dysphagia**, people may complain of a feeling of choking and coughing late in the swallow. The swallowing process can be impaired by Parkinson's disease, achalasia, scleroderma, strictures, gastroesophageal reflux disease (GERD), and masses. Some medications (such as tetracycline, potassium, iron, nonsteroidal anti-inflammatory drugs [NSAIDs], vitamin C, alendronate, and quinidine) may also cause irritation. Diagnosis is based on history, observation, barium swallow, double-contrast upper gastrointestinal (GI) series, endoscopy, manometry (for abnormality), pH monitoring (for GERD), and videography (to assess risk of aspiration). Management includes adopting an upright position when eating; placing the food in the unaffected side of the mouth if sensory deficit is evident; taking small bites of food; adjusting food temperature (cold facilitates movement in the mouth and laryngeal swallowing, while warm facilitates other swallowing); and modifying the diet (with soft food and thickened liquids).

Stages of Alzheimer's Disease

Alzheimer's disease may be staged in a number of ways. There is no specific test for Alzheimer's disease. Staging is based on a combination of a physical examination, history (often provided by family or caregivers), and mental assessment. The seven-stage classification system (developed by Barry Reisberg, MD) is used by the Alzheimer's Association:

- **Stage 1** is preclinical. There is no evident impairment, although slight changes may be occurring within the brain.
- **Stage 2** involves very mild cognitive decline. Patients may misplace items and forget thoughts or words. However, impairment is not usually noticeable to others or evident on medical examination.
- **Stage 3** is defined by mild, early-stage cognitive decline with short-term memory loss and problems with reading retention and name recall. The patient may have trouble handling money, planning, and organizing. The patient may also misplace items of value.
- **Stage 4** of Alzheimer's disease is defined by moderate cognitive decline with decreased knowledge of current affairs and/or family history. The patient exhibits social withdrawal and has difficulty with complex tasks. This stage is more easily recognized on examination and may persist for 2 to 10 years. During this stage, the patient may be able to manage most activities of daily living and hygiene.

- **Stage 5** is defined by moderately severe cognitive decline. Brain changes are evident; the cerebral cortex and hippocampus shrink and the ventricles enlarge. Patients are obviously confused and disoriented regarding date, time, and place. Patients may have difficulty using and/or understanding speech and managing activities of daily living. They may forget their address and telephone number. Individuals at this stage of the disease may dress inappropriately, forget to eat and lose weight, or eat a poor diet. They may be unable to do simple math, such as counting backward by twos.
- **Stage 6** of Alzheimer's disease is defined by moderately severe cognitive decline; the brain continues to shrink and neurons die. Patients are profoundly confused and unable to care for themselves. Individuals at this stage may undergo profound personality changes. Patients may confuse fantasy and reality. They may fail to recognize family members and experience difficulty toileting. Patients at this stage of the disease tend to pace obsessively or wander away. Patients may exhibit sundowner's syndrome, a disruption of the waking/sleeping cycle. Individuals with this syndrome tend to become restless and wander about at night. Patients may develop obsessive behaviors, such as tearing items, pulling at the hair, or wringing of the hands. This stage (with stage 7) may be prolonged, lasting one to five years.
- **Stage 7** is defined by very severe cognitive decline. During this stage, most patients are wheelchair bound or bed bound. Most patients lose the ability to speak beyond a few words. They exhibit urinary and bowel incontinence and may be unable to sit unsupported or hold their head up. They choke easily and have increased weakness and rigidity of muscles.

General Management of Patients with Alzheimer's Disease or Cognitive Impairment Patients

Patients with **Alzheimer's disease** and **cognitive impairment** become easily confused. Therefore, a regular schedule should be maintained for the patient if possible. Simple choices may be overwhelming for the patient, and caregivers should avoid having the patient make unnecessary choices. Directions should involve only one or two simple steps. Clothes without zippers or buttons may be easiest for the patient and caregivers to manage. Patients may resist bathing. In this case, Comfort Bath disposable washcloths may be used; one part of the body is washed at a time. For example, the face and arms may be washed in the morning and the trunk and legs at night. If the patient wants to pace, he or she should be allowed to do so if possible. Attempting to stop the patient from pacing rarely succeeds and will cause the patient distress. It may be helpful to take the patient outside for a walk.

Supportive Care for Patients with Alzheimer's Disease or Cognitive Impairment

Patients with **Alzheimer's disease** or **cognitive impairment** may be disruptive and difficult to manage. Caregivers may become irritated, impatient, and angry. They often need to be reminded that patients are not deliberately being difficult. Patients are often disruptive because they can't express their needs or wants. Careful observation may give a clue about what is causing the disruptive behavior. The patient may be comforted by simple activities, such as folding clothes or coloring. Some patients, especially women, are comforted by holding dolls or stuffed animals. The caregiver should hold the patient's hand or arm while walking. This action provides a feeling of security and prevents the patient from bolting if something frightening occurs. Busy places often confuse and agitate patients with Alzheimer's disease or cognitive impairment, and such places as large department stores should be avoided.

Non-Alzheimer's Dementias

The following are **non-Alzheimer's dementias:**

- *Creutzfeldt-Jakob disease* is a rapidly progressing dementia causing memory impairments, behavioral changes, and loss of coordination.
- *Dementia with Lewy bodies* involves a cognitive and physical decline similar to Alzheimer's disease, but symptoms may fluctuate frequently. This form of dementia may involve visual hallucinations, muscle rigidity, and tremors.
- *Frontotemporal dementia* may cause marked changes in personality and behavior. The dementia is characterized by difficulty using and understanding language.
- *Mixed dementia* is a combination of Alzheimer's and another type of dementia. Symptoms of the dementias interact.
- *Normal-pressure hydrocephalus* is characterized by ataxia, memory loss, and urinary incontinence.
- *Parkinson's dementia* may involve impairments in the following domains: making decisions, concentrating, learning new material, understanding complex language, and sequencing. The patient may be inflexible and exhibit short- or long-term memory loss.
- *Vascular dementia* has symptoms similar to Alzheimer's disease, but memory loss may be less pronounced.

Parkinson's Disease

Parkinson's disease (PD) is an extrapyramidal movement motor system disorder. It results from loss of brain cells that produce dopamine. Typical symptoms include tremor in the face and extremities, rigidity, bradykinesia, akinesia, poor posture, and lack of balance and coordination. These symptoms cause increasing problems with mobility, speaking, and swallowing. Some individuals with Parkinson's disease may suffer depression, mood changes, and dementia. Unilateral tremors in an upper extremity are usually evident. Diagnosis methods include the cogwheel rigidity test (passive range of motion causes an increase in muscle tone and ratchetlike movements in the affected extremity), a physical and neurological examination, and a complete medical history.

Treatment includes administration of dopaminergic drugs (levodopa, amantadine, and carbidopa) and anticholinergic drugs (trihexyphenidyl and benztropine). In cases of drug-induced Parkinson's, the drugs causing the disorder must be discontinued. Drug therapy tends to decrease in efficacy over time, and symptoms may worsen. Discontinuing the drugs for one week may cause the symptoms to worsen initially, but functioning may improve when drugs are reintroduced.

Ischemic Stroke

Strokes result when there is interruption of the blood flow to an area of the brain. The two primary types are ischemic and hemorrhagic. Approximately 80 percent are **ischemic strokes**, resulting from blockage of an artery supplying the brain. Thrombosis is the formation of a blood clot in a blood vessel. Thrombosis in a large artery, usually resulting from atherosclerosis, may block circulation to a large area of the brain. This condition occurs most frequently in the elderly and may occur suddenly or after a transient ischemic attack. A lacunar infarct (penetrating thrombosis in a small artery) is most common in those with diabetes mellitus and/or hypertension. An embolism (wandering blood clot) passes through the circulatory system and lodges in the brain, most commonly in the left middle cerebral artery. A cardiogenic embolism results from cardiac arrhythmia or surgery. An embolism usually has a sudden onset and often occurs with no warning signs. A cryptogenic stroke has no identifiable cause.

Hemorrhagic Stroke

Approximately 20 percent of strokes are hemorrhagic. **Hemorrhagic strokes** result from a ruptured cerebral artery. They cause an interruption in the supply of oxygen and nutrients. In addition, they cause edema, which results in widespread pressure and damage. An intracerebral hemorrhage involves bleeding from an artery in the central lobes, basal ganglia, pons, or cerebellum into the brain matter. Intracerebral hemorrhage may result from atherosclerotic degenerative changes, hypertension, brain tumors, anticoagulation therapy, or use of some illicit drugs, such as crack and cocaine. Onset is often sudden and the condition may be fatal. An intracranial aneurysm occurs in ballooning cerebral artery ruptures, most commonly at the circle of Willis. An arteriovenous malformation (AVM) is a tangle of dilated arteries and veins without a capillary bed. This is a congenital abnormality. Rupture of AVMs is a cause of stroke in young adults. A subarachnoid hemorrhage is bleeding in the space between the meninges and brain. It results from aneurysm, AVM, or trauma. This type of hemorrhage compresses brain tissue.

Symptoms of Strokes in Relation to the Area of the Brain Affected

Right Hemisphere

Strokes most frequently occur in the right or left hemisphere. The exact location and the extent of brain damage affect the presenting symptoms. If the frontal area on either side of the brain is involved, memory and learning deficits are usually evident. Some symptoms are unique to specific areas and help to identify the area involved.

A stroke in the **right hemisphere** results in paralysis or paresis on the left side and a left visual field deficit that may cause spatial and perceptual disturbances. People with this type of damage may have difficulty judging distance. Fine motor skills may be adversely affected, resulting in trouble dressing or handling tools. People may become impulsive and exhibit poor judgment, often denying any impairment. Left-sided neglect (lack of perception of things on the left side) may be evident. Depression, short-term memory loss, and difficulty following directions are often evident. Language skills usually remain intact.

Left Hemisphere, Brain Stem, and Cerebellum

A **left-hemisphere stroke** results in paralysis or paresis on the right side and a right visual field deficit. Depression is common and people often behave in a slow, cautious manner, requiring repeated instruction and reinforcement for simple tasks. Short-term memory loss and difficulty learning new material or understanding generalizations is common. Difficulty with mathematics, reading, writing, and reasoning may be evident. Aphasia (expressive, receptive, or global) is common.

A **brain-stem stroke** frequently causes death because the brain stem controls respiration and cardiac function. Individuals who survive may have a number of problems, including respiratory and cardiac abnormalities. Strokes may involve motor impairment, sensory impairment, or both.

The cerebellum controls balance and coordination. **Strokes in the cerebellum** are rare but may result in ataxia, nausea, vomiting, headaches, and dizziness or vertigo.

Sleep Disorders

Sleep disorders affect all age groups, but they are especially prevalent in the older adult population. Older adults often take longer to fall asleep at night and awaken more frequently than younger adults. They also sleep more often during the day. Approximately 50 percent of older adults have insomnia, while 65 to 70 percent have combined sleep disorders. Sleep disorders include sleep apnea, insomnia, circadian rhythm disorders, and sleep-related movement disorders.

Patients may not report sleep disorders but may present with vague complaints of feeling tired, lethargic, and depressed. Sleep disorders may be related to pain; incontinence; urinary frequency; obesity; neurodegenerative diseases; dyspnea; depression; anxiety disorders; bereavement; poor sleep habits; medications (such as benzodiazepines, antidepressants, diuretics, anti-Parkinson drugs, and anticonvulsants); caffeine; and alcohol. An overnight sleep study utilizing polysomnography (PSG) and sleep diaries may aid diagnosis. Treatment includes bright-light therapy in the evening to keep the individual awake and medication to induce sleep. The patient may be advised to keep the bedroom dark at night, keep set times for sleeping and arising, avoid excessive napping, eliminate caffeine, reduce noise at night, and increase daytime activity. Treatment for restless legs syndrome or sleep apnea may be required.

Pathophysiology Across the Lifespan: Psychological

Intellectual Disabilities in Older Adults

Vision, Hearing, and Dental Concerns

Adults with **intellectual disability** or a developmental disorder now have a life expectancy of approximately 66 years. However, the life expectancy of younger adults with intellectual disability is approximately 76 years. Adults with intellectual disability pose challenges for health-care providers. The most common cause of intellectual disability is Down syndrome. Older adults with intellectual disability often have associated medical conditions. *Vision impairment* related to cataracts, nystagmus, hyperplasia, corneal abnormalities, and refractive disorders are very common in this population and often remain uncorrected. Severe intellectual disability is positively correlated with severity of ocular disorders. About 50 percent of individuals older than age 50 with Down syndrome have cataracts. *Hearing loss* is very common in individuals with Down syndrome (70 percent of individuals age 59 and under). *Poor dental care* in adults with intellectual disability is common as these individuals may not care for their teeth properly. All people with intellectual disability should have a complete dental exam.

Thyroid, Obesity, Osteoporosis, and Mental Health Concerns

Thyroid dysfunction is common with intellectual disability and is often not diagnosed. Therefore, all people with intellectual disability should have their thyroid tested.

Approximately 48 percent of intellectually disabled individuals are **obese**, and this puts them at increased risk for cardiovascular disease.

Osteoporosis is common in people older than age 50 often because of poor diet and immobility. It may be associated with osteoarthritis.

Review Video: Osteoporosis
Visit mometrix.com/academy and enter code: 421205

Mental health disorders are more common among individuals with intellectual disability than among individuals in the general population. These disorders include mood disorders (such as bipolar disorder) and schizophrenia. Behavioral disorders (such as aggression, agitation, and sleep disturbances) are also more common among individuals with intellectual disability. Patients may engage in self-injurious behavior. By age 65, approximately 20 percent of individuals with non-Down syndrome intellectual disability have dementia, but this number increases to 52 percent by age 88. Individuals with Down syndrome exhibit signs of dementia earlier, with about 42 percent exhibiting dementia by age 50.

SCHIZOPHRENIA

Schizophrenia is a related group of psychiatric illnesses. The subtypes of the disorder include paranoid, disorganized, catatonic, undifferentiated, and residual. Symptoms vary widely but include positive symptoms and negative symptoms. Positive symptoms include delusions and hallucinations, and negative symptoms include flat affect and lack of motivation. Comorbidities, such as obsessive-compulsive disorder, depression, and substance abuse are common. Patients may have suicidal tendencies. In older adults, psychosis is often less severe. However, some cognitive impairment is common at all ages and is a persistent problem with chronic schizophrenia. There are approximately 300,000 older adult schizophrenics in the United States; about two-thirds of these are in nursing homes. However, only 15,000 are in psychiatric hospitals, suggesting that cognitive impairment is the bigger problem in older adults. Treatment for schizophrenia includes typical antipsychotics (chlorpromazine, haloperidol, loxapine) and atypical antipsychotics (olanzapine, clozapine, risperidone). Atypical antipsychotics are more effective at reducing negative symptoms. All medications are associated with significant side effects, including tardive dyskinesia, but atypical antipsychotics have fewer side effects. Studies suggest that atypical antipsychotics may be better tolerated by older adults.

Review Video: Anti-Psychotic Drugs: Clozapine, Haloperidol, Etc.
Visit mometrix.com/academy and enter code: 369601

DEPRESSION

Depression is associated with conditions that decrease quality of life, such as heart disease, neuromuscular disease, arthritis, cancer, diabetes, Huntington's disease, stroke, and diabetes. Some drugs (diuretics, Parkinson's drugs, estrogen, corticosteroids, cimetidine, hydralazine, propranolol, digitalis, and indomethacin, for example) may also precipitate depression. Depressed patients experience mood changes, sadness, loss of interest in usual activities, fatigue, appetite changes, weight fluctuations, anxiety, and sleep disturbance. Depression affects about 19 percent of adults older than age 55. Further, it affects approximately 37 percent of older adults who have comorbid conditions. Older adults have the highest rate of suicide and are at risk. Depression often goes undiagnosed, so screening for at-risk individuals should be performed routinely. Treatment includes TCAs and selective serotonin reuptake inhibitors (SSRIs). SSRIs have fewer side effects and are less likely to cause death with an overdose. Older adults may take longer to respond to medication than younger adults. Treatment includes counseling, addressing the underlying cause, and instituting an exercise program.

BIPOLAR DISORDER

Bipolar disorder is an affective disorder characterized by mood swings ranging from depression to mania. The disorder includes several subtypes: bipolar I, bipolar II, cyclothymia, rapid cycling, and mixed state. Comorbid conditions include substance abuse, thyroid disorders, suicidal tendencies, obsessive-compulsive disorder, post-traumatic stress disorder, and dementia. Individuals with late-onset bipolar disorder (occurring after the age of 50) tend to exhibit less severe symptoms than those with early onset bipolar disorder. Symptoms include severe mania, hypomania, normal mood, mild to moderate depression, and severe depression. Symptoms may be triggered by environmental factors, such as medication, stress, substance abuse, sleep disorders, and changes of season. The disorder is treated by various medications (mood stabilizers, anticonvulsants, and atypical antipsychotics). Antidepressants are contraindicated. Treatment with one drug (mood stabilizer) is the goal for older adults because of the potential for adverse effects and drug interactions. Electroshock treatment is effective for older adults in the depressed state.

The half-life of drugs is increased in older adults because of reduced renal clearance, so it is often necessary to administer lower doses. Careful monitoring is necessary.

Pathophysiology Across the Lifespan: Integumentary

Pressure Ulcers

Pressure ulcers are also called decubitus ulcers. They result primarily from pressure, but there are a number of other **contributing factors**:

- *Pressure intensity*. A capillary closing pressure of (10-32 mm Hg) is the minimum pressure needed to cause the collapse of capillaries. The collapse of capillaries contributes to the development of pressure ulcers by reducing tissue perfusion. Failure to change position while sitting or lying down can result in this pressure being exceeded.
- *Duration of pressure*. Low pressure for prolonged periods and high pressure for short periods can both result in pressure ulcers.
- *Tissue tolerance*. Tissue tolerance is the ability of the skin to tolerate and redistribute pressure. High tissue tolerance prevents anoxia. Extrinsic and intrinsic factors both have an effect on tissue tolerance. Extrinsic factors include shear, friction, and moisture. Shear is a situation in which the skin stays in place but the underlying tissue slides. Friction happens when the skin moves against bedding or other objects. Intrinsic factors include poor nutrition, advanced age, hypotension, stress, smoking, and low body temperature.

Risk Factors

A list of common risk factors for **pressure ulcers** has been compiled by the Centers for Medicare & Medicaid Services (CMS). Many individuals have more than one risk factor. Older adults should be assessed for the following **risk factors**:

- Impairment or decreased mobility that prevents a person from changing position.
- Comorbid conditions that affect circulation or metabolism (such as renal disease, diabetes, and thyroid disease).
- Drugs that interfere with healing (corticosteroids, for example).
- Impaired circulation (including generalized atherosclerosis or arterial insufficiency of lower extremity).
- Patient refusal of care (positioning, hygiene, nutrition, hydration, skin care).
- Cognitive impairment that prevents patients from reporting discomfort or cooperating with care.
- Fecal and/or urinary contamination of skin related to incontinence.
- Undernutrition, malnutrition, and/or dehydration.
- Presence of healed ulcers (healed ulcers that were stage III or IV may deteriorate and break down again).

Staging

Revised regulations for the care of pressure sores in long-term care facilities were established by the Centers for Medicare & Medicaid Services (CMS) in November 2004. A standardized **staging system** was developed by the **National Pressure Ulcer Advisory Panel**:

- A **stage I** ulcer is an area of intact skin with red or purple discoloration. The skin may be warmer or cooler than normal. The area may be abnormally firm or soft in consistency. The affected area may itch or may be painful.

- **Stage II** is a superficial ulcer that may appear as an abrasion, blister, or slight depression. There is a partial-thickness skin loss that involves the epidermis and/or dermis.
- **Stage III** is a deep, full-thickness ulceration of the skin. The subcutaneous tissue may be damaged or necrotic. The ulceration may extend into the fascia, and there may be tunneling of adjacent tissue.
- **Stage IV** is a deep, full-thickness ulceration of the skin. The damage and necrosis of the tissue extend to muscle, bone, tendons, and joints.

Contribution of Shear and Friction to the Development of Pressure Ulcers

Shear occurs when the tissue in the deep fascia over the bony prominences stretches and slides while the overlying skin remains in place. This action damages vessels and tissue and often results in undermining. Shear is one of the most common causes of ulcers. Ulcers that result from shear are often referred to as pressure ulcers, but they are technically somewhat different. Shearing often occurs with pressure. Elevation of the head of the bed more than 30 degrees is the most common cause of shearing. The skin is held in place against the sheets while the body slides down the bed, resulting in pressure and damage to the sacrococcygeal area. The blood vessels are damaged and thrombosed, leading to undermining and deep ulceration.

Friction is a significant cause of pressure ulcers. Pressure acts in conjunction with gravity to cause shear. Friction alone causes damage only to the epidermis and dermis. This results in abrasions or denouement, which is referred to as sheet burn. Friction and pressure can act together form ulcers.

Skin Cancers

Basal Cell Carcinoma

Basal cell carcinoma occurs most frequently in Caucasians between the ages of 40 and 79. Most lesions develop on the face, scalp, ears, neck, arms, or hands. Lesions may recur after treatment but rarely metastasize. Lesions appear waxy at first and then ulcerate and become crusty. Treatments include electrodessication and curettage, cryosurgery, chemotherapy, laser therapy, and excision.

Squamous Cell Carcinoma

This type of lesion occurs in areas that are exposed to the sun or in areas of chronic inflammation or ulceration. The risk of metastasis is considered moderate (2-5%). At first, the lesions are indurated and erythematous, but they ulcerate and crust with time. Treatment includes excision, cryosurgery, or radiotherapy.

Malignant Melanoma

There are several types of malignant melanomas: *superficial, lentigo maligna, nodular*, and *acral lentigines*. Malignant melanoma is the most serious type of skin cancer with the highest risk of morbidity and mortality. The incidence of melanoma increases with age. Melanomas often develop from moles and are irregular in shape. Melanomas are invasive and treatment involves excision. In advanced cases, palliative care is given.

Sun Exposure

For many years, patients were advised to protect their skin from all **sun exposure** in order to prevent skin damage that could lead to skin cancer. However, this behavior in conjunction with a decrease in milk drinking has resulted in an increased incidence of vitamin D deficiency in all ages. This is fueling a debate between physicians who believe that some sun exposure is warranted and others who insist that all exposure is harmful. Recent guidelines suggest that approximately 20 minutes of sun exposure daily with the arms exposed (avoiding direct sun from 10 AM to 2 PM) is a safe level of exposure and will prevent vitamin D deficiency. Sunburns should be avoided. Dark-skinned patients may tolerate more time in the sun without burning. For longer periods of time, sunscreen should be applied to all exposed areas of skin. Individuals who are fair and prone to burning must be especially careful. Skin cancers, including squamous cell carcinoma, basal cell carcinoma, and malignant melanoma, are on the rise in older adults.

Herpes Zoster

Herpes zoster is commonly called **shingles**. Shingles is caused by the varicella zoster virus, which remains in the nerve cells after a case of childhood chickenpox. The virus remains dormant until it is reactivated. This occurs most commonly in older adults who are immunocompromised. Initial symptoms include burning pain and redness. Painful blisters then develop along sensory nerves. The blisters often develop on a path from the spine around to the chest. However, blisters may develop on the head and face. Facial nerve involvement can result in loss of taste and hearing. Eye involvement can cause blindness. The lesions eventually crust over and heal in 2-4 weeks; however, in some cases, the affected individual may experience persistent postherpetic neuralgia for 6-12 months. The lesions contain live virus. Contact with the virus can cause chickenpox. To prevent the development of shingles, it is recommended that individuals older than age 60 receive the herpes zoster vaccine (single dose). Treatment for shingles includes analgesia (acetaminophen), acyclovir, and Zostrix (capsaicin cream) to reduce incidence of postherpetic neuralgia.

Scabies

Scabies is caused by a microscopic mite called *Sarcoptes scabiei,* variety hominis. The mite tunnels into the skin. This causes the development of small raised lines a few millimeters long. Although mites prefer warm areas of the body (for example, between the fingers), they can infest any area of the body. The burrowing of the mites causes intense itching. Scratching the skin can result in excoriation and secondary infections. A generalized red rash develops in some affected individuals. Scabies spreads through person-to-person contact. Staff members can spread the infection among patients. The incubation time after infection is six to eight weeks; itching usually begins in about 30 days. In most cases, only about a dozen mites are involved in an infection. However, a severe form of scabies, called Norwegian or crusted scabies, can occur in the elderly or in individuals who are immunocompromised. This type of scabies does not cause as much itching; however, the lesions can contain thousands of mites, making this type highly contagious. Treatment includes scabicides or oral medication (ivermectin) and antihistamines. Antibiotics are administered for secondary infection.

Atopic Dermatitis

Atopic dermatitis is commonly referred to as **eczema**. It is a superficial skin disorder that is chronic and inflammatory. Eczema is related to allergies and associated with xerosis, which is dry skin with impaired barrier function. It is associated with dry or cold weather, central heating (which dries the air), and the use of skin cleaners. The condition causes the skin to become red and itchy. Vesicles may develop, ooze, and crust. The skin may be rough, cracked, and scaly. Over time, the skin may darken and thicken. Lichenification, the appearance of markings from chronic scratching, may develop. To control the condition, triggers must be identified and eliminated. Treatment includes the application to weepy lesions of wet compresses soaked in aluminum acetate, lubrication of the skin three to four times each day with hypoallergenic creams, the application of topical corticosteroids for acute flare-ups, and the administration of antihistamines at night to reduce itching.

Contact Dermatitis

Contact dermatitis is a localized skin inflammation that results from contact with an allergen or irritant. The inflammation manifests as a rash that may blister and itch. The condition is commonly caused by contact with one of the following: poison oak, poison ivy, latex, benzocaine, nickel, and preservatives. However, there are many other substances and products that can cause contact dermatitis. The causative agent must be identified before treatment. A patient history must be taken to determine possible allergic reactions. A skin patch test may be performed. Corticosteroids may be administered to control inflammation and itching. Oatmeal baths may sooth the skin. Caladryl lotion is used topically to relieve itching. Antihistamines are used to reduce inflammation. Any lesions should be cleansed gently. The lesions should be evaluated for signs of secondary infection. If a secondary infection is present, antibiotics are administered. The rash should be left uncovered. The patient should be warned to avoid the allergen or irritant in the future.

Burn Injuries

American Burn Association's Burn Classification System

The **American Burn Association** classifies burns as minor, moderate, and major based on the percent of total body surface area (TBSA) affected. The criteria vary depending on the age of the burn victim.

- *Minor burns* cover less than 10 percent of the TBSA in an adult, cover less than 5 percent of the TBSA in a child or older adult, or involve a full-thickness burn that covers less than 2 percent of the body.
- *Moderate burns* cover 10 to 20 percent of TBSA in adults, cover 5 to 10 percent of TBSA in a child or older adult, or involve a full-thickness burn covering 2 to 5 percent of the body.
- *Major burns* cover more than 20 percent of the TBSA in an adult, cover more than 10 percent of TBSA in a child or older adult, involve a full-thickness burn covering more than 5 percent of TBSA; are the result of high-voltage exposure; involve known inhalation; involve the face, eyes, ears, perineum or joints; or are associated with a significant injury.

Classifications

Most burn injuries to older adults occur as a result of domestic accidents with cigarettes or stoves. About 50 percent are flame burns, 20 percent scalding injuries, 10 percent flammable liquid burns, 1 to 2 percent chemical burns, and 1 to 2 percent electrical burns. Burn injuries are often associated with impaired cognition, impaired mobility, and alcohol abuse. Burns are often deeper in older adults because the skin is thinner and healing is slower. Injuries are classified as first-, second-, and third-degree burns according to the depth of tissue affected.

- *First-degree burns* are superficial (epidermis).
- *Second-degree burns* (partial-thickness) are more serious and extend through the dermis.
- *Third-degree burns* (full-thickness) are the most severe burns and affect vasculature, muscles, and nerves.

Complications

Neurological, gastrointestinal, and endocrine/metabolic system complications of burn injuries are discussed below:

- **Neurological**: Encephalopathy may develop from lack of oxygen, decreased blood volume, and sepsis. Hallucinations, alterations in consciousness, seizures, and coma may result.
- **Gastrointestinal**: Ileus and ulcerations of the gastrointestinal mucosa often result from poor circulation. Ileus usually resolves within 48 to 72 hours, but if it returns, it is often indicative of sepsis.

- **Endocrine/metabolic**: The sympathetic nervous system stimulates the adrenal glands to release epinephrine and norepinephrine to increase cardiac output and cortisol for wound healing. The metabolic rate increases significantly. Electrolytes, especially phosphorus, calcium, and sodium, are lost with fluid loss from exposed tissue. There is also an increase in potassium levels. An imbalance in electrolyte levels can be life threatening if the burns cover more than 20 percent of total body surface area (TBSA). Glycogen depletion occurs within 12 to 24 hours. Protein breakdown and muscle wasting occur without sufficient intake of protein.

Burn injuries, especially major burns, can affect all organs and body systems, including the *cardiovascular system*, *urinary tract*, and *pulmonary system*. Cardiac output may drop by 50 percent as the permeability of the capillaries increases with vasodilation and fluid leaks from the tissues. Decreased blood flow causes the kidneys to increase the production of antidiuretic hormone (ADH), which increases oliguria. Blood urea nitrogen (BUN) and creatinine levels rise. Cell destruction in the kidneys may block tubules, and hematuria may result from hemolysis. Injury to the pulmonary system may result from smoke inhalation.

Pulmonary injury is a leading cause of death from burns and is classified according to degree of damage:

- **First-degree**—singed eyebrows and nasal hairs with possible soot in airways and slight edema.
- **Second-degree (at 24 hours)**—stridor, dyspnea, and tachypnea with edema and erythema of the upper airway.
- **Third-degree (at 72 hours)**—worsening symptoms if the patient is not intubated. Bronchorrhea and tachypnea with edematous, secreting tissue if the patient is intubated.

Pathophysiology Across the Lifespan: Hematologic

Anemia

Anemia is an abnormally low level of normal red blood cells or hemoglobin. Anemia is often caused by hemorrhage, hemolysis, hematopoiesis, or iron deficiency (in menstruating women). Anemia causes a decrease in oxygen transportation and a decrease in perfusion. This causes the heart to increase cardiac output. The blood becomes less viscous, and peripheral resistance decreases. More blood is pumped to the heart. The turbulence that results from the increased blood flow can cause a heart murmur and, perhaps, heart failure. Symptoms of anemia include general malaise and weakness, loss of appetite, pallor, shortness of breath on exertion, headache, dizziness, depression, decreased attention span, slowed cognitive processes, shock symptoms (with severe blood loss), tachycardia, hypotension, and poor peripheral circulation. Treatment includes identification of the cause, blood or blood components as indicated, oxygen, and intravenous fluids. A splenectomy may be performed for hemolytic anemias.

Effects of Leukemia

Blood and Bone Marrow

In about 80 percent of cases, **leukemia** in older adults is acute myelogenous leukemia (AML). This condition may be associated with a history of radiation or chemotherapy. However, most cases are idiopathic. The cancer cells compete with normal cells for nutrition. Older adults often exhibit the following signs and symptoms: fever, malaise, pallor, weakness, and confusion. In every type of leukemia, all cells are affected because the cancer cells in the bone marrow depress the formation of all elements. This has the following results: a decrease in production of erythrocytes (red blood cells [RBCs]), resulting in anemia; a decrease in neutrophils, resulting in increased risk of infection; a decrease in platelets, with subsequent decrease in clotting factors and increased bleeding (nosebleeds are common); and an increased risk of physiological fractures because of a weakening of the periosteum.

ORGANS, THE CNS, AND METABOLISM

There are numerous **effects of leukemia**. The liver, spleen, and lymph glands are infiltrated, resulting in enlargement and fibrosis. Infiltration of the central nervous system (CNS) results in increased intracranial pressure, ventricular dilation, and meningeal irritation. These reactions cause headaches, vomiting, papilledema, nuchal rigidity, and coma progressing to death. Hypermetabolism is exhibited. This deprives cells of nutrients and results in anorexia, weight loss, muscle atrophy, and fatigue. Treatment (chemotherapy) is more difficult in older adults who may not tolerate the resulting pancytopenia. Bone marrow transplantation is usually performed only in individuals younger than age 65. Infections requiring antibiotic therapy are common with leucopenia. Such infections compromise already-weakened patients. Regardless of the aggressiveness of treatment, older adults often relapse within a year and die one to two years following diagnosis. Therefore, treatment options depend on age, general condition, and potential outcome. Palliative care is often indicated.

Pathophysiology Across the Lifespan: Pain

NOCICEPTIVE PAIN

There are two primary types of pain: nociceptive (acute) pain and neuropathic (chronic) pain. These two types of pain may occur together. **Nociceptive pain**, also called acute pain, is the normal nerve response to a painful stimulus. Trauma that causes nociceptive pain can cause severe inflammation and damage to nerve endings. Nociceptive pain level is related to the type of injury and the extent of injury; the greater the injury, the greater the pain. It may be procedural pain (related to wound manipulation and dressing changes) or surgical pain (related to cutting of tissue). Nociceptive pain may be continuous or cyclic, depending upon the type of injury. Nociceptive pain is usually localized to the area of injury and resolves over time as healing takes place. This type of pain is often described as aching or throbbing. It generally responds to analgesia. If it is not controlled, over time nociceptive pain can lead to changes in the nervous system, resulting in chronic neuropathic pain.

NEUROPATHIC PAIN

Neuropathic pain is chronic pain. Neuropathic pain often results from a primary lesion in the nervous system or a dysfunction related to damaged nerve fibers. Neuropathic pain is associated with conditions such as diabetes, cancer, or traumatic injury to the nervous system. This type of pain occurs frequently in individuals with chronic wounds. The pain is often described as burning, stabbing, electric, or shooting. The pathology causing the pain is often not reversible. Pain may be visceral (diffuse or cramping pain of internal organs). Visceral pain is caused by injuries to internal organs. Neuropathic pain is often diffuse rather than localized. Neuropathic pain may also be somatic pain (involving muscles, skin, bones, and joints). Neuropathic pain is often more difficult to assess than nociceptive pain because the damage may alter normal pain responses. Neuropathic pain often responds better to antidepressants and antiseizure medications than to analgesics.

Review Video: Neuropathic Pain
Visit mometrix.com/academy and enter code: 780523

Individual Determinants of Health

Genetic or Familial Risks

Assessing family history for **genetic or familial risks** is an important part of disease prevention because, in some cases, early identification and intervention may reduce future health risks. Creating a genogram with the family is helpful. A thorough history should be broad and include assessment of the following:

- Early onset disorders, such as cardiovascular disease, hypertension, or Alzheimer's disease
- Progressive neurological or neuromuscular diseases
- Diabetes Mellitus
- Mental illness, such as depression, bipolar disorder, and schizophrenia
- Intellectual disability, including Trisomy 21 (Down syndrome)
- Any unusual disabilities or abnormalities, such as birth defects

Once risk factors are determined, the question of screening tests arises. If there is a possibility that a child is a carrier, then screening is usually deferred until the child can give informed consent. Screening is done for adults or for children with parental permission when it is in the best interests of the child, allowing for appropriate care and intervention.

Genetic Predictive Testing

Genetic predictive testing identifies a person with a genetic disorder that may manifest at a later date (such as Huntington's disease) or with an increased risk of developing a disease (such as breast cancer). Referral for genetic testing may be advised for familial cancer, retinoblastoma, familial adenomatous polyposis (which can cause colon cancer), cystic fibrosis, Huntington's disease, and amyotrophic lateral sclerosis. Identifying those at risk for developing cancer is especially important so that close monitoring and/or preventive measures can be taken. Familial cancer accounts for about 5-10% of cancers. The BRCA1 breast cancer gene has been mapped to chromosome 17q and the gene for BRCA2 on chromosome 13q. People carrying the abnormal gene have an 80-90% chance of developing breast/ovarian cancer. These women should be counseled about their options and the importance of close monitoring and surgical options. Tests are not available for all diseases with a genetic component (diabetes, hypertension, pyloric stenosis, spina bifida, psychiatric disorders, and Alzheimer's disease), but more genes are being identified.

Personal Risk Factors

An important aspect of the nursing process is identifying those with increased **risk factors**. Risk may relate to things that one can change, such as smoking, drinking, and poor diet, or things that one cannot change, such as age and genetic predisposition. One problem with trying to convince people to change behaviors to decrease risk is that they do not receive immediate feedback from changing behavior and may resist changes even when aware of risk. For example, if people quit smoking, they may extend their lives in the long run, but they may see no immediate results and, in fact, may miss the satisfaction they received from smoking and may suffer withdrawal. Therefore, convincing people to reduce risk requires educating them about the risks and what the risk factors mean to them individually, reinforcing and supporting changes in behavior, and acting as a role model.

Comorbidities

Comorbidities are secondary diseases that coexist with the primary disease. According to the US Department of Health and Human Services, approximately 60% of hospitalized patients have comorbidities. Some diseases are frequently linked to comorbidities. For example, COPD is often associated with cardiovascular disease and stroke, and diabetes with hypertension and heart failure. Comorbidities may have a profound effect on treatment and outcomes. The most common comorbidities (with approximate percentages) for those hospitalized include:

- Hypertension: 30%
- COPD: 12%
- Diabetes: 12%
- Fluid/electrolyte imbalance: 12%
- Iron deficiency/anemia: 8%
- CHF: 6%
- Hypothyroidism: 6%
- Depression/bipolar disorder: 5%
- Neurological disorder: 4%
- Obesity: 4%

Comorbidities vary according to age. In those <18 and >80, fluid and electrolyte disorders from dehydration or excess fluids predominate, while hypertension is most common for those >18. Diabetes is the next most common disorder for those <80. Between adolescence and age 64, both obesity and depression are common. Drug abuse is increasingly common in children, adolescents, and adults to age 44, while alcohol abuse is common in those 18 to 64.

Risk Factors for Malnutrition

There are a number of **risk factors for malnutrition:**

- *Hypermetabolism* resulting from various diseases, such as AIDS, and trauma, stress, or infection.
- *Weight loss*, especially sudden or loss of 10% of normal weight over a 3-month period.
- *Low body weight* of <90% of ideal body weight for age.
- Low Body Mass Index (BMI) of <18.5.
- *Immunosuppressive drugs*, which interfere with the absorption of nutrients.
- *Malabsorption* of nutrients caused by diseases, such as chronic failure of kidneys or liver.
- *Changes in appetite* that decrease intake of nutrients.
- *Food intolerances,* such as lactose intolerance, resulting from lack of enzymes needed to completely digest food so that it can be absorbed into the blood stream from the small intestine.
- *Dietary restrictions,* such as limiting of protein with kidney failure.
- *Functional limitations* such as inability to feed oneself.
- Lack of teeth or dentures, limiting intake.
- *Alterations of taste or smell* that render food unpalatable.

Poor Hygiene

Poor hygiene increases the risk of disease and infection. Poor hygiene is often attributable to physical impairment (such as poor vision or decreased mobility), depression, or cognitive impairment (Alzheimer's disease or substance abuse). Some adults may require assistance with hygiene. Older adults don't need daily baths, but they should bathe two to three times weekly. Grab bars, shower or tub seats, tub mats, handheld showers, and proper heating (to avoid chilling the patient) can facilitate more frequent bathing. The use of mild soap and bath oil may help prevent drying of the skin. Individuals with dementia are often fearful of tubs and showers and may find a sponge bath or Comfort Bath with premoistened, warmed towelettes preferable. Clothing that is easy to manipulate (such as pull-on pants) and clothes with Velcro closures may make it easier for older adults to change clothes and encourage bathing. Thick-handled toothbrushes or electric toothbrushes may facilitate mouth care.

Psychophysiological Stress Model

The **Psychophysiological Stress Model** was developed by **Toth** as a method of discussing how stress impacts physical health and affective behavior. In a setting where a patient is recovering from an illness, an increase in stressors may have an impact on whether the patient has detrimental health effects or a relapse in symptoms. Stress occurs when the autonomic nervous system is stimulated to the point that it makes a person alert to certain stressors, whether real or perceived. This model states that not only can certain disease processes cause illness, but that negative outcomes can also develop as the result of multiple stressors. Stress has a physiological impact on the body, including affecting vital signs and oxygen consumption; therefore, it can lead to disruptions in physiological health. Additionally, stress causes psychological disturbances, including anxiety or depression, which is linked to many negative physical health outcomes.

Roy's Adaptation Model

The **Roy Adaptation Model** was developed by **Callista Roy** in 1970. Adaptation refers to human integration into the surrounding environment, and successful adaptation improves quality of life, health, and well-being. Ultimately, human adaptation is the goal of nursing. The concepts of Roy's Adaptation Model include that a person is a being that interacts with the environment. In order to cope with changes in the surrounding environment, the person uses biological, psychological, and social mechanisms. There are four components of the model: the person, the environment, health, and nursing. The person must be able to adapt to have a positive response to environmental changes. The environment consists of the internal and external focal points, the context or the situation involved, and the effects of the situation. Health is inherent to each person and each individual has a healthy self that falls somewhere on a health and wellness continuum. Good health involves well-being and a continued pursuit of wholeness for the person. Nursing promotes healthy living by promoting adaptation for the patient to the environment.

Stress-Related Erosive Syndrome

Stress-related erosive syndrome (SRES—stress ulcers) occurs most often in individuals with critical illnesses (individuals with severe or multiorgan trauma, mechanical ventilation, sepsis, severe burns, and head injury with increased intracranial pressure). Stress causes changes in the gastric mucosal lining and a decrease in perfusion of the mucosa. These changes cause ischemia. Hemorrhage occurs in more than 30 percent of individuals with SRES, with a mortality rate of 30 to 80 percent. This makes prompt identification and treatment critical. The lesions associated with SRES tend to be diffuse and are more difficult to treat than peptic ulcers. Symptoms include coffee-grounds emesis, hematemesis, and abdominal discomfort. There are prophylactic treatments for those at risk of the disorder. Sucralfate (Carafate) protects mucosa against pepsin. Famotidine (Pepcid), nizatidine (Axid), ranitidine (Zantac), and cimetidine (Tagamet) reduce gastric secretions. Treatment for active bleeding includes intra-arterial infusion of vasopressin and intra-arterial embolization. Over sewing of ulcers or total gastrectomy is performed if bleeding persists.

Anxiety Disorders

Anxiety disorders affect approximately 18 percent of the general population and about 11 percent of individuals older than age 50. Generalized anxiety disorder and panic disorder are classified as anxiety disorders.

Generalized anxiety disorder is usually a chronic condition that manifests early in life. Symptoms include chronic worry, sleep disorders, restlessness, impaired concentration, fatigue, and depression (in 47%). A panic attack is an autonomic response. **Panic disorder** involves acute episodes (attacks) of tachycardia, dyspnea, diaphoresis, faintness, and weakness. In older adults, autonomic response to anxiety may be muted and the symptoms of panic attack less pronounced and more nonspecific (weak, light-headed, slight increase in pulse/respiration). Anxiety is predictive of increased cognitive impairment and lower pain tolerance. Individuals with chronic medical conditions are more likely to become anxious. During acute episodes, supportive care in a quiet environment should be provided. The nurse should remain with the patient and provide reassurance in a calm voice. The patient should be reoriented without being asked to make decisions. Long-term treatment includes deep-breathing exercises, progressive muscle relaxation, and cognitive behavioral therapy. Medications include selective serotonin reuptake inhibitors (SSRIs) and serotonin-norepinephrine reuptake inhibitors (SNRIs).

Psychological Crisis in Older Adults

Older adults must deal with many stressful situations as they age, especially those in nursing homes. They are as likely to suffer from psychiatric and psychological problems as younger adults; however, older adults (especially >70) are much less likely to seek psychiatric or psychological treatment that might prevent a **psychological crisis.** It is the subjective response to stress that precipitates a crisis rather than the stressful event itself. Many older adults cope well with changes in their lives, but some, such as people with depression, chronic illness, impaired cognition, extended bereavement, and substance abuse, are at increased risk. Also, at increased risk are those who have had to cope with a major change in role. The **4 categories of factors that contribute to crisis** include the following:

- *Biological*: Illness, sensory deficits, impaired mobility.
- *Environmental*: Decreased income, retirement, and change in residence.
- *Psychological*: Bereavement, cognitive impairment.
- *Sociocultural*: Role change.

Managing Nonviolent Psychological Crisis

Psychological crisis can be difficult to diagnose. Older adults often seek help for nonspecific physical ailments (such as headache or upset stomach) rather than specifically for anxiety or depression. When assessing an older adult, a history should always be taken. Taking a history of the complaint can bring out information that may indicate stress. The assessment should also include screening for depression because depression is highly correlated with crisis. The Geriatric Depression Scale (GDS) is used to screen for depression in older adults. Bereavement and substance abuse may also precipitate a crisis. Older adults faced with loss of memory often become very frightened and anxious. Older adults faced with changes in role experience stress. Intervention aims at reducing or eliminating stressors when possible. Older adults may benefit from cognitive-behavioral psychotherapy that teaches coping skills. Engagement in social or recreational activities may alleviate stress. In some cases, antidepressant drugs may be indicated. During treatment, the patient should be assisted to develop both short-term goals (take a one-hour nap in the afternoon, for example) and long-term goals (such as to learn relaxation techniques) to reduce stress.

Human Sexuality

Human sexuality is important to adults of all ages. Adults need and often crave intimacy with others, including sexual intimacy. The intimacy needs of adults should be addressed by healthcare providers directly during history and physical exams as patients may be embarrassed or reluctant to ask questions. Nurses should not avoid the topic because of personal anxiety and should respect different attitudes and behavior. Assessment should be done in private, ensuring confidentiality. Questioning should progress from general topics ("Do you have a good relationship with your partner?") to more specific questions related to sexual issues ("Is intercourse uncomfortable for you?"). Older or disabled adults may need to know how to deal with physical or environmental limitations. Some adults engage in risky sexual behavior, putting them at increased risk of HIV or STDs, so discussing sexual issues provides an opportunity for education and counseling.

High-Risk Sexual Behavior in Young Adults

High-risk sexual behavior in young adults is often coupled with other health-risk behaviors, such as drinking and drug use, and people are having sex at younger ages. About 47% of high school seniors have had sex, with many beginning as young as 10-12 years. Risk factors include poverty, single-family homes, lack of supervision, and siblings or peers who are sexually active. Those who have sex before age 15 are especially vulnerable often having multiple partners and unprotected sex, leading to sexually transmitted diseases (STDs) and pregnancy. They are emotionally vulnerable and often can't deal effectively with relationships. *Intervention* should begin early with age-appropriate honest sex education. Abstinence education, while the ideal, has not been successful in changing the sexual behavior of teenagers or young adults with studies showing that many of those signing pledges to remain virgins are already sexually active. All those who are sexually active should be advised regarding the use of condoms, birth control, and protection from STDs in a non-judgmental manner.

Intimacy in Nursing Homes

The need for **intimacy** doesn't end when older adults enter nursing homes, but there can be many obstacles to the expression of intimacy in nursing homes. The patient may have serious health problems that limit physical intimacy. Many rooms house two patients, and lack of privacy is an issue. Most facilities have only single beds available for patients. Even if the patient is in a private room, staff members are in and out of rooms frequently, interfering with privacy. Nurses and other staff may have stereotypical negative attitudes toward older adults and sexuality. Every effort should be made to overcome obstacles and allow partners/spouses private time with patients. Even if sexual intercourse is not possible, the partners can hold and caress each other and express their caring. Curtains can be drawn to provide privacy or a notice can be placed on the door ("Family time").

Human Sexuality Among Gay and Lesbian Older Adults

The gay rights movement began in 1969. Therefore, many older adults came to maturity at a time when prejudice and discrimination against *gays* and *lesbians* was overt, tolerated, and sometimes legislated. Because of this, many older adults are not open about their sexuality and may be reluctant to discuss their concerns. The nurse can open the lines of communication by asking patients directly if they have sex with the same gender while showing respect for the individual. Nurses and other healthcare providers should be aware that most gay and lesbian organizations are geared toward younger members, so there is a dearth of social services aimed at the older population.

Environmental Determinants of Health

Environmental Risk Factors

When assessing a patient, it's important to consider that **environmental factors** may place the patient at increased risk or may be a factor in disease. There are a number of different types of environmental factors:

Factors	Examples	Effects
Toxic chemicals	Lead, arsenic, muriatic acid, sulfuric acid, ammonia, lime	May result in poisoning (lead, arsenic) or burns (acids, ammonia, lime)
Physical objects	Guns, cars, knives, equipment	Accidents, gunshot wounds, stabbings, various injuries
Biological organisms	Bacteria, fungi, viruses	Infections
Temperature variations	Heat, cold	Burns, dehydration, heat stroke, hypothermia, frostbite
Ambient noise	Sirens, loud music, traffic noise, work-related noise	Hearing loss/deafness
Psychosocial	Increased stress	Anxiety, hypertension

Environmental Assessment

Environmental factors should be assessed within the actual environment if at all possible. If not, careful questioning of the patient and drawing diagrams and floor plans with the patient can be useful, especially when showing the patient needed modifications. Asking the patient to do drawings may also be helpful. Family members may also assist with the assessment, providing useful information. Some patients, especially the elderly, may be reluctant to admit that the home is cluttered or that they are unable to maintain the home environment in a sanitary condition. Brochures and handouts about home safety and assistive devices should be provided to the patient as well as contact names and numbers for equipment needed in the home. A checklist should be compiled of all necessary changes or additions with specific details, such as "Install 18-inch grab bar across from toilet." In some cases, a social worker or occupational therapist should visit the patient.

Area Specific Assessment

Environmental assessments are very helpful when developing a care plan to provide for care and safety. Rooms should be assessed according to their function:

- *The entryway* should be free of obstacles and surfaces should be even. Handrails and/or ramps may be needed for those who are unsteady or wheelchair bound.
- *Stairs/steps* should have handrails, non-skid surfaces, and contrast markings for each step.
- *The living area* should be comfortable and furniture arranged for convenience. Chairs should be firm enough for people to stand from easily.
- *Bedrooms* should have a night light and phone near the bed. Bed should be positioned close to the nearest bathroom if possible. Beds should be at the appropriate height for easy access and be of appropriate firmness.
- *Bathrooms* may require grab bars, a hand-held shower, an elevated toilet seat, and a tub seat.
- *Kitchen* items may need to be moved for convenient access. A sturdy step stool may be necessary. Unsafe equipment/tools should be removed.

Elements

Some elements of **environmental assessment** are not specific to rooms in the house but are general needs that must be met in order for people, especially the elderly or disabled, to remain safe:

- *Environmental hazards* such as piles of papers or junk on the floors, loose carpet or rugs, and cluttered pathways can cause falls and must be cleared, organized, or repaired.
- *Lighting* should be adequate enough for reading in all rooms and stairways.
- *Heat and air conditioning* must be adequate. The young and the elderly are especially susceptible to heat and cold injury.
- *Sanitation* should ensure that health hazards, such as rotting food or infestations of cockroaches, do not exist.
- *Animals* should be cared for adequately with access to food, water, toileting, and routine veterinary care.
- *Smoke/chemicals* in the environment, such as cigarette smoke or cleaning materials, may pose a hazard.

Use of Smoke Alarms

A **smoke alarm** is one of the best protections against death by fires in the home, but older adults die in fires at rates that are 2.5 to 3 times that of younger people for a variety of reasons:

- Hearing impairment may prevent older adult from hearing the smoke alarm.
- Limited mobility may prevent their responding to the fire alarm.
- Reluctance to deal with new technology may cause them to avoid getting a smoke detector.
- Access to the smoke detector may be difficult so that batteries are not changed.
- There may be an insufficient number of smoke alarms for the size of the home.

Smoke alarms should be checked regularly to make sure they are functioning and placed where the older adult can reach them. Special smoke alarms for the hearing impaired should be used if the older adult has difficulty hearing the alarm. These alarms combine audible alarms and high intensity strobe lights to alert people to smoke.

Environment and Medications for Alzheimer's Disease or Cognitive Impairment

Environment

Any unnecessary clutter should be removed from dressers, drawers, and bookshelves. Items, furniture, and rooms should be labeled if the patient is still able to read. For example, the patient's bedroom door should be labeled. If the patient is unable to read, pictures can be posted showing the use of the room or item. Dangerous items, such as knives, scissors, and matches, should be secured so that they are not accessible to the patient. If the patient is unable to climb over a gate, a child's gate can be used to block off dangerous areas.

Medications

In the early stages of their disease, patients may be able to manage medications if they are prepared in medication containers. However, the use of all medications should be monitored to ensure that they are used as directed. The caregiver should dispense medications if necessary. It may be necessary to disguise medications in food.

Cultural Differences/Issues

Often healthcare providers who strive to be culturally competent are unaware that patients/families have very different perspectives about issues central to their health. According to the National Center for Cultural Competence there are a number of specific **cultural differences/issues** that healthcare providers should understand the following:

- Attitudes about illness and the cause of illness may be very different from one culture to another.
- Understanding of general health, mechanisms of healing, and issues of wellness may be very diverse.
- Attitudes about healthcare providers may range from very positive to very negative.
- The manner of help seeking for medical problems may vary, and healthcare providers may not recognize help-seeking behavior when it is not direct.
- Attitudes about traditional and non-traditional treatment influence the individual's medical choices.
- Attitudes of healthcare workers may project biases to which the patients are subjected.
- The current health system is often not culturally or linguistically diverse, so patient needs may be overlooked.

Cultural Competence

Ethnicity

The CNS must have **cultural competence related to ethnicity.** Patients who are from diverse ethnicities are sometimes treated differently by healthcare providers, resulting in less-than-optimal care. It is incumbent upon nurses to ensure that all patients and their families receive equal quality care, but with delivery of care tailored to meet the individual needs of the patients. This begins with asking other staff to assess their own attitudes, and then conducting an open discussion about differences to help people gain self-awareness and determine if their ideas are based on stereotypes or lack of knowledge. The care plan should be formatted to specifically address diversity issues so discussions of diversity and preferences are part of the care plan development, not an addendum. The original assessment should include questions about family, country of birth, education level, religious preferences, and native language, with explanations as to why the questions are asked, establishing a relationship of trust and respect that encourages the patient or family to express individual differences.

Linguistic Barriers

Linguistic barriers often compromise patients' access to care and compliance with treatment, especially if the family are non-English speaking or have poor English skills. If the healthcare institution or practice draws from a minority population, the healthcare provider should consider proactive steps to resolving the issue of language barriers, such as hiring bilingual staff, taking language classes, providing translated materials such as treatment guidelines and pamphlets, or symbol-based signs. Many healthcare providers depend on family members, often children, to translate, but this is not a good solution, as children often lack the maturity to assume this responsibility and may also lack the vocabulary or understanding to translate effectively, leading to serious misunderstandings. Interpreters should have training in medical vocabulary. In some cases, volunteers can be trained as translators. Another solution is to pool translation resources among a number of practices or institutions so costs are manageable.

Issues of Cultural Competence

There are a number of issues related to **cultural and spiritual competence** in communicating with patients/family:

- *Eye contact:* Many cultures use eye contact differently than is common in the United States. Individuals from these cultures may avoid direct eye contact, considering it rude. They may look away to signal disapproval, or look down to signal respect. Careful observation of the way family members use eye contact can help to determine what will be most comfortable for the patient/family.
- *Distance*: Some cultures stand close to others (<4 feet) when speaking (e.g., Middle Easterners and Hispanics) and others stand at a further distance (>4 feet) (e.g., Northern Europeans and many Americans). There is considerable difference relating to concepts of personal space among cultures. Allowing the family to approach or observing whether they tend to move closer, lean forward, or move back can help to determine a comfortable distance for communication.
- *Time*: Americans tend to be time-oriented, and expect people to be on time, but time is more flexible in many cultures, so scheduling may require flexibility.

Beliefs and Traditions Regarding Death

Individual beliefs and traditions regarding death vary widely, and these affect how the patient and family deal with the end of life. The nurse should discuss these issues with the patient and/or family in order to ensure their needs are met. Those with strong spiritual beliefs may want spiritual advisors (priests, shamans, ministers, monks) present to provide support or perform rituals. People who have no belief in an afterlife may face death with resolution or may be frightened at the thought of the total end of their existence. Those who believe in reincarnation may find comfort in the thought of their rebirth but may also fear karma for the mistakes they made in this life. Some people believe in a loving God and others a vengeful God, so some may feel that they will be in a loving place after death while others fear they will suffer torment for their sins. The nurse should remain supportive and allow patients and families to express their feelings, fears, and concerns.

Hmong Patients

The **Hmong**, originally from Laos, have settled in a number of areas across the United States and often cling to their traditions, so nurses who serve Hmong populations should have an understanding of Hmong traditions. There is variation among the Hmong people as with all groups. More traditional families may shun Western medicine and rely solely on healers, while Christian Hmong may rely only on Western medicine. However, many Hmong people straddle both the traditional and Western worlds.

The *eldest male* in the family makes the decisions for the family and is deferred to by other family members, so the nurse should ask who should receive information about the patient.

Communication should be polite and respectful, avoiding direct eye contact, which is considered rude.

Respect is shown to elders by bowing the head slightly when entering the room and presenting items with both hands.

Considerations when treating **Hmong patients** (in addition to issues related to the eldest male, communication, and respect) include:

- Disagreeing is considered rude so "Yes" may mean "I hear you" and NOT "I agree with you."
- The Hmong believe that illness occurs when the spirit, soul, and body are out of balance and may want a traditional healer, a shaman, to treat the spiritual cause of the disease. Hmong believe that both spiritual and physical worlds exist and that a person has a number of souls and sickness occurs when one or more souls are lost or taken by other spirits. These souls must be reclaimed for healing to occur.
- Many Hmong use herbs to treat various ailments, but some herbs may interfere with medical treatment, so patients/families should be questioned closely about the use of herbs. Explaining that some medications contain herbal treatments and that the patient could receive too much may encourage people to provide this information.

Mexican Patients

Many areas of the country have large populations of **Mexican** and Mexican-Americans. As always, it's important to recognize that cultural generalizations don't always apply to individuals. Recent immigrants, especially, have cultural needs that the nurse must understand:

Most Mexicans are Catholic and may like the nurse to make arrangements for a priest to visit.

Large extended families may come to visit to support the patient and family, so patients should receive clear explanations about how many visitors are allowed, but some flexibility may be required.

Language barriers may exist as some may have limited or no English skills, so translation services should be available around the clock.

Mexican culture encourages *outward expressions of emotions*, so family may react strongly to news about a patient's condition, and people who are ill may expect some degree of pampering, so extra attention to the patient/family members may alleviate some of their anxiety.

Caring for **Mexican** patients requires understanding of cultural differences:

- Some immigrant Mexicans have very little formal education, so medical information may seem very complex and confusing, and they may not understand the implications or need for follow-up care.
- Mexican culture perceives time with more flexibility than American, so if patients/family must be present at a particular time, the nurse should specify the exact time (1:30 PM) and explain the reason rather than saying something more vague, such as "after lunch."
- People may appear to be unassertive or unable to make decisions when they are simply showing respect to the nurse by being deferent.
- In traditional families, the males make decisions, so a woman may wait for the husband or other males in the family to make decisions about treatment or care.
- Families may choose to use folk medicine instead of Western medical care or may combine the two.
- Children and young women are often sheltered and are taught to be respectful to adults, so they may not express their needs openly.

MIDDLE EASTERN PATIENTS

There are considerable cultural differences among **Middle Easterners,** but religious beliefs about the segregation of males and females are common. It's important to remember that segregating the female is meant to protect her virtue. Female nurses have low status in many countries because they violate this segregation by touching male bodies, so families may not trust or show respect for the nurse who is caring for their family member. Additionally, male patients may not want to be cared for by female nurses or doctors, and families may be very upset at a female being cared for by a male nurse or physician. When possible, these cultural traditions should be accommodated.

In Middle Eastern countries, males make decisions, so issues for discussion or decision should be directed to males, such as the spouse or son, and males may be direct in stating what they want, sometimes appearing demanding.

If a male nurse must care for a female patient, then the family should be advised that *personal care* (such as bathing) will be done by a female while the medical treatments will be done by the male nurse.

Caring for **Middle Eastern** patients requires understanding of cultural differences:

- Families may practice strict dietary restrictions, such as avoiding pork and requiring that animals be killed in a ritual manner, so vegetarian or kosher meals may be required.
- People may have language difficulties requiring a translator, and same-sex translators should be used if at all possible.
- Patients may be accompanied by large extended families that want to be kept informed and with whom patients consult before decisions are made.
- Most medical care is provided by female relatives, so educating the family about patient care should be directed at females (with female translators if necessary).
- Outward expressions of grief are considered as showing respect for the dead.
- Middle Eastern families often offer gifts to caregivers. Small gifts (candy) should be accepted graciously, but for other gifts, the families should be advised graciously that accepting gifts is against hospital policy.
- Middle Easterners often require less personal space and may stand very close.

ASIAN PATIENTS

There are considerable differences among different **Asian** populations, so cultural generalizations may not apply to all, but nurses caring for Asian patients should be aware of common cultural attitudes and behaviors:

- Nurses and doctors are viewed with respect, so traditional Asian families may expect the nurse to remain authoritative and to give directions and may not question the nurse's directions or remarks; therefore, the nurse should ensure that they understand by having them review material or give demonstrations and should provide explanations clearly, anticipating questions that the family might have but may not articulate.
- Disagreeing is considered impolite. "Yes" may only mean that the person is heard, not that the listener agrees with the person. When asked if they understand, they may indicate that they do even when they clearly do not to avoid offending the nurse.
- Asians may avoid eye contact as an indication of respect.

Caring for **Asian** patients requires understanding of cultural differences:

- Patients/families may not show outward expressions of feelings/grief, sometimes appearing passive. They also avoid public displays of affection. This does not mean that they don't feel, just that they don't show their feelings.
- Families often hide illness and disabilities from others and may feel ashamed about illness.
- Terminal illness is often hidden from the patient, so families may not want patients to know they are dying or seriously ill.
- Families may use cupping, pinching, or applying pressure to injured areas, and this can leave bruises that may appear as abuse, so when bruises are found, the family should be questioned about alternative therapy before assumptions are made.
- Patients may be treated with traditional herbs.
- Families may need translators because of poor or no English skills.
- In traditional Asian families, males are authoritative and make the decisions.

Religious-Based Nutritional Needs of Specific Populations

Religious-based nutritional needs for the following populations are as follows:

- **Muslims**
  - Eating pork or carnivorous animals and drinking alcoholic beverages are prohibited.
  - Animals must be slaughtered with halal methods.
  - During the month of Ramadan, people in good health are expected to fast from before dawn until after sunset.
- **Jews**
  - Eating meat of land animals that do not chew their cud or have cloven hooves is prohibited, so pigs and rabbits are forbidden. Shellfish are forbidden. Birds of prey are prohibited, and some people avoid turkey.
  - All food, wine, dishes, and utensils must be kosher.
  - Animals must be slaughtered according to kosher traditions.
  - Meat and dairy products are separated for cooking, served on separate dishes, and must be eaten at different meals.
- **Hindus**
  - Eating beef is prohibited.
  - Some castes may also avoid meat of other animals; many are vegetarian.
  - Some castes avoid eggs or eat only those fertilized and may also avoid onions and garlic.

Nutritional Needs of Vegetarians and Vegans

The **nutritional needs of vegetarians and vegans** are as follows:

- **Vegetarians**
  - Ovolactovegetarians eat plant-based diet, no meat products, but does eat eggs and dairy products.
  - Ovo-vegetarians eat eggs but no dairy products.
  - Lactovegetarians eat dairy products, but no eggs.
  - Semi vegetarians may include chicken or fish in diet, but no red meat.
  - Note: Some foods contain animal products and are avoided by most vegetarians, including marshmallows, gelatin, gum, and many prepared foods.

- **Vegans**
    - Eat no animal products of any kind, including meat, dairy products, eggs, or honey.
    - Primary sources of protein and iron are beans, lentils, spinach, and soy products, such as tofu.
    - May require vitamin B12 supplementation or nutritional yeast.
    - Primary sources of calcium include green leafy vegetables and fortified soymilk, rice milk, or orange juice.

Intergenerational Issues of the Silent Generation and Baby Boomers

Intergenerational issues may occur outside of the family, but they can cause significant conflict when they occur within the family, especially if an older adult lives with younger generations. While individuals differ widely, as a group, older adults tend to be more religious and conservative than younger adults. Attitudes toward sexuality, equality, race, lifestyle, music, and religion may be divergent to the point that conflicts occur. General characteristics related to different generations include the following:

- *Silent Generation* (born before WWII): These individuals tend to be rule-oriented and cautious. They value trustworthiness. Keeping one's word is important. They are practical and make decisions based on interest and opportunity.
- *Baby Boomers* (born 1943-1960): These individuals tend to be more self-centered, but they are also proactive and committed to ideas/causes. They tend to be resistant to compromise with others. They are focused on self-expression and introspection. This generation enjoyed prosperity to a greater degree than previous generations and came to expect that it would continue. They also had more access to health care and more medical tools (e.g., antibiotics, chemotherapy, and radiation).

Intergenerational Issues Among Generation X and the Millennial Generation

Intergenerational issues are often related to the general characteristics related to different generations (in addition to the Silent Generation and Baby Boomers):

- *Generation X* (born in the 60s and 70s): These individuals tend to be independent in thoughts and lifestyle, are creative, and adapt well to change, but may overlook ethical concerns in their quest for achievement. This generation was influenced by divorce more than preceding generations. They seek balance and like to remain open to new opportunities.
- *Millennial (Y) generation* (born 1980-2000): These individuals tend to believe they can be successful and are hardworking and confident in their abilities but may overlook the feelings and skills of others. They believe in the power of achievement and tend to make decisions as a family and are often more open to diversity (e.g., sexual preference, gender, race, and culture) than previous generations.

Abuse and Neglect

Elder Abuse

There are many different types of **elder abuse:** physical (such a hitting or improperly restraining), sexual, psychological, financial, and neglect. Elder abuse may be difficult to diagnose, especially if the person is cognitively impaired, but *symptoms* may include the following: fearfulness, disparities in reports of injuries between patient and caregiver, evidence of old or repeated injuries, poor hygiene and dental care, decubiti, malnutrition, undue concern with costs on caregiver's part, unsupportive attitude of caregiver, and caregiver's reluctance or refusal to allow patient to communicate privately with the CNS. Self-abuse can also occur when patients are not able to adequately care for themselves. *Diagnosis* of elder abuse includes a careful history and physical exam, including direct questioning of the patient about abuse. *Treatment* includes attending to injuries or physical needs (this can vary widely) and referral to adult protective services as indicated. Reporting laws regarding elder abuse vary somewhat from one state to another, but all states have laws regarding elder abuse; in 42 states, reporting of abuse by heath workers is mandatory.

Risks

Age and disability increase the **risks of elder abuse**. People older than age 80 are more than twice as likely to suffer abuse as younger adults. Abuse takes place in both the home and in institutions. At home, older adults with dementia are often abused by family members. Caregivers often lose patience and become frustrated, especially if the patient's behavior is belligerent, combative, or disruptive. Five to fourteen percent of those with dementia are victims of elder abuse. One to three percent of individuals in the general population are victims of elder abuse. Elder abuse of individuals with dementia can be very difficult to diagnose, as the patient is usually unable to report the abuse. In fact, even older adults who are not cognitively impaired may be afraid to report abuse because they depend on their abuser to care for them. Older adults who are dependent on caregivers for assistance with activities of daily living (ADLs) are particularly at risk for abuse and neglect. Abusers often suffer from depression and/or substance abuse and may be financially dependent on the victim.

Physical and Psychological Abuse

There are a number of different **types of elder abuse**. *Physical abuse* is an active form of abuse (a type of domestic violence). It is almost always associated with *psychological abuse*. Older adults may suffer various types of assaults, including slapping, punching, kicking, hair pulling, and shoving. The physical abuse of an older adult is often committed by a family member (often an adult child) or another caregiver. Caregivers may make frequent threats to hit the older adult if he or she doesn't cooperate with the caregiver's plan. The caregiver may brandish a weapon. In addition, the caretaker may tell the person to commit suicide. Ongoing intimidation may make cause terror and anxiety. Sometimes, caregivers threaten to injure pets or family members, increasing the patient's fear. Patients may be forcibly confined, forced into seclusion, and/or force-fed to the point that they choke on food. Physical symptoms are consistent with domestic abuse. Psychological symptoms include anxiety, paranoia, insomnia, low self-esteem, avoidance of eye contact, and nervousness in the presence of the caregiver, who is often reluctant to leave the patient alone.

Abuse and Neglect of Basic Needs

Neglect of basic needs is a common problem of older adults who live alone or with reluctant or incapable caregivers. In some cases, passive neglect may occur because an elderly spouse is trying to take care of a patient and is unable to provide the care needed. Active neglect is intentional and reflects a lack of caring. Active neglect may border on negligence and abuse. Indications of neglect include lack of assistive devices needed for mobility (such as cane or walker); lack of needed glasses or hearing aids; poor dental hygiene and dental care and/or missing dentures; inadequate food/fluid/nutrition, resulting in weight loss; inappropriate and unkempt clothing (for example, the lack of a sweater or coat during the winter and dirty or torn clothing); and a dirty, messy environment. In addition, the patient may be left unattended for prolonged periods of time (sometimes confined to a bed or chair) or left in soiled or urine-/feces-stained clothing.

FINANCIAL ABUSE

As older adults become unable to manage their own financial affairs, they become increasingly vulnerable to financial abuse. This is especially true if the adult has cognitive impairment or physical impairments that impair mobility. **Financial abuse** includes outright stealing of property or persuading the patient to give away possessions, forcing the individual to sign away property, emptying the individual's bank and savings accounts, stealing the individual's credit cards, convincing the individual to invest money in fraudulent schemes, and taking money from the individual for home renovations that are not done. Indications of financial abuse may be unpaid bills, unusual activity at ATMs, unusual credit activity, inadequate funds to meet needs, disappearance of items from the home, change in the provision of a will, and deferring to caregivers regarding financial affairs. Family members or caregivers may move permanently into the patient's home and take over without sharing costs.

SEXUAL ABUSE

Sexual abuse of older adults occurs when the person receiving sexual attention is forced to participate or unable to consent to sexual intimacy. Patients may be unable to consent to sexual activity due to cognitive impairment or other illness. Types of sexual abuse include physical (fondling, kissing, and rape); emotional (exhibitionism); and verbal (sexual harassment, using obscene language, and threatening). Women in their seventies or eighties who are confined to nursing homes are the most frequent targets of sexual abuse. Sexual abuse may also occur in home environments, but it is harder to detect. Most abusers of women in nursing homes are males older than age 80 who reside in the same nursing home. The most common form of abuse is sexualized kissing and fondling of the genitals. Older adults do behave sexually, and in some cases, what appears to be abuse between residents is, in fact, consensual sexual activity. Caregivers have raped or otherwise sexually abused patients, and this exercise of power over another person is always illegal abuse.

ASSESSMENT OF DOMESTIC VIOLENCE

According to the guidelines of the Family Violence Prevention Fund, assessment for **domestic violence** should be done for all adolescent and adult patients, regardless of background or signs of abuse. While females are the most common victims, there are increasing reports of male victims of domestic violence, both in heterosexual and homosexual relationships. The person doing the assessment should be informed about domestic violence and be aware or risk factors and danger signs. The interview should be conducted in private (special accommodations may need to be made for children <3 years old). The CNS's office, bathrooms, and examining rooms should have information about domestic violence posted prominently. Brochures and information should be available to give to patients. Patients may present with a variety of physical complaints, such as headache, pain, palpitations, numbness, or pelvic pain. They are often depressed and may appear suicidal and may be isolated from friends and family. Victims of domestic violence often exhibit fear of spouse/partner, and may report injury inconsistent with symptoms.

Family Violence Prevention Fund Steps to Identifying Victims of Domestic Violence

The **Family Violence Prevent Fund** has issued guidelines for identifying and assisting victims of domestic violence. There are 7 steps:

1. **Inquiry***:* Non-judgmental questioning should begin with asking if the person has ever been abused—physically, sexually, or psychologically.
2. **Interview***:* The person may exhibit signs of anxiety or fear and may blame himself/herself or report that others believe he/she is abused. The person should be questioned if he/she is afraid for his/her life or for children.
3. **Question***:* If the person reports abuse, it's critical to ask if the person is in immediate danger or if the abuser is on the premises. The interviewer should ask if the person has been threatened. The history and pattern of abuse should be questioned, and if children are involved, whether the children are abused. Note: State laws vary, and in some states, it is mandatory to report if a child was present during an act of domestic violence as this is considered child abuse. The CNS must be aware of state laws regarding domestic and child abuse, and all nurses are mandatory reporters.
4. **Validate***:* The interviewer should offer support and reassurance in a non-judgmental manner, telling the patient the abuse is not his/her fault.
5. **Give information***:* While discussing facts about domestic violence and the tendency to escalate, the interviewer should provide brochures and information about safety planning. If the patient wants to file a complaint with the police, the interviewer should assist the person to place the call.
6. **Make referrals***:* Information about state, local, and national organizations should be provided along with telephone numbers and contact numbers for domestic violence shelters.
7. **Document***:* Record keeping should be legal, legible, and lengthy with a complete report and description of any traumatic injuries resulting from domestic violence. A body map may be used to indicate sites of injury, especially if there are multiple bruises or injuries.

Injuries Consistent with Domestic Violence

There are a number of characteristic **injuries** that may indicate **domestic violence,** including ruptured eardrum; rectal/genital injury (burns, bites, or trauma); scrapes and bruises about the neck, face, head, trunk, arms; and cuts, bruises, and fractures of the face. The pattern of injuries associated with domestic violence is also often distinctive. The bathing-suit pattern involves injuries on parts of body that are usually covered with clothing as the perpetrator inflicts damage but hides evidence of abuse. Head and neck injuries (50%) are also common. Abusive injuries (rarely attributable to accidents) are common and include bites, bruises, rope and cigarette burns, and welts in the outline of weapons (belt marks). Bilateral injuries of arms/legs are often seen with domestic abuse. Defensive injuries are indicative of abuse.

Defensive injuries to the back of the body are often incurred as the victim crouches on the floor face down while being attacked. The soles of the feet may be injured from kicking at perpetrator. The ulnar aspect of hand or palm may be injured from blocking blows.

Comprehensive Assessment

Preparation for the Interview

Prior to a **patient interview**, the nurse should review previous medical records and have a clear idea of the purpose of the interview. The nurse should outline questions. If possible, the patient should be interviewed alone or should be asked if he/she wants family members present. If the patient is cognitively-impaired, then the family may need to provide information; however, as much as possible, the information should come directly from the patient or from the nurse's observations of the patient as family members may over-estimate or under-estimate the patient's functional ability. Privacy must be assured, taking care to draw curtains, close doors, or conduct the interview in a private setting. The nurse should sit close to the patient, face to face, and speak directly to him/her. Some patients who are hearing impaired use lip-reading to help with understanding, so the nurse should speak slowly and clearly.

Interview Techniques

There are a number of factors that are important to a good **interview**:

- *Initial introductions:* The nurse should make introductions by his/her full name and explain his/her roles and the purpose of the interview, asking the patient how he/she wishes to be addressed and avoiding using familiar terms, such as "dear," which may be considered condescending. The nurse should stress the confidential nature of the interview and explain who will receive the information.
- *Interview structure:* The interview may be somewhat unstructured, guided by patient responses, or may be very structured with the nurse asking a list of questions, but the nurse must remain flexible while still guiding the discussion in order to accommodate different communication styles.
- *Appearance:* The nurse should be professionally dressed and wearing a clear nametag. The patient's appearance should be observed non-judgmentally for clothes (loose/tight clothes may indicate weight change), cleanliness (dirty clothes/skin/hair may indicate cognitive or physical impairment or poverty), and demeanor (calm, fidgeting, nervous).

Eliciting Information

Both verbal and non-verbal responses should be observed during an interview. Patients may look away or become tense if they are not telling the truth or don't want to answer a particular question. Information elicited during an interview should include not only the patient's facts but also the patient's attitude and concerns. Using therapeutic questioning technique is essential for **eliciting information:**

- Ask information questions (as opposed to yes/no) with "who," "what," "where," "when" and "how," but avoid questions with "why" if possible:
- Instead of "Why do you continue to eat sugar?" ask, "What sugar substitutes have you tried?"
- Ask brief clarifying questions: "How long were you in the hospital?"
- Provide a list of options: "Is your headache throbbing, stabbing, or dull?
- Rephrase/reflect to encourage clarification:
- Patient: "My husband had the same surgery and died a month later."
- Nurse: "You're afraid you might die from this surgery?"

Comprehensive Adult Assessment Across the Lifespan

Comprehensive adult assessment across the lifespan is as follows:

- **History (Hx)** - Acute or chronic medical conditions, surgeries, allergies, and immunizations
- **Socio-economic status** - Employment, financial status, marital status, children, military service, education, use of seat belts and helmets, hobbies and related hazards, religious preferences/restrictions, availability of caregivers or support persons

- **Family hx.** - Diseases, problems, age at death, and cause of death
- **Physical** - Complete review of systems, VS, hearing and vision tests, laboratory testing (CBC, UA, chemistry panel)
- **Substances** - Tobacco, alcohol, drug use (prescription, OTC, and illicit)
- **Sexuality** - Activity, high-risk behavior, and contraception
- **Functional status** - Ambulation, balance, transfers, and ability to manage ADLs
- **Nutrition** - Eating habits, fluid intake, and nutrition
- **Mental status** - Memory, executive function, and comprehension
- **Psychological status** - Outlook, depression, agitation, anxiety, relationship problems, and sleep impairment
- **Quality of life** - Pain management, independence/dependence, and satisfaction
- **Problems** - Specific complaints and/or needs

DYSPHAGIA

Dysphagia occurs in about 10% of noninstitutionalized older adults and even more in hospitalized patients. Difficulty swallowing is evident with solids and thin liquids. Symptoms include chest tightness or pain, regurgitation, choking, esophageal reflux (especially when supine), and aspiration pneumonia. Weight loss and dehydration may result. Assessment questions include:

- Have you ever choked when eating or drinking? When? How frequently?
- Does your mouth feel too dry to chew your food?
- Do you ever experience drooling you can't control?
- Does food sometimes get stuck in your mouth or fall out of your mouth when you are trying to eat?
- Do you ever regurgitate or spit up food after you finish eating?
- Do you have to clear your throat frequently?
- Is sitting upright while you are eating a problem for you?

If the patient says yes to any of these questions or has symptoms indicating possible dysphagia, then further testing is indicated. Diagnostic studies may include observed swallowing of a variety of thin to thick liquids, endoscopy, and videofluoroscopic radiography.

SPIRITUALITY

A **spiritual assessment** allows the healthcare provider to assess the spiritual needs of the patient. The assessment should begin with a statement that spirituality is important to many people and a request to ask questions about spiritual matters, as some people consider religion very private. The **FICA format (Puchalski)** is an effective assessment.

F	Faith/belief	Do you feel you are religious or spiritual? Do your beliefs help you cope? If patients deny religious or spiritual beliefs: Is there something you feel gives your life meaning?
I	Importance	How important is your belief system? Do your beliefs influence your acceptance of treatments or choices dealing with illness? How important do you believe your religion or spiritual beliefs are in your regaining heath?

C	Community	Do you identify with a particular religious or spiritual community or church? Do you feel this community is supportive? Do you have family and friends who are important to you and supportive of you?
A	Address during care	How would you like your healthcare providers to address your spiritual needs?

Support Systems

Assessment of support systems discovers the support the patient is receiving, as well as support that may be available. Support may take a variety of forms.

Family	Do you have family living nearby? Are you close to your family? Does your family provide you assistance and/or support? Would your family be able to help you?
Friends	Do you have close friends you can depend on? Do you see your friends often or talk to them? Do your friends provide any assistance to you? Would your friends able to help you?
Religion	Do you have a church/temple/synagogue that provides you support? Is this support primarily spiritual? Does this institution provide any type of social services?
Computer	Do you belong to any message boards or chat rooms? Have you established supportive relationships with any members?
Community resources	Do you have hired personnel that can provide support? Are you aware of community resources, such as Meals-on-Wheels or home health agencies? Is this resource one that you can consider?

Auscultation, Palpation, and Percussion

Auscultation

This procedure involves the use of a stethoscope to listen to the movement of air or fluid within the body. The sounds are characterized according to intensity (loudness), frequency (pitch), and quality. Auscultation is commonly used to assess the functioning of the heart and lungs. It is also used to determine if circulatory impairment (bruit) is present and to listen to bowel sounds.

Palpation

Palpation involves using the fingertips to evaluate the characteristics of a particular part of the body. Hardness, temperature, swelling, size, and mobility can be assessed by palpation. Care should be taken when palpating the area over the liver; excessive pressure should be avoided. In some cases, sound may be felt as vibrations.

Percussion

Percussion is a technique in which the fingers of one hand are laid flat against the skin and tapped with the fingertips of the other hand. This causes sound to resonate. Percussion is most commonly used to assess organ size or changes in tissue density. Care should be used over the liver, spine, and bladder.

Assessment of the Chest, Abdomen, and Genitalia

Older patients may have a decreased respiratory force and cough reflex and may be short of breath. **Chest inspection** may have to be modified as a consequence. Inspection may take longer in order to allow the patient to rest between deep breaths.

Abdominal inspection should be done with care. Older adults may have a decreased sensation of pain on deep palpation. There is less cushioning for the liver, so the area should be palpitated gently to prevent damage to the tissue.

Genitalia should be examined, but older adults may be embarrassed, so the nurse should explain the need for the procedure. Older women often have vaginal atrophy with decreased lubrication, so a smaller speculum should be used, and it should be well lubricated. Perianal pruritis is common in older adults, but they are often embarrassed to talk about it. The nurse should ask if there is any itching in the area.

Assessment and Pain Scale

Pain is subjective and may be influenced by the individual's pain threshold (the smallest stimulus that produces the sensation of pain) and pain tolerance (the maximum degree of pain that a person can tolerate). The most common current pain assessment tool is the 1-10 scale:

0	no pain
1-2	mild pain
3-5	moderate pain
6-7	severe pain
8-9	very severe pain
10	excruciating pain

However, there is more to pain assessment than a number on a scale. Assessment includes information about onset, duration, and intensity. Identifying what triggers pain and what relieves it can be very useful when developing a plan for pain management. Different patients may show very different behavior when they are in pain. Some may cry and moan with minor pain and others may exhibit little difference in behavior when truly suffering; thus, judging pain by behavior can lead to the wrong conclusions.

Positioning, Sensory Impairment, and Extremities in Patient Assessment

Positioning

Many adults have mobility problems, a limited range of motion, and difficulty maintaining certain positions. Physical limitations differ for different patients. Each patient should be positioned in the most comfortable position. Changes of position should be minimized.

Sensory Impairment

Sensory impairments include deficits in vision, hearing, and sense of touch. These problems should be assessed early. If deficits are known, accommodations should be made. If the patient wears a hearing aid, the nurse should request that the patient wear it during the exam. The room should be quiet and free of distraction.

Extremities

Extremities should be examined using modified movements. Force must not be used. For example, care should be taken when pushing a limb into flexion or extension. The nurse should not ask the patient to do things that put too much stress on the limbs. For example, the patient should not be asked to do deep bends. Older patients may have decreased range of motion, slower reflexes, and poor balance. The nurse should always ensure that the limbs are supported during inspection.

Psychological, Social, and Sensory Functions

Functional status assessment concerns the ability to do self-care, self-maintenance, and engage in physical activities, but other factors may interfere with optimal functioning:

- *Psychological function* assesses anxiety, worry, grief, and depression. Those with depression may be at increased risk of physical disability or may neglect self-care.
- *Social function* assesses support from family or friends, the need for a caregiver, financial resources, mistreatment or abuse, the ability to drive, and the presence of advance directives.
- *Sensory function* assesses the presence of cataracts, glaucoma, myopia, presbyopia, astigmatism, macular degeneration, or eye disorders that make it difficult for people to read medication labels or do self-care. The need for audio materials or enlarged print should be assessed. Hearing is evaluated for hearing deficits and high and low frequency hearing loss as well as waxy buildup in the ear canals.

Assessment

Functional status assessment concerns the ability to perform self-care and self-maintenance and to engage in physical activities. However, other factors may interfere with normal functioning. Tests of *psychological function* assess anxiety, worry, grief, and depression. Those with depression may be at increased risk of physical disability or may neglect self-care. Tests of *social function* assess support from family or friends, the need for a caregiver, financial resources, mistreatment or abuse, the ability to drive, and the presence of advance directives. Tests of *sensory function* assess the health of the sensory systems. These tests look for signs and symptoms of cataracts, glaucoma, myopia, presbyopia, astigmatism, macular degeneration, or eye disorders that make it difficult for people to read medication labels or do self-care. It should be determined if the adult needs audio materials or enlarged print. Hearing is evaluated in both ears for hearing deficits and high- and low-frequency hearing loss as well as waxy buildup in the ear canals.

Assessing Current and Historical Functional Abilities

Functional abilities should be assessed while the adult is engaged in active behaviors. The adult should be asked to demonstrate the ability to sit, stand, get on and off of the toilet, walk, bend down, listen, read, answer questions, and remove shoes, shirt, or jacket and put them on again. Ideally, this should be in the home environment, but this is not always possible. Careful questioning by the nurse about distances and type of facilities in the home environment can help with approximating the type of activities required. The adult being assessed can walk up and down a hallway, for example, to approximate walking from the car to the front door. A careful history of functional ability can pinpoint the timing of any changes. Again, specific questioning should be used. For example, the nurse could ask, "When did you begin to use a cane?" or "How old were you when you stopped using the tub?"

Initial Nutritional Assessment

Nutritional assessment should be done within the first 24 hours of care for hospitalized patients and at first visit for others to ensure that nutritional requirements are met. The history and physical exam should include the following information about the previous 3 months:

- Changes in food intake, including number of meals eaten daily
- Weight loss (or gain)

- Episodes of depression or stress that may relate to dietary intake
- A sample of a usual daily menu should be developed.

Additional screening should include the following:

- Daily number of protein, fruit, grain, and vegetable servings
- Usual fluid intake, including type, amount, and frequency
- Method of feeding, independent or assisted
- Mobility
- Mental status
- Body Mass Index (BMI), midarm circumference, and calf circumference
- Living status (independent or dependent)
- Prescription and non-prescription drugs
- Pressure sores or other wounds or skin problems

Physical Assessment for Nutrition Deficits

The **physical assessment** is an important part of nutritional assessment to determine malnutrition or problems with self-feeding:

- *Hair* may be dry and brittle or thinning.
- *Skin* may show poor turgor, ecchymosis, tears, pressure areas, ulcerations, abrasions, or other compromises.
- *Mouth* may show dry mucous membranes. Lips may have cheilosis, cracking at the corners, and scaly lips (riboflavin deficiency). Gums may be swollen or bleeding, teeth loose or needing care, or dentures poorly fitting. Tongue may be inflamed, dry, cracked, or have sores.
- *Nails* may become brittle. Spoon shaped or pale nail bed indicates low iron.
- *Hands* may be crippled or arthritic, making eating difficult.
- *Vision* may be compromised so that people can't see to prepare food or have difficulty feeding them.
- *Mental status* may be impaired to the point that people can't understand diet instructions or prepare or eat meals.
- *Motor skills* may decrease, including hand-mouth coordination or ability to hold utensils.

Body Mass Index

The **Body Mass Index (BMI)** formula is a measurement that uses height and weight as an indicator of obesity/malnutrition. This cannot be used alone to diagnose obesity because body types differ. Women often have more body fat than men. Tables are available to make calculations simple, but the BMI can be calculated manually using either metric or English units:

$$BMI = \frac{Weight\ in\ kilograms}{(Height\ in\ meters)^2} = \frac{(Weight\ in\ pounds) \times 703}{(Height\ in\ inches)^2}$$

Resulting scores for adults age 20 and over are interpreted according to this chart:

- Below 18.5: Underweight.
- 18.5-24.9: Normal weight.
- 25.0-29.9: Overweight.
- 30 and above: Obese.

MNA®, Nutritional Screening Initiative ®, and Subjective Global Assessment®

The MNA® (Mini-Nutritional Assessment) by Nestle Nutrition is designed for nutritional assessment of those over age 65 and is only valid for that population. It is a screening and assessment tool to determine the risk for malnutrition and comprises 15 questions about dietary habits and 4 measurements, including Body Mass Index (BMI) using height and weight, mid-arm and calf circumference.

The Nutritional Screening Initiative® is another tool for geriatric patients and screens for dietary information as well as social and environmental factors, such as whether the person eats alone, prepares meals, drinks alcohol, and has sufficient income.

The Subjective Global Assessment® assesses nutritional status by a thorough history and physical examination. The history assesses weight change, dietary intake, gastro-intestinal symptoms and functional impairment. The results of this assessment tool are evaluated subjectively, and scores are assigned to determine if malnutrition risks are normal to severe.

In-Depth Cultural Needs Assessment

An **in-depth cultural assessment** should provide information about a patient's language and cultural experiences in order to provide more culturally-sensitive care. The interviewer should remain flexible and consider that the person may not be willing to share sensitive information at the initial interview. Areas covered in the assessment should include:

- *Language*: preference, language spoken in the home and with friends; *Immigration status*: country of origin, entry into US, reasons for immigration
- *Ethnic/cultural background*: personal description of ethnicity/culture; *Spiritual beliefs and/or practices*: religion or spiritual beliefs, rituals, healing and healers
- *Role of family*: definition of family, family system (patriarchal, matriarchal, equal, homosexual)
- *Trauma and/or discrimination*: treatment, intolerance, acts of discrimination, natural disasters, human disasters, and loss, including deaths
- *Social networks*: friends or family, community organizations, activities
- *Understanding of health problem*: general health literacy and medication use
- *Perception of barriers*: personal, systemic, and cultural
- *Socioeconomic concerns*: food, finances, healthcare, entertainment, hobbies, and vacations

Age/System Specific Assessment for Older Adults

Considerations in **age/system specific inspection** of older adults include the following:

- **Positioning** is an issue for many older adults who may have limited range of motion and/or difficulty sitting or lying in certain positions based on their individual physical limitations. Positioning must be adjusted accordingly to the position most comfortable for the patients, and changes of positions should be minimized.
- **Sensory impairment** (e.g., decreased vision, hearing, and sense of touch) should be assessed early and if deficits are known, accommodations made available. If the patient wears a hearing aid, the nurse should request that the patient wear it during the exam. The room should be quiet and free of distraction.
- **Extremities** should be examined using modified movements that are not overly vigorous, such as pushing a limb into flexion or extension. The nurse should avoid having patients hop on one foot or do deep bends because of decreased ROM, reflexes, and balance and should always provide support of the limbs during inspection.

- **Thermoregulation** is altered in adults, who are less tolerant of temperature changes so the patient should be kept warm and comfortable during an exam.
- **Skin** is often friable and bruises easily, so it should be handled with care, avoiding excessive palpation. The skin should be examined for lesions or indications of pressure. The skin of older adults often has benign lesions, including acrochordons (skin tags), actinic keratoses, cherry hemangiomas, dermatofibromas, lentigines (liver spots), nevi (moles), sebaceous hyperplasia, and seborrheic keratoses. Some of these (such as actinic keratoses) are pre-cancerous and should be examined carefully as they may become squamous cell or basal cell carcinoma. Malignant melanoma can occur at any age, and lesions most commonly occur on the torso, head, and neck of males and legs of females.
- **Chest** inspection may need to be adapted because patients often have decreased respiratory force and cough reflex and may have shortness of breath. Inspection may take longer in order to allow the patient to rest between deep breaths.
- **Abdominal** inspection should be done carefully. Older adults may have decreased sensation of pain on deep palpation. There is less cushioning for the liver, so the liver edges should be palpated gently to prevent damage to the tissue.
- **Genitalia** should be examined, but older adults may be very sensitive, so the nurse should explain the need for the exam. Older women often have vaginal atrophy with decreased lubrication, so the speculum should be of a smaller size and well lubricated. Perianal pruritus is common with older adults, but they are often embarrassed to talk about it, so the nurse should ask if there is any itching.
- Changes in the **genitourinary system related to aging** include the following:
    - *Renal dysfunction:* 30-40% of functional nephrons are lost, decreasing kidney size and resulting in decreased ability to concentrate urine. The filtration rate decreases, making processing of excess fluids difficult. Excess potassium may be secreted, leading to dehydration.
    - *Neurological degeneration:* Breaks in neural pathways interfere with messages sent to and from the brain so that sensations, such as a full bladder, may take longer to be perceived. The incomplete nerve pathways may result in bladder spasms from contractions of the detrusor muscle.
    - *Muscular atrophy:* Bladder and sphincter muscles lose tone, resulting in shrinkage of the muscles and less effective ability to contract and relax, resulting in more frequent urination and incontinence. Pelvic floor and sphincter muscles may atrophy, resulting in incontinence.
    - *Mechanical obstruction:* An enlarged prostate or prolapse of the uterus or bladder can create an obstruction that interferes with the ability to urinate.
    - *Nocturnal urine production* increases, and this may result in nocturia and enuresis.

PHYSICAL DISABILITIES

VISUAL IMPAIRMENT

Visual impairment is unrelated to intelligence or hearing, so the nurse should speak with age-appropriate vocabulary in a normal tone of voice, facing the patient so the nurse can observe facial expression. Depending on the degree of visual impairment, the patient may not be able to see gestures or materials; so alternate forms of materials (Braille handouts or enlarged text) or manipulatives must be considered. The field of vision may be impaired so that the patient sees shapes or has better vision in some areas than others, and the nurse should try to position herself/himself for the patient's advantage. The nurse should also announce his/her presence, explain actions and movement ("I'm putting your dressing supplies in the drawer."), announce position ("I'm at your right side."), and always tell the patient if the nurse is going to touch him/her ("I'm going to draw blood from your right arm").

Hearing Impairment/Deafness

Hearing impaired patients may have some hearing and may use hearing aids while **deaf** patients typically have little or no hearing. Some patients are able to use lip reading to various degrees, so the nurse should always face the patient (at 3-6 feet) and speak slowly and clearly, using gestures (not excessively) to augment speech:

- *Hearing impaired:* Assistive devices (e.g., hearing aids and writing materials) should be available and used during communication. Use a normal tone of voice and speak in short sentences. Minimize environmental noises.
- *Deaf*: If patients are deaf, sign language interpreters should be used for important communication (face the patient, not the interpreter). Assistive devices, such as writing materials, TDD phone/relay service, should be available for use. Always announce your presence on entering a room by waving, clapping, tapping the foot (whatever works best for the patient). Ensure alarms have visual feedback (lights). Do not chew, smoke, or eat while speaking to the patient.

Cognitive Impairment

Assessing patients with **cognitive impairment** can be challenging, and patients may have very different and individual responses, so observation of the patient must serve as a guide. Patients may be apprehensive and frightened, so the nurse should maintain a friendly normal tone of voice and should speak with the patient often to establish rapport even if the response is not clear. The nurse should always ask the patient before touching his/her things. Initiating communication by talking about familiar things (e.g., family, pictures, and the past) may be comforting for the patient. If responses are unclear or inappropriate, the nurse can say, "I didn't understand that" but should not laugh or indicate frustration. The nurse should face the patient and maintain eye contact to help the patient stay focused. Patients may get up and move away or go for a walk, and the nurse should not try to restrain the patient but should ask if he/she can walk with the person.

Problem-Focused Assessment

Problem-Based Assessment

Adults often present with a myriad of health problems, so a **problem-based assessment**, focusing on finding a solution to particular problems can be effective. Problem-based assessment requires a thorough history, including questioning family and caregivers when appropriate, to create a problem list. This approach does not preclude a complete exam, which might identify problems that the patient has neglected, but the focus remains on the problem list generated. The list should be prioritized to ensure that the most critical issues (blood in the stool) are thoroughly assessed before less critical issues (occasional insomnia). Once a problem is identified, then differential diagnoses are determined. With older adults and some younger adults, there may be a combination of physical and psychosocial elements to a problem. For example, urinary problems may relate to dehydration, lack of mobility, poor hygiene, medications, or disease. Appropriate diagnostic tests, further assessments, and interventions are completed as needed to diagnose and resolve problems.

Pain Assessment in Advanced Dementia Scale

Patients with cognitive impairment or an inability to verbalize pain may not be able to indicate the degree of pain, even by using a face scale with pictures of smiling to crying faces. The **Pain**

Assessment in Advanced Dementia (PAINAD) scale may be helpful. Careful observation of non-verbal behavior can indicate that the patient is in pain:

- *Respirations*: Patients often have more rapid and labored breathing as pain increases with short periods of hyperventilation or Cheyne-Stokes respirations.
- *Vocalization*: Patients may remain negative in speech or speak quietly and reluctantly. They may moan or groan. As pain increases, they may call out, moan or groan loudly, or cry.
- *Facial expression:* Patients may appear sad or frightened and may frown or grimace, especially on activities that increase pain.
- *Body language:* Patients may be tense and fidget or pace. As pain increases, they may become rigid, clench their fists, or lie in the fetal position. They may become increasingly combative.
- *Consolability*: Patients are less distractible or consolable with increased pain.

Assessment of Alzheimer's Disease

There are a number of methods for **staging Alzheimer's disease.** Staging is done by a combination of physical exam, history (often provided by family or caregivers), and mental assessment as there is no definitive test for Alzheimer's. The 7-stage classification system (developed by Gary Reisberg, MD) is used by the Alzheimer's Association:

Stage 1	This is pre-clinical with no evident impairment, although slight changes may be occurring within the brain.
Stage 2	This involves very mild cognitive decline with some misplacing of items and forgetting things or words, but impairment is not usually noticeable to others or found on medical examination.
Stage 3	This involves mild, early-stage cognitive decline with short-term memory loss, problems with reading retention, remembering names, handling money, planning, and organizing. The individual may misplace items of value.
Stage 4	This involves moderate cognitive decline with decreased knowledge of current affairs or family history, difficulty doing complex tasks, and social withdrawal. This stage is more easily recognized on exam and may persist for 2-10 years, during which the patients may be able to manage most activities of daily living and hygiene.
Stage 5	This involves moderately-severe cognitive decline as the cerebral cortex and hippocampus shrink and the ventricles enlarge. Patients are obviously confused and disoriented to date, time, and place. Patients may have difficulty using/understanding speech and managing activities of daily living. They may forget address and telephone number. They may dress inappropriately, forget to eat and lose weight, or eat a poor diet. They may be unable to do simple math, such as counting backward by 2s.
Stage 6	This involves moderately severe cognitive decline as the brain continues to shrink and neurons die. Patients are profoundly confused and unable to care for themselves and may undergo profound personality changes. They may confuse fiction and reality. They may fail to recognize family members, experience difficulty toileting, and begin to pace obsessively or wander away. Sundowner's syndrome, in which the person has disruption of waking/sleeping cycles and tends to get restless and wander about at night, is common. Patients may develop obsessive behaviors, such as tearing items, pulling at the hair, or wringing hands. This stage (with stage 7) may be prolonged, lasting 1-5 years.

Stage 7	This involves very severe cognitive decline during which most patients are wheelchair bound or bedbound. Most patients lose the ability to speak beyond a few words. They are incontinent (urine and feces) and may be unable to sit unsupported or hold their head up. They choke easily and have increased weakness and rigidity of muscles.

MMSE and Mini-Cog

Patients with evidence of dementia or short-term memory loss, often associated with Alzheimer's disease, should have their cognition assessed. The **Mini-mental state exam (MMSE)** or the **Mini-cog test** is commonly used. Both require the patient to carry out specified tasks.

The **MMSE** consists of the following:

- Remembering and later repeating the names of 3 common objects.
- Counting backward from 100 by 7s or spelling "world" backward.
- Naming items as the examiner points to them.
- Providing the location of the examiner's office, including city, state, and street address.
- Repeating common phrases.
- Copying a picture of interlocking shapes.
- Following simple 3-part instructions, such a picking up a piece of paper, folding it in half, and placing it on the floor.

The **Mini-cog** consists of the following:

- Remembering and later repeating the names of 3 common objects.
- Drawing the face of a clock with all 12 numbers and the hands indicating the time specified by the examiner.

Trail Making Test

The **Trail Making Test** (Parts A and B) assesses brain function and indicates increasing dementia. It is useful for detecting early Alzheimer's disease, and those who do poorly on part B often need assistance with ADLs. The patient is given a demonstration of each part before beginning:

- **Part A** has 25 sequentially-numbered scattered circles across the page, and the patient is advised to use a pencil/pen to draw a continuous line to connect in ascending order the circles (starting with 1 and ending with 25).
- **Part B** is slightly more complex and has circles with numbers (1 to 12) and circles with letters (A to L) scattered about the page. The patient is advised to draw a continuous line alternating between numbers and letters in ascending order (1-A-2-B....).

The test is scored according to the number of seconds required for completion:

- A: 29 seconds is average, and >78 indicates deficiency.
- B: 75 seconds is average and >273 seconds indicates deficiency.

Digit Repetition Test and Time and Change Test

The **Digit Repetition Test** is used to assess attention. The patient is told to listen to numbers and then repeat them. The nurse starts with two random single-digit numbers. If the patient gets this sequence correct, the nurse then states 3 numbers and continues to add one number each time until the patient is unable to repeat the numbers correctly. People with normal intelligence (without intellectual disability or expressive aphasia) can usually repeat 5 to 7 numbers, so scores ≤ 5 indicate impaired attention.

The **Time and Change Test** assesses dementia in adults and is effective in diverse populations. Patients are shown a clock face set at 11:10 and have 1 minute to make 2 attempts at stating the correct time. The patient is then given change (7 dimes, 7 nickels, and 3 quarters) and asked to give the nurse $1.00 from the coins. The patient has 2 minutes and 2 tries to make the correct change. Failing either or both tests is indicative of dementia.

Confusion Assessment Method

The **Confusion Assessment Method** is used to assess the development of delirium and is intended for use by those without psychiatric training. The tool covers nine factors. Some factors have a range of possibilities, and others are rated only as to whether the characteristic is present, not present, uncertain, or not applicable. The tool provides room to describe abnormal behavior. Factors assessed include onset, attention, thinking, level of consciousness, orientation, memory, perceptual disturbances, psychomotor abnormalities, and the sleep-wake cycle. Delirium is indicated if there is an acute onset with fluctuating attention, disorganized thinking, or altered consciousness.

- **Onset**: Acute change in mental status
- **Attention**: Inattentive, stable, or fluctuating
- **Thinking**: Disorganized, rambling conversation, switching topics, illogical
- **Level of consciousness**: Altered, ranging from alert to coma
- **Orientation**: Disoriented (person, place, time)
- **Memory**: Impaired
- **Perceptual disturbances**: Hallucinations, illusions
- **Psychomotor abnormalities**: Agitation (tapping, picking, moving) or retardation (staring, not moving)
- **Sleep-wake cycle**: Awake at night and sleepy in the daytime.

Abnormal Involuntary Movement Scale

The **Abnormal Involuntary Movement Scale (AIMS)** is a tool used to evaluate patients for tardive dyskinesia. *Tardive dyskinesia* is a movement disorder caused by some antipsychotic medications. Before or after the formal examination, the patient is observed at rest (as in the waiting area) for comparison. The examination procedure includes having the patient perform a number of activities, such as sitting in specific positions, opening his or her mouth, sticking out his or her tongue, standing, and walking while the nurse rates a number of movements on a scale of 0 (none) to 4 (severe). The severity of facial and oral movements, extremity movements, and trunk movements is rated. A score of 2 or higher in two or more movements or a score greater than 3 in one movement is positive for tardive dyskinesia. The overall severity is then assessed (based on the above scores), including patient's degree of incapacitation and patient's awareness of abnormal movements. The last part of the exam asks about dental status.

Barthel Index of ADLs

The **Barthel Index of Activities of Daily Living** is a tool to assess the functional ability of older adults. It is used to assess the person's disabilities and need for assistance. There are 10 categories that are scored from 0 to 10-15 (100-point scale) or 0 to 1-3 (20-point scale) with scores indicating complete dependence, need for assistance, or complete independence. Higher scores indicate independence. This scale is sometimes modified by institutions, so it may vary somewhat. The 10 categories usually include the following:

- Feeding (includes need to cut food)
- Mobility
- Personal grooming
- Toileting (getting on and off of toilet, wiping, and managing clothes)
- Urinary control
- Fecal control
- Ascending and descending stairs
- Ambulatory status on level ground (or if wheelchair bound, the ability to propel the wheelchair)
- Transferring, sitting up in bed
- Bathing

Index of Independence of Activities of Daily Living and Palliative Performance Scale

The **Index of Independence of Activities of Daily Living (Katz Index)** tool is a checklist that does not use scores, but the person is evaluated in 6 areas (bathing, dressing, toileting, transfer, continence, and feeding) to provide an assessment of the person's need for assistance and progression of disease and/or disability.

The **Palliative Performance Scale** assesses the functional ability of older adults receiving palliative care. Categories are assessed by percentage of ability 0% (death) to 100% with lower percentages indicative of functional impairment. The scores are used as a guide to determine probable life expectancy with 60-100% at 108 days, 30-50%, 41 days, and 10-20%, 6 days, although survival rates have been primarily correlated with cancer rather than other terminal illness. Categories include the following:

- Ability to ambulate
- Activity level and evidence of disease
- Self-care
- Intake
- Level of consciousness

IADL

Instrumental Activities of Daily Living (IADL) is an assessment tool to measure 8 activities necessary for an adult to function independently. This tool helps to determine the need for supportive services. Scores are assigned as 0 (cannot do independently) or 1 (minimal or adequate degree of ability), so the total score ranges from 0 to 8 with a higher score indicating more independence in care. Abilities that are measured include the following:

- Telephone use (Ability to look up numbers and/or call numbers).
- Shopping for food, clothes, or needed items
- Food preparation (Plans diet and prepares food)
- Housekeeping (Ability to perform all or part of household duties
- Laundry (Can wash all or some of personal clothes and linen)
- Transportation availability (Ability to drive or use public transportation)
- Medication (Ability to be responsible for managing prescriptions and taking medications)
- Financial responsibility (Ability to keep track of finances, pay bills, and budget correctly)

Braden Scale

The **Braden scale** is used to assess a patient's risk of developing pressure sores. The scale has been clinically validated and is widely used. The scale rates six different areas on a scale of 1 to 4. The subscores from all areas are added together to create a total score. The patient's risk of developing pressure sores is determined by the total score. The best (and highest) score is 23. Lower ratings indicate a higher risk of developing pressure sores. If the patient has a score of 16 or lower, prevention protocols should be initiated. The worst score obtainable is 6: This patient has a very strong possibility of developing pressure sores.

The first four assessment areas of the **Braden scale** are sensory perception, moisture, activity, and mobility. Patients are rated on a scale of 1 to 4:

- **Sensory perception**
    - Completely limited (unresponsive to pain or has limited ability to feel)
    - Very limited (responds to painful stimuli and moans)
    - Slightly limited (responds to verbal commands but has limited communication)
    - No impairment
- **Moisture**
    - Moist constantly
    - Very moist (linen change required each shift)
    - Occasionally moist (linen change required each day)
    - Rarely moist
- **Activity**
    - Bed bound
    - Chair bound
    - Walks occasionally (short distances)
    - Walks frequently
- **Mobility**
    - Completely immobile
    - Very limited (makes occasional slight position changes)
    - Slightly limited (makes frequent slight position changes)
    - No limitations

The last two areas assessed by the **Braden scale** are usual nutrition pattern and friction and shear. Patients are rated on a scale of 1 to 4:

- **Usual nutrition pattern**
    - Very poor (eats less than half of meals, inadequate protein intake, and inadequate hydration)
    - Inadequate (eats about half of food with three protein serving or not enough liquid or
    - tube feeding)
    - Adequate (eats less than half of meals and four protein servings)
    - Excellent
- **Friction and shear** (three parameters only)
    - Problem moving (skin frequently slides down the sheets, needs help to move)
    - Potential problem (moves weakly or needs some assistance, skin slides somewhat during moves)
    - No apparent problem

Norton Scale

The **Norton scale** assesses risk for pressure ulcers based on scores in five categories. Each category is rated on a scale from 1 to 4. The scores for all categories are added together. A higher number indicates higher risk. A score of 14 or greater indicates that the patient is at high risk. The scale is used for periodic assessment (on a daily or weekly basis) so that patients at risk can be identified quickly and interventions instituted.

Condition	1	2	3	4
Physical	Good	Fair	Poor	Very poor
Mental	Alert/ responsive	Apathetic	Confused	Stuporous
Activity	Ambulatory	Walks with help	Nonambulatory/ chair bound	Bedridden
Mobility	Full mobility	Slightly limited	Very limited	Immobile
Incontinence	None	Occasionally	Urinary incontinence	Fecal and urinary incontinence

Geriatric Depression Scale

The **Geriatric Depression Scale (GDS)** is a self-assessment tool to identify older adults with depression. The test can be used with those with normal cognition and those with mild to moderate impairment. The test poses 15 questions to which patients answer "yes" or "no." A score of more than five depressively tended answers is indicative of depression:

- Are you basically satisfied with your life?
- Have you dropped many of your activities and interests?
- Do you feel your life is empty?
- Do you often get bored?
- Are you in good spirits most of the time?
- Are you afraid that something bad is going to happen to you?
- Do you feel happy most of the time?
- Do you often feel helpless?
- Do you prefer to stay at home rather than going out and doing new things?
- Do you feel you have more problems with memory than most?
- Do you think it is wonderful to be alive now?
- Do you feel pretty worthless the way you are now?
- Do you feel full of energy?
- Do you feel that your situation is hopeless?
- Do you think that most people are better off than you are?

CAGE Tool

The **CAGE** tool is used as a quick assessment tool to determine if people are drinking excessively or are problem drinkers. Moderate drinking, (2 drinks per day for adult males and 1 drink a day for females and older adults), unless contraindicated by health concerns, is usually not harmful to people, but drinking more than that can lead to serious psychosocial and physical problems. One drink is defined as 12 ounces of beer/wine cooler, 5 ounces of wine, or 1.5 ounces of liquor.

C	Cutting down	Do you think about trying to cut down on drinking?
A	Annoyed at criticism	Are people starting to criticize your drinking?
G	Guilty feeling	Do you feel guilty or try to hide your drinking?
E	Eye opener	Do you increasingly need a drink earlier in the day?

"Yes" on one question suggests the possibility of a drinking problem while "yes" on two or more indicates a drinking problem, and the patient should be provided information about reducing drinking and appropriate referrals made.

Diagnostic Testing

LABORATORY TESTING FOR NUTRITIONAL ASSESSMENT

Laboratory testing for **nutritional assessment** includes:

- **Total protein: Normal values: 5-9g/kL.** The dietary requirement for wound healing is 1.25-1.5 g/kg per day.
- **Albumin**:
  - Normal values: 3.5-5.5 g/dL
  - Mild deficiency: 3-3.5 g/dL
  - Moderate deficiency: 2.5-3.0 g/dL
  - Severe deficiency: <2.5 g/dL.

  Levels below 3.2 correlate with increased morbidity and death. Dehydration (poor intake, diarrhea, or vomiting) elevates levels, so adequate hydration is important to ensure meaningful results.

- **Prealbumin**:
  - Normal values: 3.5-5.5 g/dL
  - Mild deficiency: 3-3.5 g/dL
  - Moderate deficiency: 2.5-3.0 g/dL
  - Severe deficiency: <2.5 g/dL.

  Prealbumin is a good measurement because it quickly decreases when nutrition is inadequate and rises quickly in response to increased protein intake. Protein intake must be adequate to maintain levels of prealbumin.

- **Transferrin:**
  - Normal values: 200-400 mg/dL.
  - Mild deficiency: 150-200 mg/dL.
  - Moderate deficiency: 100-150 mg/dL.
  - Severe deficiency: <100 mg/dL.

  Transferrin levels alone are not always reliable measurements of nutritional status as they may vary with other disorders.

ABGs

Arterial blood gases (ABGs) are monitored to assess effectiveness of oxygenation, ventilation, and acid-base status, and to determine oxygen flow rates. Partial pressure of a gas is that exerted by each gas in a mixture of gases, proportional to its concentration, based on total atmospheric pressure of 760 mm Hg at sea level. Normal values include:

- Acidity/alkalinity (pH): 7.35-7.45.
- Partial pressure of carbon dioxide ($PaCO_2$): 35-45 mm Hg.
- Partial pressure of oxygen (PaO_2): ≥80 mg Hg.
- Bicarbonate concentration (HCO_3-): 22-26 mEq/L.
- Oxygen saturation (SaO_2): ≥95%.

The relationship between these elements, particularly the $PaCO_2$ and the PaO_2 indicates respiratory status. For example, $PaCO_2$ >55 and the PaO_2 <60 in a patient previously in good health indicates respiratory failure. There are many issues to consider. Ventilator management may require a higher $PaCO_2$ to prevent barotrauma and a lower PaO_2 to reduce oxygen toxicity.

Review Video: Blood Gases
Visit mometrix.com/academy and enter code: 611909

Red Blood Cell Values and Morphology

Red blood cells (RBCs or erythrocytes) are biconcave disks that contain hemoglobin (95% of mass), which carries oxygen throughout the body. The heme portion of the cell contains iron, which binds to the oxygen. RBCs live about 120 days after which they are destroyed and their hemoglobin is recycled or excreted. Normal values of red blood cell count vary by gender:

- Males >18 years: 4.5-5.5 million per mm^3.
- Females >18 years: 4.0-5.0 million per mm^3.

The most common disorders of RBCs are those that interfere with production, leading to various types of anemia:

- Blood loss
- Hemolysis
- Bone marrow failure

The morphology of RBCs may vary depending upon the type of anemia:

- Size: Normocytes, microcytes, macrocytes.
- Shape: Spherocytes (round), poikilocytes (irregular), drepanocytes (sickled).
- Color (reflecting concentration of hemoglobin: Normochromic, hypochromic.

Laboratory Tests

Various laboratory tests are listed and described below:

- **Hemoglobin:** Carries oxygen and is decreased in anemia and increased n polycythemia. Normal values:
    - Males >18 years: 14.0-17.46 g/dl.
    - Females >18 years: 12.0-16.0 g/dl.

- **Hematocrit:** Indicates the proportion of RBCs in a liter of blood (usually about 3 times the hemoglobin number). Normal values:
  - Males >18 years: 45-52%.
  - Females >18 years: 36-48%
- **Mean corpuscular volume (MCV):** Indicates the size of RBCs and can differentiate types of anemia. For adults, <80 is microcytic and >100 is macrocytic. Normal values:
  - Males > 18 years: 84-96 μm^3.
  - Females >18 years: 76-96 μm^3.
- **Reticulocyte count:** Measures marrow production and should rise with anemia. Normal values:
  - 0.5-1.5% of total RBCs.
- **C-reactive protein:** Increases with inflammation in the body.
  - Normal values: 2.6-7.6 μg/dL.
- **Erythrocyte sedimentation rate (sed rate):** a non-specific test that decreases with inflammation. Values vary according to gender and age:
  - <50: Males 0-15 mm/hr. Females 0-20 mm/hr.
  - >50: Males 0-20 mm/hr. Females 0-30 mm/hr.

WBC Count and Differential

White blood cell (leukocyte) count is used as an indicator of bacterial and viral infection. WBC is reported as the total number of all white blood cells. Normal WBC for adults: 4,800-10,000. Acute infection: 10,000+, 30,000 indicate a severe infection. Viral infection: 4,000 and below. **The differential** provides the percentage of each different type of leukocyte. An increase in the white blood cell count is usually related to an increase in one type and often an increase in immature neutrophils, known as bands, referred to as a "shift to the left", an indication of an infectious process:

- **Immature neutrophils (bands):**1-3%: Increase with infection.
- **Segmented neutrophils (segs):**50-62%: Increase with acute, localized, or systemic bacterial infections.
- **Eosinophils:** 0-3%: Decrease with stress and acute infection.
- **Basophils:** 0-1%: Decrease during acute stage of infection.
- **Lymphocytes:** 25-40%: Increase in some viral and bacterial infections.
- **Monocytes:** 3-7%: Increase during recovery stage of acute infection.

Coagulation Profile

The elements of the coagulation profile are as follows:

- **Prothrombin time (PT)**
  - Normal = 10-14 seconds.
  - Increases with anticoagulation therapy, vitamin K deficiency, ↓prothrombin, DIC, liver disease, and malignant neoplasm.
- **Partial thromboplastin time (PTT)**
  - Normal = 30-45 seconds.
  - Increases with hemophilia A & B, von Willebrand's, vitamin deficiency, lupus, DIC, and liver disease.

- **Activated partial thromboplastin time (aPTT*)***
  - Normal = 21-35 seconds
  - Similar to PTT, but decreases in extensive cancer, early DIC and after acute hemorrhage. Monitors heparin dosage.
- **Thrombin clotting time (TCT) or Thrombin time (TT)**
  - Normal = 7-12 seconds (<21)
  - Used most often to determine dosage of heparin. Prolonged with multiple myeloma, abnormal fibrinogen, uremia, and liver disease.
- **Bleeding time**
  - Normal = 2-9.5 minutes (Ivy method on the forearm).
  - Increases with DIC, leukemia, renal failure, aplastic anemia, von Willebrand's, some drugs, and alcohol.
- **Platelet count**
  - Normal = 150,000-400,000 per microliter.
  - Increased bleeding <50,000 and increased clotting >750,000.

Liver Function Studies

Liver function studies consist of the following:

- **Bilirubin** – Shows the liver's ability to conjugate/excrete bilirubin:
  - Direct 0.0-0.3 mg/dL,
  - Total 0.0-0.9 mg/dL,
  - Urine bilirubin 0.
- **Total protein** – Shows if the liver is producing normal protein levels:
  - Total Protein7.0-7.5 g/dL:
  - Albumin: 4.0-5.5 g/dL.
  - Globulin: 1.7=3.3 g/dL.
  - Albumin/globulin (A/G) ratio: 1.5:1 to 2.5:1
- **Alkaline phosphatase** – Indicates biliary tract obstruction (in absence of bone disease)
  - Alkaline phosphatase: 17-142 adults (varies with method)
- **AST (SGOT)/ ALT (SGPT)** – Increase in liver cell damage.
  - AST: 10-40 units
  - ALT 5-35 units.
- **Serum ammonia** – Increases in liver failure.
  - Ammonia: 150-250 mg/dL

*Will also see increase/abnormalities in lipids, cholesterol and clotting labs.

Renal Function Studies

Renal function studies include the following:

- **Specific gravity**:1.015-1.025: Determines kidney's ability to concentrate urinary solutes.
- **Osmolality (urine)**:350-900 mOsm/kg/24 hr: Shows early changes when kidney has difficulty concentrating urine.
- **Osmolality (serum)**:275-295 mOsm/kg: Gives a picture of the number of solutes in the blood.

- **Uric acid**:3.0-7.2 mg/dL: Increase with renal failure.
- **Creatinine clearance (24-hour)**:75 to 125 mL/min.: Evaluates the amount of blood cleared of creatinine in 1 min. Approximates the GFR.
- **Serum creatinine**:0.6-1.2mg/dL: Increase with decreased renal fx, urinary tract obstruction, and nephritis.
- **Urine creatinine**:11-26 mg/kg/24 hr: Product of muscle breakdown. Increase with decreased renal fx.
- **Blood urea nitrogen (BUN)**:7-8 mg/dL (8-20 mg/dL >age 60): Increase indicates impaired renal function, as urea is end product of protein metabolism.
- **BUN/creatinine ratio**: 10:1: Increases with hypovolemia. With intrinsic kidney disease, the ratio is normal though increased BUN/Creatinine.

Urinalysis

The elements measured in a urinalysis are as follows:

- **Color**: Urine is usually pale yellow/amber. Urine darkens when it is concentrated or when other substances are present.
- **Appearance**: Urine is usually clear but may be slightly cloudy.
- **Odor**: The odor should be slight. Bacteria may impart a foul smell.
- **Specific gravity**: The specific gravity of urine is between 1.015 and 1.025 but may increase if protein levels increase or if there is fever, vomiting, or dehydration.
- **pH**: The pH of urine usually ranges from 4.5 to 8 (average 5-6).
- **Sediment**: Urine may contain red cell casts from acute infections, broad casts from kidney disorders, and white cell casts from pyelonephritis. Leukocytes at a concentration of greater than 10 per ml^3 are present in the case of urinary tract infection.
- **Glucose, ketones, protein, blood, bilirubin, and nitrates**: These values should all be negative. Urine glucose may increase with infection. Frank blood may be caused by some parasites and diseases but also by some drugs, smoking, excessive exercise, and menstrual fluids. Increased red blood cells may result from lower urinary tract infections.
- **Urobilinogen**: Values of urobilinogen range from 0.1 to 1.0 units.

Glucose and Hemoglobin A1c

Glucose is manufactured by the liver from ingested carbohydrates and is stored as glycogen for use by the cells. If glucose intake is inadequate, glucose can be produced by the breakdown of muscle and fat tissue. This can lead to increased wasting. High levels of glucose are indicative of diabetes mellitus. Fasting blood glucose levels are used to diagnose and monitor glucose levels:

- Normal values: 70-99 mg/dL
- Impaired: 100-125 mg/dL
- Diabetes: >126 mg/dL

A number of different conditions are associated with increased glucose levels: stress, renal failure, Cushing's syndrome, hyperthyroidism, and pancreatic disorders. Some medications (such as steroids, estrogens, lithium, phenytoin, diuretics, and tricyclic antidepressants) may increase glucose levels. Other conditions (adrenal insufficiency, liver disease, hypothyroidism, and starvation, for example) can decrease glucose levels.

Hemoglobin A1c is composed of hemoglobin A plus a glucose molecule. Hemoglobin holds on to excess blood glucose, so hemoglobin A1c level is used primarily to monitor long-term diabetic therapy. The normal value is less than six percent and a value of greater than seven percent is elevated.

Differential Diagnosis

The **differential diagnosis** involves determining the actual cause of a patient's symptoms when they could be caused by more than one disease or condition. When a patient presents for treatment and has symptoms, the provider must form a differential diagnosis to outline what underlying pathology is causing the symptoms. Forming the differential diagnosis is accomplished through taking the patient's history, performing a physical exam, and ordering tests such as laboratory or radiology measures. The results of these tasks will point to aspects of certain diseases that will narrow down the field of potential causes of the symptoms or even provide an actual diagnosis when other possible pathological etiologies have been eliminated. Forming a differential diagnosis involves critical thinking skills, an ability to interpret data, and recognition of symptoms common to a number of different diseases that could be the cause of the symptoms, as well as an understanding of normal health and wellbeing.

Prioritizing Nursing and/or Differential Diagnoses

One method of **prioritizing nursing and/or differential diagnoses** is to consider consequences if treatment is delayed.

- **High** (life-threatening): acute myocardial infarction
- **Medium** (delay may cause problems): malnutrition
- **Low** (treatment can be delayed safely): chronic osteoarthritis

In many cases, prioritizing can be done by using Maslow's Hierarchy of Needs. Life-threatening needs and safety needs take priority over others, regardless of the prioritization method used.

1	**Physiological** (basic needs to sustain life—oxygen, food, fluids, sleep)	Risk for aspiration Deficient fluid volume Impaired spontaneous ventilation
2	**Safety and security** (physio-logical and psycho-logical threats)	Verbal communication impaired Latex allergy response Death anxiety
3	**Love/belonging** (support, caring, intimacy)	Risk for loneliness Anxiety Caregiver role strain
4	**Self-esteem** (sense of worth, respect, independence)	Defensive coping Disturbed body image Post-trauma response
5	**Self-actualization**	Health-seeking behaviors Spiritual distress

CDSS

Clinical decision support systems (CDSS) are interactive software applications that provide information to physicians or other healthcare providers to help with healthcare decisions. The programs contain a base of medical knowledge to which patient data can be entered so that an evidence-based inference system can provide patient specific advice. For example, a CDSS system may be used in the Emergency Department so that staff can enter symptoms into the program and, based on the information entered, the CDSS program provides possible diagnoses and treatment options. The CDSS system may be used for a variety of purposes:

- Record keeping and documentation, such as authorization
- Monitoring of patient's treatments, research protocols, orders, and referrals
- Ensuring cost-effectiveness by monitoring orders to prevent duplication or tests that are not indicated by condition/symptoms
- Providing support in physician diagnosis and ensuring treatments are based on best practices

Atypical Presentations of Disease

Atypical presentations of disease are quite common. In some cases, the first indication of a disease may be a change in appetite, lethargy, or decreased function. Women may present with different symptoms from those of males, and comorbidity with diabetes may affect presentation.

Acute Myocardial Infarction

Clinical manifestations of AMI may vary considerably, with males having the more "classic" symptom of sudden onset of crushing chest pain; older adults, females, and those under 55 often present with atypical symptoms, which can include: Nausea and vomiting; Abdominal or epigastric "burning"; Vague non-radiating chest discomfort; Heavy feeling in arms; Back pain; Fatigue or impaired sleep; Dyspnea; Flushing.

Silent MIs, with no symptoms, are much more common in females than in males. Diabetic patients may have reduced sensation of pain because of neuropathy and may complain primarily of weakness. Elderly patients may also have neuropathic changes that reduce sensation of pain. Dyspnea occurs more commonly than chest pain.

Depression

Patients may lack obvious signs of sadness or depression but present with a variety of somatic complaints, such as poor appetite, abdominal discomfort, constipation, diarrhea, and impaired sleep. They may exhibit hyperactivity and pronounced agitation.

Sepsis

Patients may lack the typical signs of fever and leukocytosis, although a left shift may be evident, but they may present with a change in mental status, poor appetite, dehydration, confusion, and impaired function, which often results in falls. Glucose levels may be abnormal.

Delirium

Instead of the abrupt agitated state common to delirium, some patients may exhibit apathy with less obvious confusion, so the condition may be misdiagnosed as dementia. Additionally, patients with atypical presentations of other diseases may present with signs of delirium, so patients with delirium should be assessed for a hidden disorder.

Nursing Theories

Erik Erikson's Theory of Psychosocial Development

Erik Erikson's theory of psychosocial development describes the development of the personality. According to Erikson, personality develops in eight stages. The first five developmental stages occur in infancy and childhood. The final three stages occur in adulthood. Each stage involves a conflict that must be resolved. Failure to resolve the conflict leads to unhealthy psychosocial development. Resolving the conflict of a particular stage leads to a sense of mastery, while failure to resolve the conflict results in a feeling of inadequacy. Erikson's stages are as follows:

- Trust vs. Mistrust (birth to 1 year)
- Autonomy vs. Shame/Doubt (ages 1 to 3 years)
- Initiative vs. Guilt (3 to 6 years)
- Industry vs. Inferiority (ages 6 to 12)
- Identity vs. Role Confusion (ages 12 to 18)
- Intimacy vs. Isolation (young adulthood)
- Generativity vs. Stagnation (middle age)
- Ego integrity vs. Despair (older adulthood)

Erikson's Theory of Child/Adult Development

Erikson's psychosocial development model covers the life span, focusing on conflicts at each stage and the virtue that is the outcome of finding a balance in the conflict. The first 5 stages relate to infancy and childhood and the last 3 stages to adulthood, but childhood development affects later adult development:

Stage	Ages	Description
Trust vs. Mistrust	Birth to 1 year	Can result in mistrust or faith and optimism
Autonomy vs. shame/doubt	1-3 years	Can lead to doubt and shame or self-control and willpower
Initiative vs. Guilt	3-6 years	Can lead to guilt or direction and purpose
Industry vs. Inferiority	6-12 years	Can lead to inadequacy and inferiority or competence
Identify vs. role confusion	12-18 years	Can lead to role confusion or devotion and fidelity to others
Intimacy vs. Isolation	Young adulthood	Can lead to lack of close relationships or love/intimacy
Generativity vs. Stagnation	Middle age	Can lead to stagnation or caring and achievements
Ego integrity vs. despair	Older adulthood	Can lead to despair (failure to accept changes of aging) or wisdom (acceptance)

Scott Peck's Theory of Development

Scott Peck's theory of development proposed four stages. Progression through these stages takes the individual from selfish child to giving elder. The stages are as follows:

1. Chaotic/Antisocial
2. Formal/Institutional
3. Skeptic/Individual
4. Mystic/Communal

In the first stage, individuals act out of self-interest: they are unprincipled. Babies and children must be taught to act in an ethical and charitable manner. In the second stage, individuals want structure. They seek institutions that provide structure. Conformity is an important trait to people in this stage. Individuals may not progress to the third stage. In stage 3, individuals begin to question the rules and beliefs of the institutions they once followed without question. Individuals who do not progress beyond this stage may become depressed and bitter. In stage 4, the individual develops a genuine spiritual belief rather than just following the rules. Not all individuals reach this stage.

Peck expanded on Erikson's stages of adult development, believing that there were 7 important tasks that were required during the last two stages of life:

Stage	Tasks	Outcomes
Middle age	Valuing wisdom vs. physical powers Socializing vs. sexualizing. Cathectic (libidinal energy) flexibility vs. cathectic impoverishment Mental flexibility vs. mental rigidity	*Negative* outcomes lead to weak relationships, inflexibility, and resistance to change. *Positive* outcomes lead to strong relationships, flexibility in lifestyle, and adaptability to change.
Older adulthood	Ego differentiation vs. work role preoccupation Body transcendence vs. body preoccupation Ego transcendence vs. ego preoccupation	*Negative* outcomes leads to feeling of loss of identity after retirement, depression, inability to accept bodily -functional changes and fear of death. *Positive* outcomes lead to meaningful life after retirement, acceptance of bodily -functional changes, acceptance of death, and feeling that life has been good.

Theories of Aging

Biological

Autoimmunity	The purpose of the immune system is to protect the body against foreign substances. The *autoimmune theory of aging* states that the immune system becomes less capable of producing the antibodies to fight disease over time. In addition, the immune system becomes less capable of distinguishing between antibodies produced by the body and proteins. As a result, the body attacks itself. Autoimmune diseases include lupus, rheumatoid arthritis, multiple sclerosis, and scleroderma.
Free radical	A *free radical* is any molecule that has unpaired electrons. This creates an unbalanced molecule with a negative charge. As a result of the extra electron, the molecule reacts with balanced molecules in an unhealthy and destructive manner. Constant damage by free radicals will kill a cell. *The free-radical theory of aging* proposes that when a large enough number of cells in an organism are killed, aging occurs. Free-radical production in the body can be increased by such things as unhealthy diet, tobacco use, and radiation exposure.
Stress	Selye believed that stress is a response of the body to any demand requiring adaptation (positive or negative). The body's response to stress is characterized as a "generalized adaptation syndrome" with 3 stages: *Alarm*: This involves the physiological "fight or flight" response. *Resistance*: The body mobilizes forces to resist threat, focusing on those organs most involved in response. Chronic resistance can lead to damage of organs/systems. *Exhaustion*: The body is overwhelmed and weakened, and organs/systems begin to deteriorate (hypertrophy of adrenal glands, ulcerations of GI tract, and atrophy of thymus gland), leading to stress-related diseases and death. The body is no longer able to cope with the effects of stress.
Wear and tear	This mechanistic view states the human body is similar to a machine that wears out over time, accounting for such things as degenerative joint disease. Once worn out, the cells and systems cannot repair themselves, and aging occurs. The cells and body systems can no longer function efficiently. This particular theory is no longer widely accepted as an explanation of aging.
Homeostatic	This theory states that the body is composed of various chemical elements that must be maintained in proper balance, and when the body is not able to maintain this homeostatic balance, aging occurs.
Programmed/Cellular	This theory postulates that all cells and organisms have a life span that is predetermined, and aging occurs as the end of the lifespan is approached.
Single organ	Some theories suggest that aging is related to changes in a single organ or system. Burnside postulated that aging is a response to lowered supply of oxygen. Others suggest that the thyroid gland and a change in the rate of metabolism may be responsible for aging.

Somatic mutation	Mutations in the cellular DNA lead to dysfunction and disease associated with aging. Although most mutations can be repaired or destroyed, extensive damage to DNA can cause changes in the sequence of genes. The mutated genes copy themselves, leading to disease and diminished functioning. Mutations can occur because of mistakes in cell division or as a result of exposure to toxins and radiation.

Accumulative Waste and Glycosylation Theories of Aging

The **accumulative waste theory of aging** states that cells accumulate more waste products than they can eliminate. The waste products in the cell can include toxins. When the toxins build to a certain level, the cell dies. Aging results when this process occurs in a critical number of cells.

The **glycosylation theory of aging** states that aging occurs as a result of the binding of glucose (which is a simple sugar) to protein. This process occurs in the presence of oxygen. The binding of glucose to the protein impairs the actions of the protein. The protein is not able to perform its functions efficiently, and aging results.

Exchange, Gerotranscendence, and Life Course Theories of Aging

According to the **exchange theory of aging**, interactions between people are based on the exchange of resources. Because older adults often do not have as many resources as younger people, interactions between younger and older individuals are often limited. This occurs because younger adults do not perceive a benefit from interacting with older adults.

The **gerotranscendence theory of aging**, formulated by Lars Tornstam, states that older adults experience a cognitive transformation as they age. According to this theory, adults tend to be materialistic when they are younger and become more spiritual as they age. With age comes a focus on external matters and improved relationships. An acceptance of death develops.

According to the **life course theory of aging**, aging is a process that involves continuing changes from infancy to old age. Changes occur in social, psychological, and biological functioning.

Abraham Maslow's Hierarchy of Needs

Abraham Maslow studied individuals he referred to as exemplary people in order to develop his hierarchy of needs. Exemplary people included the likes of Albert Einstein and Eleanor Roosevelt. ***Maslow's hierarchy of needs*** forms a pyramid, with the more basic requirements of life on the bottom of the structure. Maslow referred to the needs in the lower four levels as deficiency needs. Deficiency needs must be met first before higher needs can be attended to.

The following are the hierarchy of needs:

- Physiological needs (the base)
- Safety and security
- Belonging
- Self-esteem
- Self-actualization (the apex)

People may not progress in one direction from one need to another but movement may be in multiple directions in a lifelong process of working toward self-actualization, which requires creativity and some degree of freedom. Failure to develop toward self-actualization may result in depression and feelings of failure.

Carl Jung's Theory of Individualism

Carl Jung proposed, in his **theory of individualism**, that personality continues to develop over an individual's lifetime. Personality is composed of ego, personal unconsciousness, and collective unconsciousness. Although an individual can be introverted or extroverted, emotional health requires a balance between the two. Jung believed that people begin to question their accomplishments, values, and beliefs as they reach middle age. After middle age, people begin to turn inward. Jung believed that successful aging occurs when people value themselves more than they value external factors and when they do not become overly concerned about their physical limitations. Jung believed that it is necessary for an aging adult to accept his or her diminishing capacities in order to age successfully. Older adults must also adapt to change and loss.

Social Exchange Theory of Development

Social exchange theory is rooted in the following disciplines: structural anthropology, behavioral psychology, utilitarian economics, sociology, and social psychology. The basic tenet of social exchange theory is that an individual interacts with others in the expectation of profit. Each individual acts in a way to reap rewards and avoid punishment and develops a set of strategies to achieve these goals. Behaviors that produce the desired effect are repeated, while those that produce an unwanted effect are not repeated. This learning begins in infancy and continues throughout life. Behaviors and thought processes are, therefore, the result of interactions with society. People in a society are, in effect, trained by other members of society to behave and think in certain ways. George Caspar Homans, an American sociologist, is considered to be the founder of social exchange theory.

Havighurst's Theory of Adult Development

Havighurst believed that there are a number of tasks that need to be accomplished during each stage of development and that remaining active is important. His adult stages reflect stereotypical roles to some degree related to the 1960s when marrying young was more typical than it is now.

Stage	Tasks
Early adulthood	Tasks include finding a mate, marrying, having and children, managing a home, getting started in an occupation/profession, assuming civic responsibility and finding a congenial social group.
Middle age	Tasks include achieving civic/social responsibility, maintaining an economic standard of living, raising teenagers and teaching them to be responsible adults, developing leisure activity, accepting physiological changes related to aging and adjusting to aging of parents.
Older adulthood	Tasks include adjusting to decrease in physical strength and health, death of spouse, and life in retirement and reduced income. Other tasks include establishing ties with those in the same age group (Senior Citizen's groups/retirees), meeting social and civic obligations, and establishing physical living arrangements that are satisfactory.

Age Stratification Theory of Aging and Continuity Theory of Aging

The **age stratification theory of aging** was developed by Matilda Riley, Marilyn Johnson, and Anne Foner. The theory states that society is divided into age cohorts. The roles of the different cohorts vary, and cohorts differ in status. Individuals in the same age cohort share the same historical context. Individuals born in different eras have had different experiences. For example, individuals who were age 80 in 1950 are not the same as individuals who were age 80 in the year 2000. The events of a particular era affect development, and individuals from the same cohort have shared experiences.

Robert Havighurst, Bernice Neugarten, and Sheldon Tobin postulated that personality type correlates with successful aging. Their **continuity theory of aging** states that individuals will try to maintain the same lifestyle throughout their lives. Older adults will engage in the same activities and behaviors as they did in their youth. Older adults use strategies to maintain continuity.

Activity Theory of Aging and Disengagement Theory of Aging

The **activity theory of aging** states that remaining engaged in life and active has a positive effect on individuals as they age. Older adults can stay active in many ways even if they can't take part in all the activities that they participated in when they were younger. New roles must replace old ones. Staying involved in life has been found to be positively correlate with satisfaction with life.

The **disengagement theory of aging** was developed by Elaine Cumming and William Henry in 1961. The disengagement theory of aging states that to age successfully, an individual should withdraw from society. This disengagement relieves both the aging individual and society from unwanted responsibilities. The withdrawal from society allows the older adult time to reflect and helps keep society functioning smoothly.

Political Economy of Age Theory of Aging

Carroll Estes, James Swan, and Lenore Gerard proposed the **political economy of age theory of aging.** The political and economic requirements of society determine the way older adults are treated. Programs for older adults are designed to serve the needs of society rather than the needs of the older adults.

Role Theory of Aging

The **role theory of aging** was proposed by Irving Rosow. Each person assumes a role in society, which changes with age; each role prepares the individual for the next role. As status is influence by age, role and status may be in conflict. This results in a loss of self-esteem and sense of identity.

Subculture Theory of Aging

Rosow also proposed the **subculture theory of aging**. People in a society form subcultures based on shared interests. Individuals who do not meet inclusion criteria are excluded. Older adults form subcultures based on shared interests and are excluded from the subcultures of younger people. Physical health and mental functioning determine status within the older adult subculture.

Modernization Theory of Aging

Emile Durkheim and Max Weber developed the **modernization theory of aging.** This theory explains the changing status of older adults in the United States. According to modernization theory, the status of older adults in a society is inversely related to the society's degree of technological development. The status of older adults in a technologically advanced society is lower than in a less technologically advanced society. This is because there are fewer roles that can be filled by older adults in a technologically advanced society.

Person-Environment Fit Theory of Aging

M. Powell Lawton proposed the **person-environment fit theory**. This theory states that a person's functional competencies determine how well he or she fits into an environment. Functional competencies include ego strength, motors skills, health, cognitive ability, and sensory-perceptual ability. Functional competencies change with age, and this affects the way people interact with the environment. The loss of functional competencies makes the world a frightening place. This leads to withdrawal from society.

Reminiscence Theory and Aging

Reminiscence theory states that reminiscence has benefits for the older adult. There is evidence to suggest that older adults who reminisce are less prone to depression and are mentally healthier than those who don't reminisce. However, the type of reminiscing makes a difference. Idealizing the past or dwelling on negative memories does not have a positive effect. Reminiscence can help the older adult maintain his or her identity.

Self-Efficacy Theory and Aging

Self-efficacy theory has been applied to aging. It has been suggested that age-related differences in ability may be related to age-related differences in self-efficacy. Older individuals may be unable to perform a function because they believe that they cannot perform this function. This outcome is based on a belief rather than on fact. Higher levels of self-efficacy lead to more successful aging.

Ethical Health Care Practice

Nursing Code of Ethics

The American Nurse Association (ANA) developed the **Nursing Code of Ethics**. There are 9 provisions:

1. The nurse treats all patients with respect and consideration, regardless of social circumstances or health condition.
2. The nurse's primary commitment is to the patient, regardless of conflicts that may arise.
3. The nurse promotes and advocates for the patient's health, safety, and rights, maintaining privacy and confidentiality and protecting the patient from questionable practices or care.
4. The nurse is responsible for his/her own care practices and determines appropriate delegation of care.
5. The nurse must retain respect for self and his/her own integrity and competence.
6. The nurse participates in ensuring that the healthcare environment is conducive to providing good health care and consistent with professional and ethical values.
7. The nurse participates in education and knowledge development to advance the profession.
8. The nurse collaborates with others to promote efforts to meet health needs.
9. The nursing profession articulates values and promotes and maintains the integrity of the profession.

Autonomy and Justice

Autonomy is the ethical principle that the individual has the right to make decisions about his/her own care. In the case of children, the child cannot make autonomous decisions, so the parents serve as the legal decision maker. The nurse must keep the parents fully informed so that they can exercise their autonomy in informed decision-making.

Justice is the ethical principle that relates to the distribution of the limited resources of healthcare benefits to the members of society. These resources must be distributed fairly. This issue may arise if there is only one bed left and two sick children. Justice comes into play in deciding which child should stay and which should be transported or otherwise cared for. The decision should be made according to what is best or most just for the patients and not colored by personal bias.

Beneficence and Nonmaleficence

Beneficence is an ethical principle that involves performing actions that are for the purpose of benefiting another person. In the care of a patient, any procedure or treatment should be done with the ultimate goal of benefiting the patient, and any actions that are not beneficial should be reconsidered. As a patient's condition changes, procedures need to be continually reevaluated to determine if they are still of benefit.

Nonmaleficence is an ethical principle that means healthcare workers should provide care in a manner that does not cause direct intentional harm to the patient:

- The actual act must be good or morally neutral.
- The intent must be only for a good effect.
- A bad effect cannot serve as the means to get to a good effect.
- A good effect must have more benefit than a bad effect has harm.

Organizational Ethics

Organizational ethics is the value system at work within an organization. While almost all healthcare organizations have a code of ethics, an ethical organization embodies that code within all processes, including the following:

- Relationships with customers and the public, utilizing a code of right conduct
- Recognition of the patient's/customer's right to quality care and respect for personal religious beliefs, culture, and psychosocial values
- Openness in disclosure of information and accountability
- Adherence to regulations and best practices
- Recognition of the need to empower staff and patients/customers
- Leadership without intimidation or fear tactics
- Following standard open guidelines for organ donation and procurement and for research projects
- Maintenance of a bioethics committee to provide guidance related to ethical issues in healthcare

Patients' Rights

Patients' (families') rights in relation to what they should expect from a healthcare organization are outlined in both standards of the Joint Commission and National Committee for Quality Assurance. Rights include the following:

- Respect for patient, including personal dignity and psychosocial, spiritual, and cultural considerations
- Response to needs related to access and pain control
- Ability to make decisions about care, including informed consent, advance directives, and end of life care
- Procedure for registering complaints or grievances
- Protection of confidentiality and privacy
- Freedom from abuse or neglect
- Protection during research and information related to ethical issues of research
- Appraisal of outcomes, including unexpected outcomes
- Information about organization, services, and practitioners
- Appeal procedures for decisions regarding benefits and quality of care

- Organizational code of ethical behavior
- Procedures for donating and procuring organs/tissue

Confidentiality

Confidentiality is the obligation that is present in a professional-patient relationship. Nurses are under an obligation to protect the information they possess concerning the patient and family. Care should be taken to safeguard that information and provide the privacy that the patient deserves. This is accomplished through the use of required passwords when family call for information about the patient and through the limitation of who is allowed to visit. The nurse should not assume that family members can be apprised of an older adult's health information without that person's consent. There may be times when confidentiality must be broken to save the life of a patient, but those circumstances are rare. The nurse must make all efforts to safeguard patient records and identification. Computerized record keeping should be done in such a way that the screen is not visible to others, and paper records must be secured.

Review Video: Confidentiality
Visit mometrix.com/academy and enter code: 250384

Confidentiality Agreement and Conflict of Interest

Maintaining confidentiality of performance improvement activities and records requires that staff be informed regarding regulations and correct reporting activities. A complete understanding of this issue may allay part of the concern staff member have related to performance review. Most organizations require personnel engaging in review of medical records or participating in improvement activities to sign **confidentiality agreements** that outline privacy issues and increase awareness of confidentiality concerns. **Conflict of interest policies** should be in place in each healthcare organization to ensure that those involved in review activities should not be primary care givers or have an economic or personal interest in a case under review. In all cases, access to protected health information should be limited to those who need the information to complete duties related to direct care of performance improvement review activities.

Informed Consent

The patient or the patient's family must give **informed consent** for all treatment the patient receives or for any study in which the patient participates. The physician must give a thorough explanation of all procedures and treatment and the associated risks. Patients and/or their families should be apprised of all options and be allowed input on the treatments administered. Patients and/or their families should be made aware of all risks and any complications that might be life threatening or increase morbidity. The American Medical Association has established guidelines for informed consent. The patient and/or family must receive the following information:

- Explanation of diagnosis.
- Nature and reason for treatment or procedure.
- Risks and benefits of proposed treatment or procedure.
- Alternative options (regardless of cost or insurance coverage).
- Risks and benefits of alternative options.
- Risks and benefits of not having a treatment or procedure.

Competence and Capacity

Competence and capacity are related to the ability to give informed consent.

- **Competence** is a legal definition that refers to the cognitive ability to make informed decisions or carry out activities. Competence is a property. People are assumed to be competent and able to comprehend information and understand consequences unless declared incompetent through a judicial process. People may be judged incompetent because of psychiatric illness, mental disability, or dementia.
- **Capacity** is a medical definition that refers to the degree of capability a person has to make informed decisions, to comprehend information, and to understand consequences of accepting or refusing treatment. Capacity is an ability, not a property. Capacity may vary, depending on the circumstances including whether the patient is ill or medicated, and may change over a period of time. Capacity may be determined by physicians, but may require referral to the judicial system for a ruling of incompetence. Capacity should be considered both when a patient accepts and refuses treatment.

Need to Know

Patients have a right to expect that when they divulge personal information to a nurse that only those with a **need to know** (such as the physician and other nurses) will be provided this information. When nurses must document care, they must be sensitive to the information that they put into the written record or report because many people have access to these records. If the information is health-related, then the nurse is obligated to record this and should tell the patient. Need to know issues also relate to the patient's need to know about care and prognosis. Patients may be overwhelmed by information or, if they are cognitively impaired, confused. Older adults and families should be asked how much information they want. Some patients/families want to know all of the details, including treatment options and expected outcomes. Others want only the basic information or don't want to discuss health issues at all.

Boundary Issues

Power issues are inherent in matters associated with **professional boundaries.** Physical abuse is both unprofessional and illegal, but behavior can easily border on abusive without the patient being physically injured.

Coercion

Nurses can easily intimidate patients into having procedures or treatments they don't want. Regardless of age, patients have the right to choose and the right to refuse treatment. Difficulties arise with cognitive impairment, and in that case, another responsible adult (often a child or spouse) is designated to make decisions, but every effort should be made to gain patient cooperation. Forcing the patient to do something against his/her will borders on abuse and can sometimes degenerate into actual abuse if physical coercion is involved.

Gifts

Over time, patients may develop a bond with nurses they trust and may feel grateful to the nurse for the care provided and want to express thanks, but the nurse must make sure to maintain **professional boundaries.** Patients often offer gifts to nurses to show their appreciation, but older adults, especially those who are weak and ill or have cognitive impairment, may be taken advantage of easily. Patients may offer valuables and may sometimes be easily manipulated into giving large sums of money. Small tokens of appreciation that can be shared with other staff, such as a box of chocolates, are usually acceptable (depending upon the policy of the institution), but almost any other gifts (jewelry, money, clothes) should be declined: "I'm sorry, that's so kind of you, but nurses are not allowed to accept gifts from patients." Declining may relieve the patient of the feeling of obligation.

Personal Information

When pre-existing personal or business relationships exist, other nurses should be assigned care of the patient whenever possible, but this may be difficult in small communities. However, the nurse should strive to maintain a professional role separate from the personal role and respect **professional boundaries**. The nurse must respect and maintain the confidentiality of the patient and family members, but the nurse must also be very careful about disclosing personal information about himself/herself because this establishes a social relationship that interferes with the professional role of the nurse and the boundary between the patient and the nurse. The nurse and patient should never share "secrets." When the nurse divulges personal information, he/she may become vulnerable to the patient, a reversal of roles.

Attention

Nursing is a giving profession, but the nurse must temper giving with recognition of **professional boundaries.** Patients, especially older adults, have many needs; as acts of kindness, nurses, especially those involved in home care, often give patients extra attention and may offer to do favors, such as cooking or shopping. In this way, nurses may become overly invested in the patients' lives. While this may benefit a patient in the short term, it can establish a relationship of increasing dependency and obligation that does not resolve the long-term needs of the patient. Making referrals to the appropriate agencies or collaborating with family to find ways to provide services is more effective. Becoming overly invested may be evident by the nurse showing favoritism or spending too much time with the patient while neglecting other duties. On the other end of the spectrum are nurses who are disinterested and fail to provide adequate attention to the patient's detriment. Lack of adequate attention may lead to outright neglect.

Sexual Boundary Issues

When the **boundary** between the role of the professional nurse and the vulnerability of the patient is breached, a boundary violation occurs. Because the nurse is in the position of "authority," the responsibility to maintain the boundary rests with the nurse; however, the line separating them is a continuum and sometimes not easily defined. It is inappropriate for nurses to engage in sexual relations with patients, and if the sexual behavior is coerced or the patient cognitively impaired, it is illegal. However, more common violations with older adults include exposing a patient unnecessarily, using sexually demeaning gestures or language (including off-color jokes), harassment, or inappropriate touching. Touching, such as touching a hand or shoulder, should be done with care. Hugging may be misconstrued.

Bioethics

Bioethics is a branch of ethics that involves making sure that the medical treatment given is the most morally correct choice given the different options that might be available and the differences inherent in the varied levels of treatment. In the acute/critical care unit, if the patients, parents, and the staff are in agreement when it comes to values and decision-making, then no ethical dilemma exists; however, when there is a difference in value beliefs between the patients/parents and the staff, there is a bioethical dilemma that must be resolved. Sometimes, discussion and explanation can resolve differences, but at times the institution's ethics committee must be brought in to resolve the conflict. The primary goal of bioethics is to determine the most morally correct action using the set of circumstances given.

Ethical and Clinical Conflicts

Ethical and clinical conflicts among patients and their families and healthcare professionals are not uncommon. Issues frequently relate to medications and treatment, religion, concepts of truth telling, lack of respect for patient's autonomy, and limitations of managed care or incompetent care. Additionally, healthcare providers are in a position to easily manipulate patients/families by providing incomplete information to influence decisions, and this can give rise to ethical conflicts. Facilitation involves questioning and listening, acknowledging each person's perspective while sharing different viewpoints:

- Open communication is critical to solving conflicts. Asking what steps could be taken to resolve the conflict or how it could be handled differently often leads to compromise because it allows for exchange of ideas and validates legitimate concerns. Sharing cultural perspectives can lead to better understanding.
- Advocacy for the patients/families must remain at the center of conflict resolution.

Ethical Dilemmas

While the terms *ethics* and *morals* are sometimes used interchangeably, ethics is a study of morals and encompasses concepts of right and wrong. When dealing with **ethical dilemmas,** one must consider not only what people should do but also what they actually do as these two things are sometimes at odds. Ethical issues can be difficult to assess because of personal bias, and that is one of the reasons that sharing concerns with other internal sources and reaching consensus is so valuable. Issues of concern might include options for care, refusal of care, rights to privacy, adequate relief of suffering, and the right to self-determination. Internal sources might include the ethics committee whose charge is to make decisions regarding ethical issues. Risk management can provide guidance related to personal and institutional liability. External agencies might include government agencies, such as the public health department.

Ethical Issues Related to Treatment of Terminally Ill Patients

There are a number of ethical concerns that healthcare providers and families must face when determining the treatments that are necessary and appropriate for a **terminally-ill patient.** It is the nurse's responsibility to provide support and information to help parents/families make informed decisions:

- *Analgesia* – *Advantage*: Provide comfort. Ease the dying process *Disadvantage:* Increase sedation and decrease cognition and interaction with family. Side effects. May hasten death.
- *Active treatments* – (such as antibiotics, chemotherapy) *Advantage*: Prolong life. Relieve symptoms. Reassure family. *Disadvantage*: Prolong the dying process. Side effects may be severe (as with chemotherapy)
- *Supplemental nutrition* – *Advantage*: Relieve family's anxiety that patient is hungry. Prolong life. *Disadvantage*: May cause nausea, vomiting. May increase tumor growth with cancer. May increase discomfort.
- *IV fluids for hydration* – *Advantage*: Relieve family's anxiety that patient is thirsty. Keep mouth moist *Disadvantage*: May result in congestive heart failure and pulmonary edema with increased dyspnea. Increased urinary output and incontinence may cause skin breakdown. Prolong dying process.
- *Resuscitation efforts* – *Advantage*: Allow family to deny death is imminent. *Disadvantage*: Cause unnecessary suffering and prolong dying process

Advance Directives, DNR, and Durable Power of Attorney

In accordance to Federal and state laws, individuals have the right to self-determination in health care, including decisions about end of life care through **advance directives** such as living wills and the right to assign a surrogate person to make decisions through a **durable power of attorney**. Patients should routinely be questioned about an advanced directive as they may present at a healthcare organization without the document. Patients who have indicated they desire a **do-not-resuscitate** (DNR) order should not receive resuscitative treatments for terminal illness or conditions in which meaningful recovery cannot occur. Patients and families of those with terminal illnesses should be questioned as to whether the patients are Hospice patients. When dealing with a DNR request or request for withdrawal from life support, staff should provide the patient with palliative care rather than taking curative measures. Palliative measures include pain control and/or oxygen and emotional support for the patient and family. Religious traditions and beliefs about death should be treated with respect.

Organ Donation

People of any age can **donate organs and/or tissue**, including the following:

- Organs
- Stem cells
- Blood/platelets
- Tissue
- Whole body

There are different types of donations:

- *Whole body*: Usually organs cannot be donated separately and the body is donated intact.
- *Living donor*: Organs are donated by a living individual (one kidney, one lobe of liver, one lobe of lung, part of intestine, blood, stem cells).
- *Donation after cardiac or brain death*: Solid organs must be transplanted between 6-72 hours after removal although tissues can be frozen and banked.

Tissues and organs are screened for diseases that may infect the recipient. People who are HIV positive are restricted from donating. People may indicate they wish to be organ donors, but family members often must make the decision after a patient dies. The request for donor organs should be made with sensitivity, and no one should be coerced into approving donation.

Environment for Ethical Decision-Making and Patient Advocacy

An **environment** for ethical decision-making and patient advocacy does not appear when it's needed; it requires planning and preparation. The expectation for the institution should clearly communicate that nurses are legally and morally responsible for assuring competent care and respecting the rights of patients. Decisions regarding ethical issues often must be made quickly with little time for contemplation; therefore, ethical issues that may arise should be identified and discussed. Clearly defined procedures and policies for dealing with conflicts, including an active ethics committee, in-service training, and staff meetings, must be established. Patients and families need to be part of the ethical environment, and that means empowering them by providing patient/family information (print form, video, audio) that outlines patients' rights and procedures for expressing their wishes and dealing with ethical conflicts. Respect for privacy and confidentiality and a non-punitive atmosphere are essential.

Moral Distress

Moral distress occurs when a person acts in a manner inconsistent with personal moral values or is aware of an ethical action but unable to carry it out. Indications of moral distress can include:

- Physical problems such as insomnia, weight changes, impaired cognition, GI disturbances, fatigue, and various physical ailments
- Emotional problems such as anger, grief, depression, outburst, confusion, and frustration
- Behavioral problems such as substance abuse, gambling, inflexibility, aggression, depersonalization, and violations of boundaries
- Spiritual problems such as loss of faith or meaning in life, impaired relations with others

The **four steps** to addressing moral distress include:

1. **Asking**: personal questioning to gain awareness of moral issues.
2. **Affirming:** recognizing the reality of issues and determining to address the issue
3. **Assessing:** determining the source and severity of moral distress and evaluating the pros and cons of action
4. **Acting:** making the decision to act and taking steps to resolve moral issues while anticipating and dealing with obstacles

Engaging Resources to Resolve Issues of Moral Distress and Ethical Conflict

Ombudsman and Ethical Consult Team

The **ombudsman and ethical consult teams** can be activated by anyone with a concern, including the physician, nursing staff, patient, family, or community members, usually by simply telephoning or emailing, but procedures and availability may vary from one institution to another.

- An **ombudsman** is a person charged with advocating for the rights of the patient and for adequate patient care, and with assisting in resolving conflicts. The ombudsman may visit patients and work with staff to resolve moral distress and ethical conflicts. In many cases, the ombudsman is a trained volunteer and often serves geriatric or disabled patients and/or those in long-term care.
- An **ethical consult team** is usually composed of interdisciplinary team members who meet on request to assist with solving ethical problems. The team members also often educate other staff members, patients, and community members about ethical issues and provide recommendations and advice.

Care Conference and Chaplain

Care conferences usually involve all team members charged with care of a patient and may be activated routinely on a regular basis, such as weekly, but may meet more frequently at the request of a team member or when concerns regarding moral distress and ethical conflicts are voiced by the patient or a family member. Whenever possible, the patient or family member should attend the care conference. Conflicts often result from inadequate communication.

Chaplains provide spiritual and emotional support to patients, family, and healthcare providers. In some cases, such as in Catholic hospitals, the chaplain is a priest, but other hospitals may have chaplains who are priests, rabbis, imams, or pastors. In some cases, chaplains are not ordained but are trained in providing spiritual support. Availability and methods of contacting a chaplain vary. Some chaplains work regular hours; others are on call. In most cases, chaplains are trained to provide interfaith support.

Ethical Decision-Making Theories

There are a number of **ethical theories:**

- *Casuist:* This theory states one should compare a current ethical dilemma with similar ethical dilemmas to study outcomes and arrive at a compromise solution. In some cases, however, there may not be comparative dilemmas.
- *Deontology:* This theory states that when confronted with an ethical dilemma, people should adhere to obligations and duties. This provides some consistency, but there is no clear method of establishing the basis for deciding on obligations and duties.
- *Rights:* This theory protects and supports the rights set up by society, such as those permitted by tradition or law. Individuals may also grant rights to others. However, this theory doesn't establish an ethical basis for establishing rights.
- *Utilitarianism – Act, Rule:* This theory is based on the concept that consequences are predictable. In Act Utilitarianism, ethical decisions are those that benefit the most people, regardless of personal feelings or laws. In Rule Utilitarianism, ethical decisions must take laws and fairness into consideration.
- *Virtue:* This theory purports that when one's ethical decisions are questionable, then the person's morals and motivation (virtues) should be taken into account; however, this theory doesn't recognize that morals can change.

Problem Solving

Problem solving in any medical context involves arriving at a hypothesis and then testing and assessing data to determine if the hypothesis holds true. If a problem has arisen, taking steps to resolve the immediate problem is only the first step if recurrence is to be avoided:

1. *Define the issue.* Talk with the patient or family and staff to determine if the problem related to a failure of communication or other issues, such as culture or religion.
2. *Collect data:* This may mean interviewing additional staff or reviewing documentation, gaining a variety of perspectives.
3. *Identify important concepts*: Determine if there are issues related to values or beliefs.
4. *Consider reasons for actions:* Distinguish between motivation and intention on the part of all parties to determine the reason for the problem.
5. *Make a decision:* A decision on how to prevent a recurrence of a problem should be based on advocacy and moral agency, reaching the best solution possible for the patient and family.

Ethical Framework

An **ethical framework** may facilitate decision-making in complex healthcare situations, for example with issues related to clinical effectiveness (expensive vs cost-effective treatments), scientific advances, including issues of availability and cost, density of distribution, and external influences, such as regulations and standards.

Ethical framework	
Identify issues	Objectively describe the ethical issue, acknowledging emotional biases.
Clarify values	Determine if decision-making is affected by personal values or the values of others, and whether there is conflict in these values.
Identify influences and barriers	Consider medical condition, risk factors, socioeconomic status, religion, support systems, and barriers, such as conflicts, differing professional assessments, regulations, and control issues.
Apply principles	Use and apply ethical principles: autonomy, beneficence, nonmaleficence, justice, privacy, confidentiality, veracity, and fidelity.

Ethical framework	
Find alternative solutions	Explore alternate solutions, considering pros and cons, ethical issues, and outcomes.
Resolve conflicts	Use collaboration, compromise, and/or accommodation, rather than coercion or avoidance, to reach a solution.
Implement solution	Select and carry out a solution that you can defend as an ethical decision.
Assess process and outcomes	Assess the process of reaching an ethical solution and the outcomes.

Social Media

Ethical Issues

Social media can be effectively used in many situations to promote healthcare practice through networking, providing information about conditions, and gaining support about certain medical situations that are challenging. Social media also brings patients in for care whom are more informed about their conditions because of information available. In many ways, these are all appropriate and helpful uses, but social media can also be abused in ways that result in breaches of ethical conduct. Health professionals should monitor their time spent on social media and be very careful not to breach patient confidentiality by inadvertently giving away information about specific patients, even when seeking help or guidance for certain cases. They must remember that despite privacy settings, no one is truly anonymous for long on the Internet. Healthcare professionals must also take care that any pictures that they post on social media (especially if taken at their workplace) not have any identifying patient information, even in the background. Many people see healthcare workers as professionals, therefore healthcare professionals should use wisdom when making statements regarding health, as this may have its own ethical consequences if it provides incorrect information that could be substituted for appropriate medical care. Connecting with patients and others on social media can also have consequences that the healthcare professional should be mindful of. Healthcare organizations should consider setting social media guidelines in place to make sure that everyone on staff is aware of how social media should be handled in that organization.

Impact on Healthcare

Social media was once a tool used among a certain age group to exchange photos or messages, but after years of development and evolution, social media now has an enormous impact on healthcare. Professionals such as doctors or nurses use social media to gain information and data about health issues and current practices, and they can stay up to date on many different issues or topics. Many health care professionals use social media for professional purposes and professional networking. Social media is also important for healthcare consumers, many of whom say that the information they obtain from social media, like health-related conversations has an effect on the way they deal with health. Social media allows consumers to track, communicate, and learn about health and wellness in ways that have never been available before. This results in increased numbers of educated consumers who have support, guidance, and information at their fingertips to use whenever it is needed. Many health care organizations use social media to attract consumers to their organizations, and the number of organizations using social media is expected to increase in the future.

Resource Allocation

Resource allocation in healthcare is an ethical issue that is not easily resolved. Perspectives include:

- *Right to care*: If all patients deserve an equal right to care but resources are limited, then the task becomes one of determining ways to acquire more resources so all can be served, but this is not always possible. There is unequal geographic and economic distribution of resources.
- *Quality of life*: If limited resources are allocated according to quality of life issues, someone has to decide what qualities take precedence, but there is little consensus in healthcare. Gender, race, and ethnicity should not be factors, but it can be difficult to separate these from economic factors or social support issues.
- *Economic considerations*: With limited resources, care is often rationed according to those who have insurance or other economic means to pay for it. Medicaid and other programs to pay for care provide some balance, but these programs may not pay for expensive procedures that are available to those with more financial resources.

Planning and Implementation

Principles of Pharmacotherapeutics

Pharmacokinetics

Rate of Clearance and Volume of Distribution

Pharmacokinetics relates to the effects that the body has on a drug, and pharmacodynamics relates to the effects that a drug has on the body. Both must be considered to ensure adequate dosing to achieve the optimal response from medications. With all drugs there is an intake (dose) and a response:

Pharmacokinetics refers to the route of administration, the absorption, the dosage, the frequency of administration, the distribution, and the serum levels achieved over time. The drug's **rate of clearance** (elimination) and doses needed to ensure therapeutic benefit must be considered. Most drugs are cleared through the kidneys, with water-soluble compounds excreted more readily than protein-soluble compounds. **Volume of distribution** (IV drug dose divided by plasma concentration) determines the rate at which the drug passes into tissue. Drug distribution depends on the degree of protein binding and ion trapping that takes place.

Half-Life, Recovery Time, and Effect-Site Equilibrium

Elimination half-life is the time needed to reduce plasma concentrations to 50%. Usually, the equivalent of 5 half-lives is needed to completely eliminate a drug. Five half-lives are also needed to achieve steady-state plasma concentrations if giving doses intermittently. Context-sensitive half-life, in contrast, is the time needed to reach a specific amount of decrease (50%, 60%) after stopping administration of a drug.

Recovery time is the length of time it takes for plasma levels to decrease to the point that the person awakens. This is affected by plasma concentration.

Effect-site equilibrium is the time between administration of a drug and clinical effect (the point at which the drug reaches the appropriate receptors) and must be considered when determining dose, time, and frequency of anesthetic agents. The bioavailability of drugs may vary, depending upon the degree of metabolism that takes place before the drug reaches its site of action.

Gerontological Changes

There are a number of **changes in older adults** that affect **pharmacokinetics**:

- Absorption slows because of increased gastric pH and slower emptying time, so medication may take effect more slowly, but excess may be absorbed.
- Distribution may alter because of decreased intracellular and extracellular water, reducing distribution of water-soluble medications. Body fat increases (≤36% in men and ≤48% in women) between early adulthood and 80, so fat soluble medications (e.g., benzodiazepines) accumulate in fat and half-life is prolonged. Protein-binding alterations may change half-life as well. Decreased cardiac output and systemic illness may impact distribution.

- Metabolism is affected by a decrease in liver size (25-35%) and blood flow to the liver (≤40% by age 90). The enzymes necessary to break down medications are decreased. These changes can increase half-life 2-3 times in some medications (benzodiazepines, diazepam, and alprazolam).
- Elimination of most drugs is through the kidneys, but renal function declines in about 65% of the elderly, so half-life is extended, necessitating lower doses.

PHARMACODYNAMICS

Pharmacodynamics relates to the biological effects (therapeutic or adverse) of drug administration over time. Drug transport, absorption, means of elimination, and half-life must all be considered when determining effects. Responses may include continuous responses, such as blood pressure variations, or dichotomous response in which an event either occurs or does not (such as death). Information from pharmacodynamics provides feedback to modify medication dosage (pharmacokinetics). Drugs provide biological effects primarily by interacting with receptor sites (specific protein molecules) in the cell membrane. Receptors include voltage-sensitive ion channels (sodium, chloride, potassium, and calcium channels), ligand-gated ion channels, and transmembrane receptors. Agonist drugs exert effects after binding with a receptor while antagonist drugs bind with a receptor but have no effects, so they can block agonists from binding. The total number of receptors may vary, upregulating or downregulating in response to stimuli (such as drug administration). Dose-response curves show the relationship between the amount of drug given and the resultant plasma concentration and biological effects.

GERONTOLOGICAL CHANGES

There are a number of **changes related to aging** that affect **pharmacodynamics**:

- Central nervous system changes include changes in receptor sensitivity and in numbers of receptor sites can result in increased side effects, delirium, and behavioral changes, especially with benzodiazepines, opioids, alcohol, antipsychotics, anticholinergics, and barbiturates.
- Decrease in beta-adrenergic receptor function may necessitate an increased dosage of some medications, such as β-blockers and the vasopressor isoproterenol (Isuprel®).
- Decrease in baroreceptor function may affect the ability to increase vascular tone or cardiac output/hear rate in response to vasoactive medications, such as antihypertensives, resulting in orthostatic hypotension.
- Impaired glucose counter-regulation increases risk of hypoglycemia for those on antidiabetic medications.

ISSUES RELATING TO GERONTOLOGICAL DOSAGE

Gerontological dosage can be affected by a number of factors. Adverse drug effects occur two to three times more often in older adults than in younger adults. This is often related to polypharmacy. Since most drug trials are conducted on younger adults, information on correct dosage and drug effects in older adults is lacking. Some diseases, such as hypertension, congestive heart failure, renal failure, and diabetes, are associated with drug intolerance. In adults with these diseases, it may be necessary to use alternative medications. Drugs and nutrients may interact, impairing appetite and adversely affecting nutrition. Food and drug interactions may also alter the pharmacokinetics of nutrients or drugs, interfering with absorption, distribution, metabolism, and elimination. Mixing drugs in tube feedings or administering drugs with food increases the risk of interactions. Therefore, medications should be taken with water unless the physician instructs otherwise.

Older Adults and Problems with Various Drugs

Anticholinergics, Anticoagulants, Antidepressants, Anti-Diabetics, and Anti-Dysrhythmics

The following are problems associated with older adults and different types of drugs:

- **Anticholinergics***:* Anti-cholinergic effects are cumulative and include urinary retention, dry mouth, dry eyes, and constipation. CNS effects include sedation, confusion, hallucinations (auditory and visual), and increased risks of falls. These effects are magnified if the patient is cognitively impaired. Numerous drugs have anticholinergic effects, including some antihistamines, antidepressants, antipsychotics, cimetidine and ranitidine, antispasmodics, antidiarrheals, antiemetics, and anti-Parkinson's drugs.
- **Anticoagulants***:* Anticoagulants may cause severe bleeding in those over the age of 65. Warfarin should be used with care and at a lower dose if total protein or albumin concentration is low.
- **Antidepressants***:* Antidepressants are associated with excess sedation, so typical doses are only 16-33% of a younger adult's dose. SSRIs are safest, but Prozac® may cause anorexia, anxiety, and insomnia so should be avoided.
- **Anti-diabetics (oral):** Oral anti-diabetic agents should be started at ½ the usual dose because of the danger of hypoglycemia. First generation drugs should be avoided. Glucotrol® has fewer side effects than Diabeta®.
- **Anti-dysrhythmic***:* Alterations in pharmacokinetics mean that dosage should depend on effect rather than serum level.
- **Antipsychotics***:* Older antipsychotics, such as haloperidol, have high incidence of side effects. Atypical anti-psychotics appear to be safer with risperidone (<2mg daily) having the fewest adverse effects. The lowest possible doses should be tried first with careful monitoring of any anti-psychotic.
- **Chemotherapeutics***:* Bone marrow toxicity may be increased and hematopoietic recovery delayed.
- **Digoxin***:* A lower dose is needed with reduced renal function.
- **H_2 antagonists***:* Cimetidine (Tagamet®) is eliminated (70%) through the kidneys, so reduced renal function may result in increased CNS side effects. Cimetidine interacts with many drugs.
- **NSAIDs***:* NSAIDs, such as ibuprofen, may cause increased gastric irritation and bleeding. Acetaminophen is the preferred non-narcotic analgesic, but the dose should be <4 g per day and lower in those with liver disease.
- **Opioids***:* Codeine is preferred but may cause nausea, vomiting, and diarrhea and anticholinergic CNS effects. Meperidine may produce psychosis, and propoxyphene may have a toxic effect. Oxycodone may be used. Tramadol may be used, but the half-life may be prolonged.

Cost-Effective Drugs

The **cost of drugs** is one of the most expensive aspects of medical care for patient, so patients sometimes cannot afford treatment. Even those with insurance drug coverage or Medicare D may have considerable costs, especially with non-generic drugs. There is much pressure from drug representatives to prescribe new drugs, and patients are often influenced by direct-to-consumer advertising, but the nurse can help the patient ensure that drugs are prescribed based on evidence. Additionally, the cost versus benefit of drugs must always be considered. It is the responsibility of the nurse to act in the best interests of the patient and to educate the patient about drugs. If a less expensive drug is as effective as a more expensive or newer drug, then the nurse and patient should request that the less expensive drug be prescribed. The nurse should educate people about the use of generic drugs as a cost-saving measure, as—in most cases—these are as effective as non-generic.

Pharmacologic Interventions

Diuretics

A **diuretic** is any drug that increases the rate of urine formation and urination. This reduces preload. Increasing urine production releases fluids from the body and also reduces salt levels. Diuretics are used to treat peripheral and pulmonary edema, heart failure, some kidney diseases, and hypertension. Diuretics are usually the first medication prescribed for hypertension. Other medications are also prescribed for hypertension to be used in conjunction with diuretics. There are a number of categories of diuretics. These include loop diuretics, thiazide diuretics, and potassium-sparing diuretics. The different categories of diuretics have different mechanisms of action. Diuretics can cause adverse reactions depending on the particular diuretic.

Potassium-Sparing Diuretics

Potassium-sparing diuretics act in the late convoluted distal tubules and collecting ducts. This class of drugs inhibits the absorption of sodium but does not promote the secretion of potassium into the urine. Potassium-sparing diuretics cause the kidneys to retain potassium. If administered alone, potassium-sparing diuretics may raise potassium above normal levels. This can cause weakness, arrhythmia, and cardiac arrest. However, because these drugs are not as effective as other diuretics, they are often taken in conjunction with thiazide, which helps to balance potassium levels. Chlorothiazide is a combination of a potassium-sparing diuretic and thiazide. Side effects include dehydration, nausea, insomnia, and blurred vision. Side effects are most likely to occur at the beginning of treatment.

Loop Diuretics and Thiazide Diuretics

Loop diuretics inhibit the reabsorption of sodium and chloride in the ascending loop of Henle. Loop diuretics also interfere with the reabsorption of magnesium and calcium. Loop diuretics are short acting. Other classes of diuretics many be more appropriate for the treatment of hypertension. Loop diuretics can cause serum levels of potassium, sodium, and magnesium to decrease and calcium levels to increase. This can cause arrhythmia, weakness, and mental confusion. The risk of adverse reactions increases with increasing dosage.

Thiazide diuretics act primarily in the distal convoluted tubules and impede the reabsorption of sodium and chloride. Thiazide also causes a loss of potassium from the body and an increase in uric acid in the blood. Thiazide diuretics are often given in conjunction with potassium supplements. The effects of thiazide diuretics are long lasting; this class of drug is appropriate for treating hypertension. Side effects include dizziness, postural hypotension, blurred vision, and sun sensitivity.

Digitalis Drugs

Digitalis drugs, the most common of which is digoxin (Lanoxin), are made from the foxglove plant. These drugs are administered to increase contractility of the heart muscle, increase left ventricular output, and slow conduction through the atrioventricular (AV) node. The drug lowers a rapid heart rate and promotes diuresis. Although digoxin does not decrease the incidence of death, it does increase activity tolerance and reduce the number of hospitalizations for heart failure. It is essential not to exceed therapeutic levels (0.5-2.0 ng/mL) in order to avoid toxicity. Toxicity can occur even if therapeutic levels are not exceeded. Early signs and symptoms of toxicity include increasing fatigue, depression, nausea, and vomiting. Later symptoms include sudden changes in heart rhythm, sinoatrial (SA) or AV block, dysrhythmia, and tachycardia. Digitalis toxicity is treated by discontinuation of the medication and serum monitoring. Digoxin immune FAB (Digibind) may be administered to inactivate digoxin.

Heart Failure and Hypertension Medication

A number of different types of medication are used to treat heart failure and hypertension:

- **ACE inhibitors**, such as captopril (Capoten), enalapril (Vasotec), and lisinopril (Prinivil), reduce afterload and preload and reverse ventricular remodeling. However, they may initially cause hypotension and are contraindicated for individuals with renal insufficiency.
- **Beta-blockers**, such as metoprolol (Lopressor), carvedilol (Coreg), and esmolol (Brevibloc), decrease the heart rate, reduce hypertension, prevent dysrhythmia, and reverse ventricular remodeling. However, these drugs should not be used during decompensation. Individuals with airway disease, uncontrolled diabetes, a slow/irregular pulse, or heart block should be monitored carefully while taking beta-blockers.
- **Aldosterone antagonists**, such as spironolactone (Aldactone), reduce preload, myocardial hypertrophy, and edema. These drugs may increase blood levels of potassium because this is a potassium-sparing diuretic. Therefore, while water and sodium are excreted, potassium is retained.

Vasodilators

Smooth-muscle relaxants (vasodilators) improve heart function by dilating the arteries or veins. These agents may be administered as a treatment for pulmonary hypertension or generalized systemic hypertension. Vasodilators may be taken by individuals who cannot tolerate angiotensin-converting enzyme (ACE) inhibitors or angiotensin-receptor blockers. Dilation of arteries reduces afterload and improves cardiac output. Dilation of veins reduces preload, decreasing filling pressures. Smooth-muscle relaxants reduce peripheral vascular resistance. However, they may cause hypotension and headaches.

There are a number of types of vasodilators:

- **Sodium nitroprusside (**Nipride) dilates arteries and veins. This agent is used to reduce hypertension and afterload for heart failure. It has a fast onset of action.
- **Nitroglycerin** (Tridil) dilates veins primarily and is administered intravenously to reduce preload in acute heart failure, unstable angina, and acute myocardial infarction (MI). Nitroglycerin may also be administered after percutaneous coronary intervention (PCI) to prevent vasospasm.
- **Hydralazine** (Apresoline) dilates arteries. This drug is administered intermittently in the treatment of hypertension.
- **B-type natriuretic peptide** (BNP), available as nesiritide (Natrecor), is a new kind of vasodilator. BNP is a recombinant form of a peptide found in the human brain. BNP reduces filling pressure and vascular resistance. It increases the output of urine. BNP may cause hypotension, headache, bradycardia, and nausea.
- **Alpha-adrenergic blockers** cause vasodilation of arteries and veins by blocking alpha receptors. Side effects include orthostatic hypotension and edema from fluid retention.
- **Labetalol** (Normodyne) is a combination drug. It is a peripheral alpha-blocker and cardiac beta-blocker. This drug is used in the treatment of acute hypertension, acute stroke, and acute aortic dissection.
- **Phentolamine** (Regitine) dilates the peripheral arteries. It reduces afterload and is used to treat pheochromocytoma.

- **Selective specific dopamine DA1-receptor agonists,** such as fenoldopam (Corlopam), are peripheral dilators. They dilate renal and mesenteric arteries. These drugs can be used to treat renal dysfunction. They can also be used to treat individuals at risk for renal insufficiency.
- **Calcium channel blockers** are primarily arterial vasodilators. These agents may cause dilation of the peripheral and/or coronary arteries. Side effects include fatigue, flushing, abdominal and peripheral edema, and indigestion.
- **Dihydropyridines,** such as nifedipine (Procardia) and nicardipine (Cardene), are primarily arterial vasodilators. These drugs dilate both coronary and peripheral arteries and are administered in the treatment of acute hypertension.
- **Benzothiazines,** such as diltiazem (Cardizem), and phenylalkylamines, such as verapamil (Calan, Isoptin), dilate coronary arteries primarily. These agents are used to treat angina and supraventricular tachycardia.
- **ACE inhibitors** cause vasodilation by limiting the production of angiotensin. These drugs may cause a large drop in blood pressure, so individuals taking ACE inhibitors must be carefully monitored. These are first-line agents in the treatment of acute hypertension and heart failure and are also administered to prevent nephropathy in patients with diabetes.
- **Captopril** (Capoten) and **enalapril** (Vasotec) are administered to reduce afterload and preload in cases of heart failure.

ANTIDYSRHYTHMICS

Antidysrhythmics are drugs that control dysrhythmia by acting on the conduction system, the ventricles, and/or the atria. There are four classes of antidysrhythmic drugs and some unclassified antidysrhythmics:

- Class I includes three subtypes of sodium channel blockers (quinidine, lidocaine, and procainamide).
- Class II includes beta-blockers (esmolol and propranolol).
- Class III drugs slow repolarization (amiodarone and ibutilide).
- Class IV includes calcium channel blockers (diltiazem and verapamil).

Unclassified drugs include adenosine. Different drugs are used for specific dysrhythmias. Antidysrhythmic drugs are used to treat paroxysmal supraventricular tachycardia, atrial fibrillation, atrial flutter, sinus tachycardia, PVCs, ventricular tachycardia, and ventricular fibrillation. All of these drugs have specific uses and are associated with adverse effects.

SIDE EFFECTS

Adenosine is used to terminate episodes of supraventricular tachycardia. The drug acts to cause a transient heart block at the atrioventricular (AV) node. Adenosine is also a vasodilator. Side effects include facial flushing, asystole, excessive sweating, and light-headedness.

Amiodarone (Cordarone) acts on the atria and ventricles and may cause a reduction in blood pressure (BP) and have adverse effects on the liver.

Digoxin (Lanoxin) acts on the conduction system. It decreases the conduction rate through the AV node. It increases the force at which the heart muscles contract. It may cause bradycardia, heart block, nausea and vomiting, and central nervous system (CNS) depression.

Diltiazem (Cardizem, Tiazac) decreases conduction through the AV node and may cause arrhythmia, bradycardia, and palpitations.

Ibutilide (Corvert) acts on the conduction system. It can cause a severe and potentially fatal arrhythmia called polymorphic ventricular tachycardia. Although this usually occurs in conjunction with QT prolongation, this is not always the case.

Esmolol (Brevibloc) acts on the conduction system and may cause a reduction in BP, bradycardia, and heart failure.

Lidocaine acts on the ventricles and may cause CNS toxicity, nausea, and vomiting.

Procainamide affects the atria and ventricles of the heart. Use of this drug may result in a reduction in BP and electrocardiogram (ECG) abnormalities (widening of QRS and QT).

Verapamil (Calan, Verelan) acts on the conduction system and may cause a reduction in BP, bradycardia, and heart failure.

Treatment for Supraventricular Tachycardia, Paroxysmal Supraventricular Tachycardia, Atrial Fibrillation, Atrial Flutter, Sinus Tachycardia, Premature Ventricular Contractions, Ventricular Tachycardia, and Ventricular Fibrillation

Supraventricular tachycardia is treated with diltiazem (Cardizem and Tiazac), esmolol (Brevibloc), propranolol (Inderal), and procainamide.

Paroxysmal supraventricular tachycardia is treated with adenosine, digoxin (Lanoxin), and verapamil (Calan, Verelan).

Atrial fibrillation is treated with digoxin (Lanoxin), diltiazem (Cardizem and Tiazac), ibutilide (Corvert), and amiodarone (Cordarone).

Atrial flutter is treated with digoxin (Lanoxin), diltiazem (Cardizem and Tiazac), ibutilide (Corvert), verapamil (Calan and Verelan), amiodarone (Cordarone), and procainamide.

Sinus tachycardia is treated with esmolol (Brevibloc).

Premature ventricular contractions are treated with lidocaine and procainamide.

Ventricular tachycardia is treated with lidocaine, amiodarone (Cardizem, Tiazac), and procainamide.

Ventricular fibrillation is treated with lidocaine.

Agents Used in Pulmonary Pharmacology

There are a wide range of agents used in **pulmonary pharmacology**. The agents used depend on the type and degree of pulmonary disease. Agents include opioid analgesics, neuromuscular blockers, and human B-type natriuretic peptides:

- *Opioid analgesics* are given to provide pain relief and sedation for those on mechanical ventilation. These agents reduce sympathetic response. Such medications include fentanyl (Sublimaze) or morphine sulfate.

- *Neuromuscular blockers* are used to induce paralysis in individuals who have not responded adequately to sedation, especially for the purposes of intubation and mechanical ventilation. Medications include pancuronium (Pavulon) and vecuronium (Norcuron). There is controversy surrounding the use of these drugs because induced paralysis has been linked to increased mortality rates, sensory hearing loss (pancuronium), atelectasis, and ventilation-perfusion mismatch.
- *Human B-type natriuretic peptides* are used to lower pulmonary capillary wedge pressure. Medications include nesiritide (Natrecor).
- *Diuretics* are used to decrease pulmonary edema. Agents include loop diuretics, such as furosemide (Lasix) and metolazone (Mykrox).
- *Nitrates* are administered for the purpose of vasodilation. Vasodilation reduces preload and afterload, which reduces the heart muscle's oxygen requirement. Nitrates include nitroglycerin (Nitro-Bid) and nitroprusside sodium (Nitropress).
- *Antibiotics* are used to treat respiratory infections, including pneumonia. Antibiotics used depend on the pathogenic agent in question and may include macrolides such as azithromycin (Zithromax) and erythromycin (E-Mycin).
- *Antimycobacterials* are used to treat tuberculosis and other mycobacterial diseases. Antimycobacterial agents include isoniazid (Laniazid, Nydrazid), ethambutol (Myambutol), rifampin (Rifadin), streptomycin sulfate, and pyrazinamide.
- *Antivirals* are used to disrupt viral replication early in a viral infection. The effectiveness of this treatment decreases with time because the replication process is already under way. Antiviral medications include ribavirin (Virazole) and zanamivir (Relenza).

Pulmonary pharmacology agents include vasopressors/inotropes, surfactants, alkalinizers, pulmonary vasodilators, and methylxanthines:

- *Vasopressors/inotropes* are used to raise cardiac output. Dopamine (Intropin) increases renal output and blood pressure. Dobutamine (Dobutrex) increases cardiac contractibility and blood pressure.
- *Surfactants* lower surface tension and prevent alveoli from collapsing. Beractant (Survanta) is made from bovine lung tissue, and calfactant (Infasurf) is made from calf lung tissue. These agents are administered by inhalation.
- *Alkalinizers* are used in the treatment of metabolic acidosis. These drugs reduce pulmonary vascular resistance by producing an alkaline pH. Medications include sodium bicarbonate and tromethamine (Tham).
- Administered by inhalation, *nitrous oxide* is used as a pulmonary vasodilator. This gas relaxes the vascular muscles and produces pulmonary vasodilation. The gas may reduce the need for extracorporeal membrane oxygenation (ECMO).
- *Methylxanthines* are used to stimulate contractions of the chest muscles and stimulate respiration. Medications include aminophylline (Aminophylline), caffeine citrate (Cafcit), and doxapram (Dopram).

Pharmacological Agents for Asthma

There are a number of pharmacologic agents used in **the treatment of asthma:**

- *Methylxanthines* (aminophylline and theophylline) stimulate muscle contractions of the chest and stimulate respirations.
- *Magnesium sulfate* is used to relax smooth muscles and decrease inflammation. These drugs may be administered intravenously or by inhalation. If given intravenously, magnesium sulfate must be administered slowly to prevent the occurrence of hypotension or bradycardia. When inhaled, the drug potentiates the action of albuterol.
- *Heliox* (helium-oxygen) is given to decrease airway resistance in cases of airway obstruction. It works to decrease respiratory effort. Heliox improves oxygenation in patients requiring mechanical ventilation.
- *Leukotriene inhibitors* are used in the long-term management of asthma and inhibit inflammation and bronchospasm.
- *Cromolyn sodium* and nedocromil may be administered to prevent asthmatic response to exercise or allergens.

Laxative Products

There are different types of **laxatives**: Stool softeners (emollients, such as Colace and Phillips' Liqui-Gels) use wetting agents, such as docusate sodium, to increase liquid in the stool. The increased liquid softens the stool. Stool softeners should not be used in conjunction with mineral oil because of increased absorption of the oil through the intestines. Hyperosmotics, which are available by prescription, contain materials that are not digestible and keep stool moist by holding fluid in the stool. Hyperosmotics (such as Kristalose and MiraLAX) soften the stool but may result in increased abdominal distention and flatus.

There are three types of **hyperosmolar laxatives**: 1) lactulose, 2) polymer, and 3) saline. *Lactulose* hyperosmotics contain a form of sugar and work similarly to saline laxatives, but more slowly, and may be used for long-term treatment. The *salines* work quickly and are used for short-term relief. The *polymers* contain polyethylene glycol, which retains fluid in the stool and is used for short-term relief. Combination drugs use two or more types of laxatives and should be used only for short-term treatment.

Insulin Types

There are different types of **insulin** with varying onsets of action. Insulin is used to metabolize glucose in individuals whose pancreases do not produce insulin. People with diabetes may need to take a combination of insulin types. Duration of action may vary according to the individual's metabolism, intake, and level of activity:

- *Humalog* (Lispro H) is a fast-acting insulin with a short duration. It acts within 5 to15 minutes after administration, peaks within 45 to 90 minutes, and lasts 3 to 4 hours.
- *Regular* (R) is a relatively fast-acting (30 minutes) insulin that peaks in 2 to 5 hours and last 5 to 8 hours.
- *NPH* (N) or *Lente* (L) insulin is intermediate-acting. It acts in 1 to 3 hours after administration, peaks at 6 to12 hours, and lasts 16 to 24 hours.
- *Ultralente* (U) is long-acting insulin that acts in 4 to 6 hours, peaks at 8 to 20 hours, and lasts 24 to 28 hours.
- *Combined NPH/Regular* (70/30 or 50/50) acts in 30 minutes, peaks in 7 to 12 hours, and lasts 16 to 24 hours.

Emergency Contraception

Females who have had unprotected sexual intercourse, consensual or rape, are at risk for pregnancy and may desire **emergency contraception.** Emergency contraception inhibits ovulation and prevents pregnancy rather than aborting a pregnancy. Because the medications contain hormones (such as ethinyl estradiol and norgestrel or levonorgestrel) in differing amounts, this treatment is contraindicated in those with a history of thromboembolia or severe migraine headaches with neurological symptoms. The criteria for administration of emergency contraception include the following:

- ≤ 72 hours since unprotected sexual intercourse
- Negative pelvic exam
- Negative pregnancy test

The regimen involves taking a first dose of 1-20 pills (depending upon the brand and concentration of hormones) and then a second dose of 1-20 pills 12 hours later. A follow-up pregnancy test should be done if the person does not menstruate within 3 weeks as the failure rate is about 1.5%. Side effects include nausea (relieved by taking medication with meals or with an antiemetic), breast tenderness, and irregular bleeding.

WHO Pain Ladder

The **World Health Organization (WHO) pain ladder** has been established as guidance for pain management. Medications are usually given every three to four hours around the clock to prevent breakthrough pain.

- **Level 1—Mild pain:** Pain management usually begins with acetaminophen or aspirin followed by NSAIDs. Adjuvant drugs may be administered. There are a number of different NSAIDs. There are individual differences in the response to drugs, so patients should be monitored carefully and medication changed if indicated.
- **Level 2—Mild to moderate pain***:* Aspirin or acetaminophen is given with codeine and adjuvant medication. Medications include hydrocodone, oxycodone, and tramadol.
- **Level 3—Moderate to severe pain:** Opioid drugs (morphine, fentanyl, and oxycodone) are given to control moderate to severe pain. Some nonopioid drugs and adjuvant drugs may also be used. Adjuvant drugs include NSAIDs, anticholinergics, anticonvulsants, antiemetics, antipruritics, and corticosteroids.

Pharmacologic Measures to Maximize Perfusion

The purpose of using **pharmacologic measures to maximize perfusion** is to reduce the risk of thrombosis.

- *Antiplatelet drugs* (for example, aspirin, Ticlid, and Plavix) inhibit clotting by interfering with the plasma membrane function. These drugs prevent the formation of clots but are ineffective at treating existing clots.
- *Vasodilators* help divert blood away from areas of ischemia. Some of these drugs, such as Pietal, dilate arteries and reduce clotting. Pietal is administered to control intermittent claudication.
- *Antilipemics* (for example, Zocor and Questran) slow the progression of atherosclerosis.
- *Hemorheologics* (such as Trental) decrease fibrinogen. This reduces blood viscosity and erythrocyte rigidity. These drugs may be used to treat intermittent claudication.
- *Analgesics* may be used to improve the quality of life. Opioids may be needed for severe pain.

- *Thrombolytics* (for example, streptokinase) may be administered to dissolve clots. The drug is injected into a blocked artery under angiography.
- *Anticoagulants* (such as Coumadin and Lovenox) prevent the formation of blood clots.

Venous Dermatitis

Venous dermatitis develops on the ankles and lower legs and can cause severe itching and pain. Without treatment the condition may deteriorate, resulting in the formation of ulcers. Therefore, treatment to address the symptoms is necessary. *Antihistamines* are administered topically to decrease itching and prevent excoriation from scratching. *Low-dose topical steroids* are administered reduce inflammation and itching. However, because they increase the risk of ulceration, steroids should be used only for short periods (2 weeks). Compression therapy using compression stockings is used to improve the venous return in the affected leg. Leg elevation is recommended when sitting. Topical antibiotics (such as bacitracin) are used to reduce the danger of infection as needed. If there is a systemic infection, oral antibiotics are administered. Hypoallergenic emollients (such as petroleum jelly) improve the skin's barrier function and should be used as a preventive measure when the acute inflammation has subsided.

Pharmacologic Treatments for Fecal Incontinence and Constipation/Fecal Impaction

Pharmacologic treatments for **fecal incontinence** include the following:

- Medications include antidiarrheals, cholinergic medications, laxatives, stool softeners, rectal stimulants, and hormones. Antidiarrheals reduce diarrhea, increase rectal muscle tone, decrease stool fluid content, and protect the lining of the intestine from irritation. Cholinergic medications reduce intestinal motility and secretions. Opium derivatives increase intestinal muscle tone and decrease motility. Laxatives treat constipation. Stool softeners increase the amount of fluid in the stool. Rectal stimulants cause bowel contractions to increase, leading to increased stool evacuation. Hormones are administered to postmenopausal women to improve incontinence.

Pharmacologic treatments for **constipation/fecal impaction** include the following:

- *Change in medications* causing constipation can relieve constipation. Additionally, use of stool softeners, such as Colace®, or bulk formers, such as Metamucil®, may decrease fluid absorption and move stool through the colon more quickly. Overuse of laxatives can cause constipation.

Pharmacologic Treatments for Urinary Incontinence

The following are medical treatments for **urinary incontinence**:

- *Antispasmodics* (Detrol, Ditropan, and Levsin): Antispasmodics are administered in the treatment of overactive bladders. These agents may cause thirst. Longer-acting preparations of these drugs have fewer side effects and may be more appropriate for some patients.
- *Antidepressants* (Tofranil): Antidepressants are administered to relax the bladder and to contract the muscles at the bladder neck.

- *Hormone replacement therapy* (HRT): HRT is used in the form of a vaginal cream, ring, or patch. Its purpose is to protect bladder and urethral mucosa. Oral estrogen may not be as effective as a topical preparation for the treatment of incontinence.
- *Antibiotics*: Infection may cause or worsen incontinence. Antibiotics are administered to treat these infections.

Food and Drug Interactions

Food and drug interactions can impact the drug's effect on the body:

- ACE inhibitors (captopril & moexipril): Avoid potassium supplements or foods high in potassium (bananas, oranges, green leafy vegetables.
- Antibiotics (quinolones and tetracyclines): Avoid milk products. Avoid vitamins and minerals containing iron and avoid caffeine.
- Anticoagulants: Avoid foods high in vitamin K (broccoli, spinach, Brussels sprouts, cauliflower, kale). Avoid vitamin E supplements.
- Antifungals: Avoid milk products and alcohol.
- Antihistamines, antidepressants, anti-anxieties: Avoid alcohol. Avoid grapefruit juice (buspirone, sertraline).
- Beta blocker (e.g., propranolol), nitrates, narcotics, NSAIDs: Avoid alcohol.
- Bronchodilators, histamine blockers: Avoid caffeine and alcohol.
- Carbamazepine, cyclosporine and tacrolimus, HIV medications, statins: Avoid grapefruit juice
- Diuretics, potassium sparing: Avoid food high in potassium.
- MAO inhibitors: Avoid alcohol and non-alcoholic substitute for beer or wine, foods high in tyramine (organ meats, cured meats, caviar, cheese products, avocados, bananas, raisins, soy, fava beans), and products containing caffeine (tea, cola, chocolate, coffee).

Polypharmacy

Adult patients, especially older adults, are at risk for **polypharmacy** (taking many drugs). This may occur when individuals take the same drug under generic and brand names or when physicians prescribe drugs for many different conditions. Problems arise when individuals take drugs for one condition that are contraindicated for another and take drugs that are not compatible. Reasons for polypharmacy include multiple prescriptions from different doctors; forgetfulness; confusion; failure to report current medications; the use of supplemental, over-the-counter, and herbal preparations in addition to prescribed medications; and failure of healthcare providers to adequately educate the patient. Patients should be encouraged to keep a list of all current medications (prescribed and otherwise) and to bring all medications with him/her to appointments. If family members are present, they should be enlisted in ensuring the patient avoids polypharmacy. Healthcare providers must take the time to discuss medications with the patient to ensure that the patient understands and must ask directly if the patient is taking any other medications. Helping the patient to make lifestyle changes, such as losing weight or quitting smoking, may reduce the need for medications.

Drug Interactions

Drug interactions occur when one drug interferes with the activity of another in the domain of either pharmacodynamics or pharmacokinetics. In a pharmacodynamic interaction, two drugs may interact at receptor sites, causing an adverse effect or interfering with a positive effect. In a pharmacokinetic interaction, the absorption and clearance of one or both drugs are altered. This may cause delayed effects, changes in effects, or toxicity. Interactions may cause problems in a number of domains. Absorption may be increased or (more commonly) decreased. This is usually related to the effects within the gastrointestinal system. Distribution of drugs may be altered due to changes in protein binding. Metabolism may be affected, causing changes in drug concentration. Drug interactions can impair biotransformation of the drug. Biotransformation usually occurs in the liver and gastrointestinal tract. Interactions affecting clearance may alter the body's ability to eliminate a drug, usually resulting in increased concentration of the drug.

Medication Dose Boxes

Medication dose boxes can improve medication compliance and ensure that the correct dose of medication is taken. Patients may have difficulty opening medicine bottles, may forget if they have taken medication, and may skip a dose or take a double dose. If the adult is taking multiple medications, the issue becomes more confusing. Most medication dose boxes can be filled with a week's worth of medications. Some boxes are harder to open than others, so the patient may have to try several types of boxes. Even patients able to manage their own medications often prefer the timesaving measure of preparing all medications for the week at one time. Some dose boxes will accommodate medications taken three to four times daily, but the day and time should be clearly marked on the individual cell. For people who have trouble remembering to take medications, there are a number of helpful electronic devices that can be programmed to give a reminder. There are dose boxes that beep and watches that signal time to take medications. Pharmacies will put easy-opening lids on pill bottles on request and some pharmacies, such as Target, will color-code bottles for different family members.

Medications That Commonly Cause Physiologic Responses

A **physiologic response** is a change that occurs as a result of a type of treatment, such as with a medication. The physiologic response of a medication may be positive, as in providing a therapeutic effect for which it was prescribed, or negative, as in untoward side effects. Many medications cause physiologic responses in the form of side effects, and some are mild, while others may be more severe. Common side effects of medications include nausea, vomiting, dizziness, headache, dry mouth, and itching. Other physiological responses that may occur and that may be life threatening include allergic reactions, such as hives, itching, swelling of the face and tongue, and breathing difficulties. Other drugs can cause effects that can be very serious, such as an increase in bleeding risk, changes in blood pressure levels, or an increased susceptibility to infection. Each drug has had thorough research and testing before being released for use, and side effects and warnings of physiologic changes should be listed on its packaging or available through a pharmacy.

Determining if a Medication is the Cause of a Pathologic Change

Administering medication is a multifaceted process, one that has the potential for complications associated with errors from the administrator as well as negative effects from the medication itself. In certain patients, a medication will produce pathologic changes as negative side effects. Determining whether medication is the cause of these changes may be difficult, especially if the symptoms overlap with other symptoms of illness. Eliminating the medication for a period of time to determine if it is the cause of the changes may not be an option for some patients who need the drugs for regular health maintenance. Close patient monitoring is important before, during, and after medication administration to determine changes in health or symptoms. The nurse who is familiar with a patient's baseline of health may be more likely to recognize if medications are causing pathologic changes. Significant changes should be reported to the physician to determine if there is an alternative treatment.

Analyzing Patient's Response to New Medication

Starting a new medication may cause an array of responses from the patient. Remembering to take the prescribed dose, refill the medication, and learning its effects often takes time. A patient who is prescribed new medications should be educated on purposes and side effects. The nurse must evaluate several aspects of the patient's response, including adherence to the medication regimen, whether side effects have developed, and if the medication is working for the problem for which it was prescribed. This must usually be done at a later time to give the medication time to achieve therapeutic levels. The nurse may discuss the medication with the patient to determine if there are any barriers to taking the medication, such as financial obstacles, unpleasant side effects, or lack of perceived need. After evaluating the patient's response, the nurse can make decisions about the need to provide further education about the importance of the medication, as well as assistance with situations where the patient is having difficulty adhering to the medication regimen.

Analyzing Patient's Response to New Therapy Regimen

An important component of nursing care is **continually evaluating the patient's response to interventions**, whether they are new medications, nursing interventions, or new therapy regimens. When a patient begins a new type of therapy, there may be a variety of responses to it. If the therapy is difficult, causes pain, interferes with his lifestyle, or otherwise causes discomfort, the patient may not appreciate the therapy and may have trouble adhering to the regimen. Alternatively, if the patient is deriving benefit from the therapy, understands the need for it, or otherwise enjoys it, it is more likely that this patient may continue to maintain the regimen. The nurse can assess the patient's response by discussing feelings about the therapy and perceived results of performing the regimen. Talking with the patient about any barriers preventing the patient from performing the therapy, and providing resources for assistance so that the patient can continue with the therapy as prescribed are positive ways to promote adherence.

Complementary and Alternative Therapies

Complementary Therapies

Complementary therapies are used as well as conventional medical treatment and should be included if this is what the patient/family wants, empowering the family to take some control. Complementary therapies vary widely, and most can easily be incorporated into the plan of care. The National Center for Complementary and Alternative Medicine recognizes the following:

- *Whole medical systems* include homeopathic, naturopathic medicine, acupuncture, and Chinese herbal medications.
- *Mind-body medicine* can include support groups, medication, music, art, or dance therapy.
- *Biologically-based practices* include the use of food, vitamins, or nutrition for healing.
- *Manipulative/body-based programs* include massage or other types of manipulation, such as chiropractic treatment.
- *Energy therapies* may be biofield therapies intended to affect the aura (energy field) that some believe surrounds all living things. These therapies include therapeutic touch and Reiki.
- *Bioelectromagnetic-based therapies* use a variety of magnetic fields.

Visualization/Therapeutic Imagery

Visualization (therapeutic imagery) is used with adults for a variety of purposes:

- Relaxation and reduction of stress
- Performance improvement
- Rehabilitation

The principles behind all of these are the same, although the focus of concentration is different. Visualization involves creating a visual image in the mind of a desired outcome and imagining or "feeling" oneself in that place or situation. For example, if the focus is on healing and recovery of an injured leg with limited range of motion, then the patient uses the senses to imagine how it "feels" to extend and flex the limb in normal range of motion and imagines walking and using the limb with the mind focused on the goal of therapy. All of the senses may be used to imagine a scene—what it looks like, smells like, feels like, and sounds like.

Methods

There are a number of methods used for **visualization.** Some include audiotapes with guided imagery, such as self-hypnosis tapes, but the adult can be taught basic techniques that include the following:

- Sit or lie comfortably in a quiet place away from distractions.
- Concentrate on breathing while taking long slow breaths.
- Close the eyes to shut out distractions, and create an image in the mind of the place or situation desired.
- Concentrate on that image, engaging as many senses as possible and imaging details.
- If the mind wanders, breathe deeply and bring consciousness back to the image or concentrate on breathing for a few moments and then return to the imagery.
- End with positive imagery.
- Sometimes, older adults are resistive at first or have a hard time maintaining focus, so guiding them through visualization for the first few times can be helpful.

Music Therapy

Music therapy is used for many different clinical purposes in occupational and physical therapy, perioperative care, geriatric care, and hospice care to do the following:

- Reduce anxiety and stress
- Control pain
- Alter moods
- Promote relaxation
- Aid sleep
- Promote alertness
- Promote activity
- Distract patient

Soothing background music is often played to help reduce stress and to help distract people from discomfort and from other background noise, such as that associated with equipment or treatments. People may listen to music, for example, during an MRI. Music has a number of physiological effects, depending on the type of music. Slow music may help decrease respiratory and heart rate and lower blood pressure as it promotes relaxation. Studies have shown that combining music and relaxation therapy is more effective than relaxation therapy alone. Fast music may help people maintain pace during exercise or stay alert. Music must be selected carefully and appropriately for the situation, keeping in mind personal preferences and ethnic background as tastes in music vary widely.

Herbal Remedies and Dietary Supplements

There are literally thousands of **herbal remedies and dietary supplements** and myriad claims of success in treating or preventing disease despite there being very little scientific evidence to support most claims. Many doctors recommend one daily multivitamin to ensure adequate vitamin intake and fish oil concentrate to reduce cholesterol, but patients often take high doses of herbal remedies and dietary supplements. This poses a number of problems. High doses of some vitamins can cause toxicity:

- *Vitamin A:* Headaches, loss of hair, liver damage, bone disorders, and birth defects
- *Vitamin C*: Diarrhea and gastrointestinal upset
- *Vitamin D:* Kidney stones, muscle weakness, and bleeding
- *Vitamin E:* Inhibits action of vitamin K
- *Niacin*: Liver damage, gastric ulcers, and increased serum glucose
- *Vitamin B_6:* Neurological damage

Herbal remedies often contain small amounts of agents found in drugs, so they can cause drug reactions and interactions. Also, patients often fail to inform their physicians when they are using alternative treatments.

Herbals

A wide variety of **herbals** are in common use. Some preparations contain ingredients similar to those found in prescription drugs, and some may interfere with absorption or utilization of prescription drugs, so herbals should be carefully reviewed during assessment:

Herbal	Uses	Adverse effects/problems
St. John's wort	Depression and anxiety	Nausea, dry mouth, headache, dizziness; May interact with antibiotics, birth control pills, antidepressants, warfarin, anticonvulsants, MAO inhibitors, antivirals, immunosuppressants and migraine drugs
Melatonin	Insomnia, Alzheimer's, cancer, ADHD, sexual disorders	Depression, lethargy, headache May interact with NSAIDS, antihypertensives, steroids, and antianxiety medications
Ginseng	Stress, cancer, high cholesterol, diabetes, and to increase immunity and strength	Headache, anxiety, insomnia, rash, breast tenderness, hypertension or hypotension, and vaginal bleeding; May interact with cardiac drugs, anticoagulants, aspirin, antidiabetic medications, diuretics, and NSAIDs
Gingko biloba	Alzheimer's, erectile dysfunction, mood elevation	GI disturbance, diarrhea, headache, muscle cramps, dizziness, seizures, increased bleeding, and skin irritation May interact with aspirin, anticoagulants, diuretics, and NSAIDs
Echinacea	Viral infections, UTIs, allergic rhinitis, and fungal infections	GI disturbance, constipation, diarrhea, dizziness, and rash May interact with immunosuppressants and steroids

INTEGRATING COMPLEMENTARY AND INTEGRATIVE THERAPIES INTO TREATMENT PLANS

Many **complementary and integrative therapies**, including massage, yoga, acupuncture, guided imagery, humor, and music therapy, pose little risk to the patient and much benefit and should be integrated into treatment plans according to patient's individual needs. These therapies are especially valuable for those with chronic disorders, such as low back pain, arthritis, anxiety, and hypertension. The nurse should assess the patient's use of complementary therapy and, when appropriate, advocate for continuing this therapy as part of the treatment plan. Additionally, the nurse can serve as a resource person for other staff and patients regarding the benefits of these therapies and help determine appropriate therapies for the patient's needs. Patients at risk because of complementary and integrative therapies, such as herbals with toxic properties, need a treatment plan to inform them and other health providers of the risks. Issues of concern include (1) the need for policies to support the use of these therapies, (2) appropriate consent forms, and (3) methods for monitoring and evaluating the therapies.

Non-Pharmacologic Interventions

DIETARY MANAGEMENT OF BOWEL DYSFUNCTION

Dietary management requires identifying foods that increase *bowel dysfunction*. This is accomplished by having the patient make a list of the foods that he or she eats in a one-week period and keep track of bowel activity. Foods to avoid are cured or smoked meats and spicy, fatty, and greasy foods, because these often cause diarrhea and fecal incontinence. Individuals who are lactose intolerant should avoid dairy products. Caffeine, alcohol, and some artificial sweeteners (such as aspartame, NutraSweet, and saccharine) can act as laxatives, so they should be avoided. However, Splenda and stevia do not usually cause a problem. Eating several small meals instead of fewer large meals may reduce bowel contractions. Increasing fiber intake to 20 to 30 grams per day results in formed stool that is easier to control; however, too much fiber can cause bloating and gas. Therefore, fiber should be slowly added to the diet. This can be accomplished by adding whole fruits, whole grains, and vegetables to the diet. Fluid intake should be at least eight glasses per day to prevent constipation and impaction.

DIETARY FACTORS RELATED TO URINARY INCONTINENCE

Dietary factors can cause urinary incontinence. Caffeine occurs naturally in coffee beans, tea leaves, and cocoa beans. Caffeine is also contained in many soft drinks, chocolate drinks, and candy. In addition, it is also an additive in many drugs (such as Excedrin, Anacin, Darvon Compound, and Fiorinal). Caffeine can increase detrusor muscle contractions, causing increased pressure that can result in urinary urgency and frequent urination. Artificial sweeteners (such as aspartame, NutraSweet, and saccharine) are bladder irritants. Citrus foods (orange juice and cranberry juice, for example) are highly acidic and irritate the lining of the bladder. Substances that irritate the bladder can worsen overactive bladder and urge incontinence. Spicy foods, such as Mexican food, Chinese food, horseradish, and chili peppers also irritate the bladder lining. Excessive fluid intake (more than 32-48 ounces per day) can exacerbate both stress and urge incontinence. Alcohol acts directly on the bladder as a diuretic.

RECOMMENDED DIETARY CHANGES TO ADD PROTEIN AND CALORIES TO THE DIET

There are a number of **dietary changes that can add protein** to the diet. Before increasing dietary protein, comorbid conditions such as diabetes or high cholesterol should be considered; some foods, such as cheese, are high in sodium and fat, which may be restricted. Methods of increasing protein include adding meat to vegetarian dishes; adding milk powder to many foods during preparation; substituting milk for water in soups, hot cereals, and cocoa; adding cheese to dishes such as pastas and casseroles; providing high-protein drinks, such as Ensure High Protein; using peanut butter on bread and apples; and adding extra eggs to dishes such as custards and meat loaf. Methods to increase *calories* in the diet include using whole milk or cream rather than low-fat or nonfat milk; adding butter, sour cream, or whipping cream to foods; and eating frequent snacks.

Dietary Fiber in Managing Constipation

Constipation is usually caused by insufficient fiber in the diet. Diets high in processed foods often contain inadequate amounts of fiber. An adequate amount of fiber is 20 to 30 grams daily. There are both soluble and insoluble forms of fiber, and both add bulk to the stool. Soluble and insoluble fibers are not absorbed by the body. Some foods contain both types. *Soluble fiber* dissolves in liquids to form a gel-like substance. This is one reason why liquids are so important in conjunction with fiber in the diet. Soluble fiber slows the movement of stool through the gastrointestinal tract. Food sources include bananas, starches (such as potatoes and bread), cheese, dried beans, nuts, apples, oranges, and oatmeal. *Insoluble fiber* changes little with the digestive process and increases the speed of stool through the colon, so too much can result in diarrhea. Food sources of insoluble fiber include oat bran, seeds, skins of fruits, vegetables, and nuts.

DASH

The National Institutes of Health and the National Heart, Lung, and Blood Institute have developed a program called **Dietary Approaches to Stop Hypertension (DASH).** Nutrient goals (based on a 2,100 calorie diet) include total fat, 27 percent of total calories; saturated fat, 6 percent; protein, 18 percent; carbohydrates, 55 percent; cholesterol, 150 mg; sodium, 1,500 to 2,300 mg; potassium, 4,700mg; calcium, 1,250 mg; magnesium, 500 mg; and fiber, 30 g. Food groups and daily servings are as follow: grains (whole grains preferred), six to eight; vegetables and fruits, four to five each; fat-free or low-fat milk/milk products, two to three; lean meat, poultry, fish six servings or less (serving = one ounce); fats and oils, two to three servings; nuts, seeds, legumes, four to five per week; and sweets and added sugars, five or less per week. Serving size depends on the food.

NDD

The **National Dysphagia Diet (NDD)** was developed by the American Dietetic Association:

- *NDD-1* (dysphagia pureed) includes foods with the consistency of pudding (such as puddings and pureed meats, fruits, and vegetables). Foods excluded from the diet include scrambled eggs, peanut butter, gelatin, yogurt with fruit, and cottage cheese. A variation of this diet is the dysphagia mixed diet. This is the NDD-1 diet with one item from NDD-2 included.
- *NDD-2* (dysphagia mechanically altered) includes moist, soft, easily chewed food, such as ground or finely diced meats, tender vegetables, soft fruit, smooth moistened cereals, scrambled eggs, pancakes, and juice (thickened if needed). Excluded foods include breads, cakes, rice, peas, corn, hard fruits and vegetables, skin of fruit/vegetable, nuts, and seeds. The mechanically softened diet is a variation of the NDD-2 diet. It is the same except that it allows bread, cakes, and rice.
- *NDD-3* (dysphagia advanced) includes foods with regular texture, including moist tender meats, breads, cake, rice, and shredded lettuce. Excluded are hard fruits and vegetables, corn, skins, nuts, and seeds.

MNT for Diabetes

Medical nutrition therapy (MNT) for diabetes includes individualized diet modifications, which may include low-fat and low-carbohydrate guidelines. Saturated fats should be restricted to less than seven percent of the total calories. Carbohydrates should be monitored through the use of carbohydrate counting or exchanges. About 45 to 65 percent of total calories should come from complex carbohydrates, and simple carbohydrates (found in sugars, pasta, potatoes, and rice) should be limited. Severely restricted carbohydrate intake (<130 mg daily) is not recommended. Sugar alcohols and nonnutritive sweeteners (such as aspartame and Splenda) are permissible. Alcohol intake should be limited to one drink per day for females and two drinks per day for males. If weight loss is an issue, women should limit intake to 1,000 to 1,200 kilocalories (kcal) per day. Men should limit their intake to 1,200 to 1,600 kcal per day. This should result in a weight loss of one to two pounds per week.

Seventh Report of the Joint National Committee on Prevention, Detection, Evaluation, and Treatment of High Blood Pressure Recommendations for Reducing Weight

The **Seventh Report of the Joint National Committee on Prevention, Detection, Evaluation, and Treatment of High Blood Pressure** has recommended a number of lifestyle changes to reduce weight:

- ***Decrease sedentary behaviors***: Long periods spent watching television, searching the Internet, playing video games, and instant messaging should be avoided. A time limit should be established to encourage physical activity.
- ***Increase exercise and physical activity***: Everyone should engage in at least 30 minutes of exercise daily (a minimum 150 minutes/week) if possible. Walking, biking, aerobic dancing, weight lifting, tennis, and exercise and dance classes are beneficial. Group activities, such as hiking, can encourage participation.
- ***Modify diet***: Food portions, dietary fat, and simple carbohydrates should be reduced. Snacking between meals should be avoided or healthy snacks (such as celery sticks) substituted.
- ***Modify beverage intake***: Consumption of high-calorie, high-carbohydrate beverages (such as sodas, juices, and flavored and sweetened water) should be reduced.

Nursing Therapeutics

Nursing therapeutics comprises all activities intended for patient care, including the Assessment and History themselves as well as outcome goals. Approaches to nursing therapeutics vary according to the guiding theory. Nursing therapeutics can include:

- **Touch therapy:** Touch is used to exchange energy, promote relaxation, reduce anxiety, manage pain, and promote healing.
- **Role supplementation:** When role insufficiency (inability to carry out roles) occurs, role supplementation provides preventive and therapeutic strategies to decrease or eliminate the role insufficiency.
- **Care:** The nurse assists patients in providing self-care and identifies self-care deficits and offers strategies to compensate.
- **Use of self:** The nurse purposefully uses the self (personality, knowledge) as part of the therapeutic process to bring about changes in the patient.
- **Symptom management:** Strategies for management of symptoms are developed, influenced by various physiological, psychological, and situational factors.
- **Transitional care:** Focus is on assisting patients transitioning from hospital to home, including coordination of care, engagement of caregivers, management of symptoms, and education to promote self-care.
- **Comfort:** While need for comfort is universal, the need for comfort during illness may vary according to disease and condition.

Nonpharmacologic Assessment and History

Nonpharmacologic assessment and history in nursing therapeutics may include a range of techniques associated with complementary medicine.

- *Massage*: Using massage to decrease pain, reduce anxiety, and promote relaxation
- *Validation therapy*: Validating the patient by empathizing with the patient's feelings and emotions rather than with behavior
- *Behavioral therapy*: Using positive reinforcement to help patients control behavior
- *Music therapy*: Using music to help relax or energize patients and reduce anxiety
- *Aromatherapy*: Using aromas to soothe patients, reduce symptoms, and promote well-being
- *Light therapy*: Manipulating light to help maintain circadian rhythm and decrease depression
- *Activity therapy*: Using activities such as dancing, exercising, walking, and participating in sports to improve physical and mental functioning
- *Reality orientation*: Using materials, such as clocks, signs, and calendars, to help orient patients
- *Reminiscence therapy*: Helping patients remember past experiences to promote pleasure and sense of well-being
- *Multisensory therapy*: Providing a variety of textures, sights, lights, smells, and sounds to stimulate the senses

Equipment

Part of nursing therapeutics is prescribing and using necessary **equipment**, which may range widely, depending on the purpose and the patient's condition. Equipment may include all durable medical equipment (DME) as well as a variety of other materials used as tools to promoting health and well-being.

- *Preventing injury:* overlays, support surfaces, footboards, padding, grab rails, support bars
- *Promoting activity:* walkers, canes, crutches, wheelchairs, monkey bars, over-bed poles.
- *Promoting independence*: grabbers, assistive devices for cooking, dressing, and other activities
- *Promoting relaxation/enjoyment*: music CDs, videos, books, games, and magazines
- *Orienting patient*: calendars, clocks, and signage
- *Assessing physical condition:* blood pressure cuff, thermometer, and stethoscope
- *Providing wound care:* scissors, gloves, PPE, dressing supplies
- *Promoting continence:* urinals, bedside commodes
- *Maintaining and improving oxygenation*: pulse oximeter, oxygen, and oxygen-delivery devices

Procedures and Treatment

The CNS may prescribe and carry out a wide range of **procedures and treatments**, in accordance with the scope of practice established by the individual state as well as the institution. The CNS in acute-care settings may perform a number of procedures that in the past were reserved for physicians. These can include such procedures as insertion of central lines and gastrostomy tubes, and wound debridement, but this varies widely from one state to another. Prescribed procedures and treatments must relate to the CNS's area of specialization. In all cases, the CNS must review the state Nurse Practice Act and the privileges accorded to the CNS. Some CNS's do not have prescriptive authority because they have not completed necessary requirements or because they are restricted by the state in which they are licensed.

Therapeutic Massage

Therapeutic massage is often included in the treatment plan for musculoskeletal disorders, such as pulled muscles, stiffness, and low back pain. Studies show that massage helps reduce pain and anxiety and may reduce blood pressure and stimulate the immune system. Techniques include:

- *Compression*: deep rhythmical compressions of the muscles to increase circulation and make muscles more pliable
- *Effleurage*: massage done in rhythmical broad strokes with the palms of the hands to relax patients
- *Friction*: massage either in line with muscle fibers or across the muscle fibers to create stretching and to reduce adhesions and scarring
- *Petrissage*: kneading massage, usually used on large muscle areas, such as the calf or thigh, to increase circulation and relax muscles
- *Vibration*: vibratory massage used for deep muscle relaxation and reduction of pain
- *Tapotement*: massage using quick rhythmic tapping to increase circulation or relieve cramped muscles
- *Trigger point*: pressure applied with a finger or thumb to areas of point tenderness to reduce spasticity and pain

Progression in Strengthening Exercises

Older adults may benefit from **strengthening exercises** to improve both strength and mobility. Many facilities offer special exercise programs for older adults. The exercises follow a progression:

- *Isometric exercises* are done with the muscle and limb in static position with no movement of the joint or lengthening of the muscle. The muscle is contracted against resistance.
- *Isotonic exercises* include movement of the joint during exercise (such as walking and weight lifting) and both shortening and lengthening of the muscles through eccentric or concentric contractions. Isotonic refers to tension, so the tension is constant during shortening and lengthening of the muscle.
- *Isokinetic exercises* make use of machines (such as stationary bicycles) to control the rate and extent of contraction as well as the range of motion. Both speed and resistance can be set, so the patient is limited by the settings of the machine.

Aquatic Exercise

Aquatic exercise can be very beneficial. Aquatic exercise can effectively increase range of motion of the arms and legs and improve balance by strengthening the trunk and abdomen. Immersion in water causes a number of physiological effects unrelated to the exercises. Physiological changes include increased cardiac and intrapulmonary blood volume with increases in pressure in the right atrium and increased volume at left ventricular diastole. In addition, there is increased stroke volume and overall cardiac output. Concurrently, there is a reduction in peripheral circulation and lung expansion, decreasing vital capacity. Heart rate often remains unchanged or remains significantly lower than when doing similar exercises outside of the water. This effect depends on the depth of the water and speed of exercise. Resistance in water increases with depth of immersion up to about the middle of the body. After this point, buoyancy counterbalances resistance. Exercising in water at waist level results in a similar heart rate and consumption of oxygen as exercising out of the water.

Cardiovascular Conditioning/Endurance Training

Cardiovascular conditioning/endurance training is especially important after injury or illness because cardiovascular/respiratory fitness can decrease rapidly with inactivity. The type of cardiovascular exercises will depend upon the site of injury and the phase of healing. The following provide examples:

- If there is an injury of a lower extremity, then non-weight bearing exercises, such as swimming, weight lifting, or upper body cycling may be indicated.
- If there is an injury to an upper extremity, then weight bearing exercises, such as climbing stairs, running, aerobics, or use of elliptical machine is more appropriate.
- Cardiac rehabilitation focuses on the whole body.
- In all cases, the type of cardiovascular conditioning should be tailored to the individual with a goal of increased heart rate of 60-90% of maximal heart rate (220 – person's age x 0.65) for 15-60 minutes ≥3 times weekly.

Exercise Considerations for Older Adults

Exercises should be tailored for the individual older adult. Warm-up exercises should be part of any exercise program and should be performed before participation in sports activities. Warm-up exercises increase circulation and muscle elasticity and prevent injury. Warm-up exercises should begin slowly and systematically involve all parts of the body. There are three types of warm-up: passive, general body wide, and specific stretching motions. Passive warm-up may include a massage or a warm shower. General body wide warm-ups may include brisk walking. Specific stretching motions should be bilateral and static. It's important to stretch and warm up all muscles, but special attention should be paid to the muscles most used in the activity. Exercise should be low to moderate in intensity to prevent injury. The duration of exercise should be increased gradually to 30 or more minutes daily (or three 10-minute periods) with a goal of daily exercise.

Mental Aerobics

Mental aerobics are exercises to maintain cognitive ability and memory skills. Those who remain active mentally have a lower incidence of Alzheimer's disease and may slow progression of dementia and prompt neurogenesis (development of new neurons). Exercises should focus on right brain, left brain, and whole brain stimulation. Older adults should start with simple exercises and then progress to more difficult ones. There are many different types of activities that are part of mental aerobics, but the goal is to exert mental effort to "exercise" the brain:

- Taking classes and learning new information
- Reading books that contain new material
- Solving puzzles (crossword, jigsaw, Sudoku, scrambled words, symbol sequence, mazes)
- Using the non-dominant hand to eat, draw, comb hair, brush teeth, or write
- Using mnemonic devices to help facilitate short and long-term memory
- Studying a new language

Bladder Diary

A Bladder diary is a complete daily record of all urinations and episodes of urinary incontinence. The diary is usually kept for 3-5 days as part of the urological assessment and includes the following:

- *Time* must be recorded to document patterns of urination.
- *Amount* of urination should be estimated (small, medium, or large) or measured as directed.

- *Intake* should be recorded to determine if fluids are contributing to incontinence or urinary problems.
- *Incontinence* should be characterized by estimations of amount. A small volume of less than 30 ml is enough to wet the underwear. A moderate volume of 30-60 ml is enough to soak the underwear with overflow down the legs. A large volume of more than 60 ml is usually enough to soak clothes and run onto the floor or furniture.
- *Incontinence* should be characterized by activity and sensation of urge at the time of incontinence to help determine the type of incontinence.

Bladder Retraining

Bladder retraining teaches people to control the urge to urinate. It usually takes about three months to strengthen a bladder muscle weakened from frequent urination. Frequent urination may cause a decreased urinary capacity. A short urination interval is gradually lengthened to every two to four hours during the daytime. The urge to void is resisted for increasingly longer periods of time. To start, the person keeps a bladder (or urination) diary for a week to establish a baseline frequency. An individual program is established with scheduled voiding times and goals. For example, if a person is urinating every hour, the goal might be every 80 minutes with increased output. When the urination goal is met consistently, a new goal is established. The progress is charted in the urination diary. The person is taught techniques to stop urination. For example, the person is instructed to sit on a hard seat or on a tightly rolled towel to put pressure on pelvic floor muscles and squeeze the pelvic floor muscles five times while breathing deeply and counting backwards from 50.

The Knack to Control Urinary Incontinence

The knack is the use of precisely-timed muscle contractions to prevent stress incontinence. It is "the knack" of squeezing up before bearing down. The knack is a preventive use of Kegel exercises. Women are taught to contract the pelvic floor muscles right before and during events that usually cause stress incontinence. For example, if a woman feels a cough or sneeze coming, she immediately contracts the pelvic floor muscles and holds until the stress event is over. This contraction augments support of the proximal urethra, reducing the amount of displacement that usually takes place with compromised muscle support, thereby preventing incontinence. It is particularly useful if used before and during stress events, such as coughing, sneezing, lifting, standing, swinging a golf club, or laughing. Studies have shown that women who are taught this technique for mild to moderate urinary incontinence and use it consistently are able to decrease incontinence by 73 to 98%.

Nocturia

Nocturia is a condition in which an individual wakes up one or more times during the night with the need to urinate. Some authorities believe that one event per night is within normal limits. Some people have to urinate five or six times each night. In about 70 percent of cases, nocturia is related to overproduction of urine at night. Nocturia is one of the most common causes of sleep deprivation. Approximately two-thirds of those older than age 50 have nocturia. Studies have shown that nocturia involving urination more than two times each night is strongly linked to depression. The goal of treatment is to reduce urination during the night. Treatment involves medication and/or fluid management. The primary treatment for nocturia is the medication desmopressin (Stimate). This drug acts as an antidiuretic hormone that reduces volume of urine by increasing concentration. This medication allows for about five hours of undisturbed sleep. It increases the first period of sleep by about two hours. Fluid management by reducing fluids in the evening can help some people.

Bowel Diary

Bowel diary is a complete daily record of all defecations and episodes of fecal or flatal incontinence. The diary is usually kept for 3-5 days as part of the intestinal assessment and includes the following:

- *Time* of each event should be carefully documented.
- *Type* of bowel movement should be noted, using the Bristol Stool Form Scale or other guide: hard lumps, sausage-shaped, cracked sausage-shaped, smooth and snake-like, soft blobs, fluffy pieces, or liquid.
- *Amount* of stool should be estimated.
- *Abnormalities* such as blood or mucous and the need for finger splinting or straining should be noted.
- *Fecal incontinence* should be characterized by amount and type and activity at the time of incontinence.
- Flatal incontinence should be noted.
- *Intake* of both food and fluids should be recorded to see if intake relates to bowel activities.
- *Medications* should all be recorded, including laxatives, vitamins, and any over-the-counter preparations.

Bowel Retraining

Bowel retraining is a behavioral modification program that helps people establish control over bowel disorders. It teaches strategies to develop a routine schedule for defecation:

- The person keeps a bowel diary for a week.
- Diet and fluid intake are modified to assure normal stool consistency. This may include increasing fiber and fluids, eating meals at scheduled times, and avoiding foods that increase bowel dysfunction.
- A schedule for defecation is established, preferably at the same time each day and about 20-30 minutes after a meal, which stimulates the gastrocolic reflex that propels fecal material through colon.
- The person is taught Kegel exercises to strengthen muscles.
- A stimulus is used to promote defecation. The stimulus may be an enema, suppository, or laxative in the beginning, but the goal is to decrease such use. Digital stimulation or hot drinks may be used.
- The person keeps a record of stool consistency and evacuation.

Kegel Exercises

Pelvic floor muscle exercises, also known as **Kegel exercises,** are used to strengthen the periurethral and pelvic muscles in order to increase control of urination and fecal elimination. Basic exercises involve tightening the muscles for about 3 seconds and then relaxing for the same period. The exercise should be repeated about 10 times, gradually increasing the time tightening the muscles to 5-10 seconds. The exercise set should be performed 3 to 4 times daily. Isolating the right muscles to tighten is important. Tightening the stomach, leg, or other muscles will not help. People should not hold their breath during the exercises because this may tighten other muscles. There are three methods to check that the pelvic floor muscles are flexing:

- Stop flow of urine in the midst of urination.
- Pull in the anus as though trying to stop from passing flatus.
- In supine position, place finger inside the vagina and squeeze as though trying to stop urine. Tightness should be felt.

Kegel exercises strengthen the pelvic floor muscles, which cross the floor of the pelvis and attach to the pubic bone and coccyx. The urethra, rectum, and vagina all open through the pelvic floor muscles, which support the pelvic organs.

- *Caution*: Avoid holding the breath or tightening the abdominal or buttocks muscles during pelvic floor exercises.
- *Procedure*: Tighten and squeeze the muscles about the rectum, vagina, and urethra and try to "lift" them inside as though trying to stop from passing gas and urine. Hold. Relax. Rest a few seconds. Repeat.
- *Schedule*: Exercises should be done at least 3 times daily. They may be done while lying down in the morning and evening and while sitting at midday.
- *1-2 weeks:* Tighten 1 second and relax 5. Repeat 10 times. Then tighten 5 seconds and relax 10. Repeat 10 times.
- *3-4 weeks:* Tighten 5-10 seconds and relax 10. Repeat 20 times.
- *5-6 weeks:* Tighten 8-10 seconds and relax 10. Repeat 20 times.

Caring for Patients with Alzheimer's Disease or Cognitive Impairment

Toileting

Urinary and fecal incontinence usually occur over time in patients with Alzheimer's disease and cognitive impairment. However, in the early stages, certain practices, such as **scheduled toileting** (every 2 to 4 hours), fluid monitoring, and reducing fluid intake after dinner can help control the problem. Stool softeners may be administered to help bowel function; however, laxatives should be avoided as they may exacerbate the problem. Constipation and diarrhea can be controlled by monitoring diet. Protective coverings should be placed over the mattress and seat cushions. Disposable pads or adult diapers may eventually be necessary. The patients may resist the use of these products; different products should be tried to find one acceptable to the patient. Inappropriate toilets such as wastebaskets should be removed if necessary. A commode may be placed in a convenient location close to a chair or the bed if necessary.

Sundowner's Syndrome

Sundowner's syndrome, also called sleep-wake cycle disruption, is a disturbance of the normal sleep-wake pattern. Some patients get up during the night and wander around the house or go through drawers or closets. They may move items around or tie them up in packages. Keeping the patient awake during the daytime can help manage the condition. In addition, turning on bright lights in the evening can help maintain the sleep-wake cycle. It may be possible to reestablish the sleep-wake cycle over one to two weeks of concerted effort. However, some people resist the process or get up at night to urinate and fail to go back to bed. Fluid restriction in the evening and/or scheduled toileting may help manage the condition. It may help to put the patient back to bed. The patient should be kept calm and relaxed at bedtime. Some patients fall asleep in a chair. In this case, a comfortable recliner placed the room may encourage the patient to sit down and fall asleep.

Wandering

Some patients with Alzheimer's disease or cognitive impairment tend to **wander**. This may be due to confusion. After getting lost, the patient may become frightened and hide. Patients should be registered with the Alzheimer's Association MedicAlert + Safe Return program. Patients enrolled in this program are given a MedicAlert bracelet, which they should wear at all times. It may be necessary to use alarms, latches, and locks to keep track of patients, but alarms may frighten the patient. It is best that the alarms sound in the caregiver's room rather than in the patient's room. Latches at either the top or bottom of a door are usually enough because patients usually don't think to look for a latch. In some cases, hanging a sheet or curtain over a doorway will prevent the patient from exiting through the door as patients in this condition often forget the door is there. Baby monitors may be used to keep track of the patient.

Maintaining Assistive Devices

There are many different assistive devices available. These include basic items (dentures, Velcro openings, elastic shoestrings, and grab bars); tools (reaching devices and special cookware, dishes, and silverware); and large pieces of equipment (oxygen tanks, wheelchairs, walkers, and commodes). **Maintaining assistive devices** can be difficult. The first step is to assist the person to make a comprehensive list of devices he or she uses and then prepare a checklist indicating what needs to be done for maintenance. This process also helps the nurse to evaluate the need for assistive devices. Different types of devices require different types of maintenance. Some devices may only need periodic cleaning (commodes and urinals). Other devices may require battery changes or servicing. If there is a caregiver, they should be informed about the maintenance of any equipment used by the patient in his or her care.

Call Bells and Personal Alarms

There are numerous call bells and personal alarms available. Most **call bells** have a push button of some type, although voice-activated devices are available. Some services make daily calls to patients and notify family or emergency services if there is no answer. One type of **personal alarm** available for has a base set and an alarm that is worn on a pendent around the neck or on a wrist strap. If the person falls or needs help, he or she presses the alarm. The alarm alerts a call center that sends assistance. There are alert alarm systems (movement sensors) that attach to the patient's clothes. These alarms are meant to prevent wandering. An alarm sounds if the person falls or gets out of the bed or chair. Movement sensors in stationary positions (such as by a doorway) sound an alarm if a patient walks or moves past the sensor. Door alarms sound when a patient tries opens a door.

Substance Use and Addictive Disorders

Substance Abuse in Older Adults

Approximately 7 percent of Americans abuse alcohol and many abuse other drugs. Alcohol and drug abuse are often linked to an underlying psychiatric disorder. Of concern **substance abuse** by the elderly often remains undiagnosed.

Commonly abused prescription drugs include narcotics and benzodiazepines. Abuse of benzodiazepine may lead to an increase in falls and auto accidents. The effects of benzodiazepine are potentiated if the drug is taken with alcohol or narcotics. Patients may experience withdrawal symptoms if the medication, especially Xanax, is stopped suddenly.

Drug abusers often have multiple prescriptions from different doctors.

Nonprescription drugs include over-the-counter sleep preparations and alcohol. Alcohol may cause symptoms similar to those of depression. Individuals who abuse alcohol may develop chronic disorders (such as cirrhosis, cardiomyopathy, and neuropathy), because many alcoholics do not eat a healthy diet and suffer from B_1 deficiency. Further, alcohol brain syndrome can develop and lead to suicide. Withdrawal may cause delirium tremens and seizures.

Illicit drugs include marijuana.

Signs of Long-Term Substance Abuse

Many people with substance abuse (alcohol or drugs) are reluctant to disclose this information, but there are a number of indicators that are suggestive of **long-term substance abuse:**

- **Physical signs**
  - Needle tracks on arms or legs
  - Burns on fingers or lips
  - Pupils abnormally dilated or constricted; eyes watery
  - Slurring of speech, slow speech
  - Lack of coordination, instability of gait
  - Tremors
  - Sniffing repeatedly, nasal irritation
  - Persistent cough
  - Weight loss
  - Dysrhythmias
  - Pallor, puffiness of face
- **Other signs**
  - Odor of alcohol/marijuana on clothing or breath
  - Labile emotions, including mood swings, agitation, and anger
  - Inappropriate, impulsive, and/or risky behavior
  - Lying
  - Missing appointments
  - Difficulty concentrating/short term memory loss, disoriented/confused
  - Blackouts
  - Insomnia or excessive sleeping
  - Lack of personal hygiene

Alcohol Addiction

All patients should be assessed for **alcohol addiction** as part of the initial physical exam. If there are health indications (abnormal liver function tests, falls, or insomnia) or social indications (family problems, divorce, or job loss) subsequent assessments should be made. There are numerous self-assessment screening tools used to measure drinking. About 33 percent of older adult alcoholics began drinking at an older age, often in response to depression. Social drinking is common in retirement facilities. Studies indicate that there may be some health benefits to the consumption of small amounts of wine, but alcohol often interacts with drugs and this can lead to complications. Therefore, the patient should not drink until the physician has reviewed the patient's medications and determined that it is safe. If the patient has a problem with alcohol, the nurse should discuss the assessment with the patient. The patient should be informed of the health consequences of drinking. The patient should be provided with information about resources (such as Alcoholics Anonymous and alcohol rehabilitation programs).

12-Step Programs

Alcoholics Anonymous was created in 1935 by Bill Wilson and Bob Smith based on 12 steps to recovery with a strong spiritual component. Other 12-step programs, such as Narcotics Anonymous, Over-eaters Anonymous, Sexual Compulsions Anonymous, and Gamblers Anonymous, all are based on the same premise that the aberrant behavior is a form of addiction, but over time there has been less emphasis on religion. Basic tenets of all of these programs include the following:

- Admitting the inability to control the compulsion/addiction
- Looking to a greater power for strength
- Using the assistance of experienced members to examine and come to terms with past errors
- Making amends
- Establishing a new code of behavior and living accordingly
- Assisting others with the same compulsion/addiction
- Twelve-step programs promote the concept that individuals with substance abuse have essentially an allergy-like response that causes them to be addicted, but even in the case where substances are not involved (Gamblers Anonymous), there is an inability to control compulsions.

Prescription Drug Addictions

Abuse of prescription drugs includes taking a lower dose than prescribed, taking a higher dose than prescribed, or taking the drugs erratically. Older adults are particularly vulnerable to abuse of prescription drugs because of easy access. Approximately a third of all prescriptions are written for older adults. Many older adults are isolated and have infrequent contact with health-care providers. For these reasons, symptoms of prescription drug abuse (such as confusion, falls, or lethargy) may be overlooked or attributed to health conditions, such as Alzheimer's disease. People who abuse alcohol often abuse prescription drugs as well, so assessment of alcohol abuse should also include assessment for drug abuse. Patients who abuse drugs may see a number of different physicians to obtain prescriptions. Narcotic analgesics (taken to control chronic pain) and central nervous system depressants (taken to reduce anxiety and improve sleep) are the most commonly abused prescription drugs. Patients often deny abuse of drugs even though the evidence of abuse is clear. Treatment may include behavioral therapy, medications to relieve withdrawal symptoms, and 12-step or other recovery programs.

Recreational Drug Use

Illicit **recreational drug use** by older adults in the United States is expected to increase 300 percent between 2001 and 2020. Currently, the incidence of recreational drug use among older adults is a relatively low 1.7 percent (up from 1 percent 10 years ago). However, this percentage is expected to increase dramatically as more long-term users from the baby boomer generation enter older age. Adding to the increase is the fact that methadone programs and better treatment for human immunodeficiency virus/acquired immune deficiency syndrome (HIV/AIDS) have prolonged the lives of illicit drug users, many of whom in the past would not have lived to an older age. The stress of dealing with aging and chronic illness causes some older adults to turn to recreational drugs to reduce stress or relieve symptoms. Marijuana, which is the most frequently abused recreational drug, is frequently taken for "health" reasons. Marijuana may impair short-term memory, executive functioning, and attention. Treatment for drug use includes behavioral therapy and 12-step programs. Programs geared toward older adults are usually more successful in treating this age group.

TOBACCO ADDICTION

Approximately 10 percent of adults older than 65 use **tobacco** (primarily cigarettes). Many more are former smokers. Older adult smokers are at particular risk for smoking-related diseases because they often have smoked for more than 40 years and are usually heavy smokers. Smoking is the cause of 90 percent of chronic obstructive pulmonary disease cases. Smokers are twice as likely as nonsmokers to die from stroke or heart attack. Smoking reduces life expectancy by 13 to 15 years, so patients of any age should be advised to quit completely. Quitting smoking can prolong life and improve the quality of life. Simply reducing the amount of tobacco used has little health benefit, and use usually increases again after a time. Many long-term smokers have numerous health problems related to smoking. Smokers may be extremely resistant to quitting in spite of the health risks because of tobacco's addictive qualities. Patients who abuse other substances (alcohol or drugs) are more likely to fall asleep while smoking than patients who do not abuse other substances and are more likely to suffer burns as a consequence.

SEX ADDICTION

Sex addiction occurs when people become fixated on sex, arousal, and thrill seeking. The act of sex becomes more important than intimacy. This addiction often causes people to seek sexual relations with multiple partners (sometimes younger), including prostitutes. Sex addiction may also take the form of masturbation in response to Internet pornography or inappropriate behavior, such as masturbating in public or exposing oneself. Sex addiction that involves multiple partners increases the danger of both getting and spreading sexually transmitted diseases (STDs). While it does not cause sex addiction, Viagra (and other such drugs) can fuel sex addiction in males. Indications of sex addiction include increasing need for sexual stimulation; inability to control sexual urges; engaging in high-risk sexual activities (such as contact with prostitutes); utilizing sexual fantasies to cope with stress; mood swings; and neglecting social obligations, family, and friends. Most people with sex addiction are reluctant to discuss their disorder. The subject should be raised with individuals with STDs or those found engaging in inappropriate behavior. The disorder is treated with behavioral therapy.

GAMBLING ADDICTION

Older adults often find it easy to gamble with the prevalence of lotteries, casinos, and Internet gambling sites. Older adults may turn to **gambling** as an outlet for frustration or stress and may not understand the dynamics of addiction before they have squandered their savings. Because of the difficulty older adults have in finding employment, they may not be able to replace the money that they lost, resulting in increasing poverty and stress. Older adults who get into debt through gambling may argue about the habit with family or friends. Older adults with cognitive impairment may not completely understand the implications of losing money gambling. Gambling problems may be difficult to identify, because older adults may hide their addiction because of embarrassment. They are often reluctant to seek counseling to help them stop gambling. Signs of gambling include an increased focus on gambling to the exclusion of other activities; physical problems such as headaches, increased anxiety, depression, bowel and bladder problems, and constant tiredness; and financial concerns and lack of basic needs (such as food and clothing).

Family and Caregiver Roles

CAREGIVER BURDEN

Caregiver burden results from the demands of caring for patients who are physically or mentally disabled, such as those with advanced Parkinson's disease or Alzheimer's. The caregiver may feel overwhelmed by responsibilities, lack of adequate rest, isolation, financial difficulties, and sheer physical exhaustion. Most caregivers are unpaid family members, such as spouses or children, and most recipients of care are >50. More than half of caregivers are women, and many live in poverty. Depression occurs in over half of caregivers, especially those providing care ≥20 hours weekly, and many caregivers provide round-the-clock care every day, with little respite. The person receiving care may live in the home of the caregiver or separately. Caregivers often lack the knowledge and skills to effectively provide care, but have no one to turn to for help. Over time, the caregiver may become increasingly depressed, angry, and resentful, and this can lead to abuse or neglect of the patient.

Assessment

Caregiver burden assessment may include a variety of self-assessment questions that the caregiver rates as occurring never (0), rarely (1), sometimes (2), frequently (3), or almost always (4). The higher the score, the more the burden. Typical questions include these:

- Does the person you care for ask for more help than necessary?
- Does caregiving rob you of time you need for yourself?
- Do your combined responsibilities of caregiving and other responsibilities cause stress?
- Are you embarrassed by the person's behavior?
- Do you feel angry when providing care?
- Do you worry about the person's future?
- Is caregiving affecting your relationship with other family members?
- Is the person too dependent on you?
- Are you stressed around this person?
- Has caregiving negatively affected your health?
- Has caregiving interfered with your social life?
- Do you avoid having friends over because of this person?
- Are you concerned about expenses related to care?
- Do you feel you have no control over your life?
- Would you like to be able to stop caring for this person?
- Do you think you should provide more or better care?

Methods for Relief

Assessing the caregiver for **caregiver burden** must be followed by proactive steps to help the caregiver cope and better manage care. **Support mechanisms include:**

- Provide support through regular contact, allowing the caregiver to express feelings and concerns.
- Make referrals to appropriate community resources, such as home health agencies, Meals-on-Wheels, and Social Services.
- Assist in identifying and finding appropriate respite care, such as adult daycare programs.
- Encourage participation in support groups for caregivers.
- Assess the patient's needs and provide basic training in care to the caregiver, such as methods to avoid choking and ways to safely transfer the patient.
- Encourage the caregiver to approach family members or friends to assist with care or sit with the patient for periods of time so the caregiver can have some time for him/herself.
- Complete an environmental assessment and provide information about improving safety measures in the home, such as installing latches, alarms, safety bars, and shower chairs, and removing barriers such as scatter rugs.

Resources for Caregivers

Knowledge

Many caregivers are unprepared for the **role of caregiver** and **lack knowledge** about the patient's disease and treatments or strategies to care for the patient. Caregivers should be provided oral and, when appropriate, printed information about the basics of the disease process, including what to expect in the future. For example, a caregiver for a parent with early-onset Alzheimer's needs to be taught about the different stages of Alzheimer's, problems that may arise, and possible interventions, both pharmaceutical and nonpharmaceutical. If the caregiver must carry out medical treatments, he or she should be instructed with demonstrations and should give return demonstrations to show mastery. The cultural needs of the caregivers must be considered. In some cultures, only women provide care, so expecting a male to provide assistance may not be realistic. Materials should be provided in the appropriate language for non-English speakers.

Respite Care

Respite care is provided to relieve the burden of the caregiver, rather than to serve the patient. Respite care is provided in a number of different ways. Under Hospice, a patient may be admitted to a skilled nursing facility for up to 5 days, but with other programs, a nurse aide may be provided to stay with the patient for a few hours while the caregiver leaves the home, or the caregiver may be provided with money to hire help in the home. Most respite programs are intended for those providing long-term care for patients with chronic or terminal diseases or dementia, usually related to Alzheimer's disease. Caregivers can easily feel overwhelmed with the constant need to provide care, especially if patients are up at night, as often occurs with Alzheimer's patients, or if they can never be left unattended for safety reasons. If no program for respite care is available, family members or friends may be willing to help.

Support Groups

Support groups play an important role in helping caregivers cope with the stress of caregiving. Groups vary widely and range from informal discussion groups to groups led by psychotherapists or nurses. Regardless of the format, support groups generally follow similar procedures:

- Caregivers describe their situations or updates to the group, usually in turn.
- The group members may question, comment, or make suggestions on dealing with issues.
- The leader helps to keep the group focused and allow everyone to participate.
- Caregivers are encouraged to express their feelings, positive and negative, without receiving criticism. The frequency and duration of meetings also varies, but monthly meetings are common, as caregivers often must arrange for someone to stay with the patient during the meeting. Support groups may be sponsored by senior citizens' organizations, the Alzheimer's Association, or religious groups. Most support groups are free of charge to participants. Nurse and therapist leaders are mandatory reporters of abuse, which sometimes occurs when caregivers become overwhelmed.

Adult Day Care

Adult day care programs provide caregivers a place to take older adults who require supervision. Programs vary widely and may be available a few hours 2 or 3 times a week or 40-50 hours weekly to allow caregivers to hold a job. The costs of the programs also vary widely, with some non-profit organizations accepting minimal payment according to income and other organizations charging fees up to about $300 week. In some cases, the primary purpose of placing an older adult in an adult day care program may be to provide socialization, but more often it is because they have physical and or cognitive impairment resulting in a need for supervision. Day care programs usually provide meals and activities. Many programs are specifically set up in a secure environment to deal with older adults with mild to moderate dementia. Many programs are without medical personnel, but some may include nursing supervision.

FAMILY SYSTEMS THEORY

Bowen's **Family Systems Theory** suggests that one must look at the person in terms of his/her family unit because the members of a family have different roles and behavioral patterns, so a change in one person's behavior will affect the others in the family. There are **8 interrelated concepts:**

- *Triangle theory:* Two people comprise a basic unit, but when conflict occurs, a third person is drawn into the unit for stability with the resulting dynamic of two supporting one or two opposing one. This, in turn, draws in other triangles.
- *Self-differentiation:* People vary in need for external approval.
- *Nuclear family patterns*: These patterns include the following: marital conflict, one spouse dysfunctional, one or more children impaired, and emotional distance.
- *Projection within a family:* Problems (emotional) are passed from parent to child.
- *Transmission (multigenerational):* Small differences in transmission from parent to child are evident.
- *Emotional isolation:* This involves reducing or eliminating family contact.
- *Sibling order:* Sibling order has an influence on behavior and development.
- *Emotional process (society):* Emotional process results in regressive or progressive social movements.

CORE PRINCIPLES TO SUPPORT SELF-CARE

Supporting self-care of individuals involves encouraging patients to make decisions and take responsibility for their actions and behavior. The **core principles to support self-care** include ensuring that patients are able to make choices for themselves in order to manage their own needs, providing appropriate communication to help them to assess their own abilities for self-care, and helping patients to gain access to information to manage their needs. Self-care core principles also include teaching patients the skills they need to care for themselves, teaching or supporting learning technology, educating patients about how to find support networks, being involved in the planning and evaluation of the services they receive, and supporting risk taking and management to increase personal choice. These core principles should be implemented by healthcare providers in a method that is helpful and supportive, recognizing the need for self-care opportunities among patient populations.

BEHAVIOR MODIFICATION AND COMPLIANCE RATE

Education, like all interventions, must be evaluated for **effectiveness**. Two determinants of effectiveness include the following:

- *Behavior modification* involves thorough observation and measurement, identifying behavior that needs to be changed and then planning and instituting interventions to modify that behavior. A CNS can use a variety of techniques, including demonstrations of appropriate behavior, reinforcement, and monitoring until new behavior is consistent. This is especially important when longstanding procedures and habits of behavior are changed.

- *Compliance rates* are often determined by observation, which should be done at intervals and on multiple occasions, but with patients, this may depend on self-reports. Outcomes are another measure of compliance; that is, if education is intended to improve patient health and reduce risk factors and that occurs, it is a good indication that there is compliance. Compliance rates are calculated by determining the number of events/procedures and degree of compliance.

Advocacy and Moral Agency

Nurse competencies under the synergy model include **advocacy/moral agency**:

- *Advocacy* is working for the best interests of the patient despite personal values in conflict and assisting patients to have access to appropriate resources.
- *Agency* is openness and recognition of issues and a willingness to act.
- *Moral agency* is the ability to recognize needs and take action to influence the outcome of a conflict or decision.

The **levels of advocacy/moral agency** include the following:

- *Level 1:* This nurse works on behalf of the patient, assesses personal values, has awareness of patient's rights and ethical conflicts, and advocates for the patient when consistent with the nurse's personal values.
- *Level 3:* This nurse advocates for the patient/family, incorporates his or her values into the care plan even when they differ from the nurse's, and can utilize internal resources to assist patient/family with complex decisions.
- *Level 5:* This nurse advocates for the patient/family despite differences in values and is able to utilize both internal and external resources to help empower the patient/family to make decisions.

Incorporating Patient Goals into Plan of Care

The plan of care is developed from information gained from patient interviews, history and physical exam, and medical records. Once a problem list is generated, the nurse must review and prioritize the list and determine **patient goals,** depending on the type of problem. Goals should be specifically related to the problem, measurable by some method, and attainable:

- Some problems (such as cardiac arrhythmias) can improve with treatment, so goals will aim toward resolution: "Pulse rate will not exceed 90 at rest."
- Other problems (such as chronic conditions) probably won't resolve, so the goals will aim toward preventing deterioration or further complications: "Patient will maintain current weight."
- Some problems (terminal cancer) cannot be resolved and deterioration of condition is inevitable, so the goal will aim toward palliation and ensuring the patient's comfort and support: "Patient will not experience breakthrough pain."

Incorporating Patients' and Families' Rights into Care Plan

Patient/family rights should be incorporated into the patient's *care plan*. To accomplish this, the care plan needs to be designed in a collaborative effort that encourages the participation of patients and family members. There are a number of different methods that can be useful to address patients' rights. Patients and families can be included on advisory committees. Additionally, assessment tools, such as patient/family surveys, can be employed to gain insight in the issues that are important to patients and their families. Because many hospital stays are now short term, programs that include follow-up interviews and assessments are especially valuable in determining if the needs of the patient/family were addressed in the care plan.

Patient Characteristics Related to Barriers to Patient Care

According to the American Association of Critical-Care Nurses' synergy method for patient care, there are a number of **patient characteristics** that must be considered in matching a staff member's competencies to the requirements of the patient and the patient's family. Resiliency is the ability to recover from a devastating illness and regain a sense of stability, both physically and emotionally. Resiliency can be strengthened by faith, a positive sense of hope, and a supportive network of friends and family. Vulnerability refers to those factors that put a person at increased risk and interfere with recovery and/or compliance. These factors include anxiety, fear, lack of support, chronic illness, prejudice, and lack of information. Stability allows a patient and his or her family to maintain a state of equilibrium despite illness and challenges. Important factors contributing to stability include motivation; values; and relief from stress, conflicts, or emotional burdens. Complexity occurs when more than one system is involved. These systems can be internal (cardiac and renal systems) or external (addicted and homeless) or some combination of both (ill with poor family dynamics).

Facilitating Decision-Making

Prioritization by Reasoning, Voting, Multivoting and Prioritization Matrix

Brainstorming interventions or solutions to problems may result in multiple possibilities, so **prioritization** is necessary to determine which intervention or solution is most important and should be attended to first.

Prioritization	
Reasoning	Many times, priorities are established by simply thinking about different options and, based on experience and knowledge, choosing the most critical to attend to first. This format is used most often for individual decision-making.
Voting	Voting is frequently used in groups to establish priorities, but a simple vote can yield inadequate results. For example, if there are 3 choices and each gets 5 votes, there is no solution. If, however, choice 1 gets 6 votes, choice two 4 votes, and choice three 5 votes, choice 1 would win, even though 9 voters feel it is not the priority.
Multivoting	This format is often used for group decisions. Once a list of possible solutions is created, members receive a number of votes, usually 1 more than half the total number of solutions, and can apply the votes as they wish—placing all votes on one solution or scattering votes. Solutions receiving few or no votes are eliminated or go to the bottom of the list, and then people vote again, as many times as necessary.
Prioritization matrix	Important criteria are selected and solutions are placed into a matrix based on criteria. Common criteria include High benefit and low cost or effort High benefit and high cost or effort Low benefit and low cost or effort Low benefit and high cost or effort Those interventions or solutions that are high benefit and low cost or effort are usually of highest priority, and those with low benefit and high cost or effort are the lowest.

Empowerment

Empowerment is necessary through all spheres of influence in decision-making. Empowerment is allowing and encouraging people to make decisions and trusting them to do so and to carry out interventions. Empowerment correlates to the individual's stage of power:

- *Powerlessness*: feeling dependent on others, manipulated, and unable to make decisions
- *Association*: feeling they have some degree of power based on their association with or emulation of those in power
- *Symbol*: believing that symbols, such as degrees or job titles, convey power
- *Reflection*: recognition of self-worth and power to make decisions, the beginning of true empowerment
- *Purpose*: believing that power comes from having values and allowing others freedom to lead and make decisions
- *Gestalt*: believing that power derives from wisdom, inner values, and strength, allowing them to assess the degree of empowerment to allow others, based on individual strengths.

Empowering Patients/Families

Empowering patients and families to act as their own advocates requires that they have a clear understanding of their rights and responsibilities. These should be given (in print form) and/or presented (audio/video) to patients and families on admission or as soon as possible:

- *Rights* should include competent, non-discriminatory medical care that respects privacy and allows participation in decisions about care and the right to refuse care. They should have clear understandable explanations of treatments, options, and conditions, including outcomes. They should be apprised of transfers, changes in care plan, and advance directives. They should have access to medical records information about charges.
- *Responsibilities* should include providing honest and thorough information about health issues and medical history. They should ask for clarification if they don't understand information that is provided to them, and they should follow the plan of care that is outlined or explain why that is not possible. They should treat staff and other patients with respect.

Therapeutic Relationship

A **therapeutic relationship** is a continuum based on a trust, caring, empathy, and acceptance. The needs of the patient are the focus, not the feelings or needs of the nurse.

- **Orientation**
    - The patient seeks or is brought in for help; needs and concerns are elicited.
    - Nurse responds to client, listens actively, and responds, explaining roles and trying to relieve the patient's anxiety while helping the patient focus on problems.
- **Identification**
    - The patient begins to identify with the nurse and increases understanding of problems; testing behavior decreases as the patient has a better understanding of roles and expectations.
    - The nurse shows acceptance and continues to assess and provide support and information.

- **Working**
    - The patient makes better use of the relationship but may engage in exploitative behavior with wide behavior shifts between dependence and independence, while showing better problem-solving skills and improved communication.
    - Nurse supports client and explores feelings at client's own pace.
- **Termination**
    - The patient establishes independence from nurse and sets new goals.
    - The nurse encourages family/community support and preventive care.

Collaboration Between Nurse and Patient/Family

The **collaboration** between the nurse and the patient and or the patient's is extremely important but is often overlooked. Nurses and health-care providers must always remember that the point of collaborating is to improve patient care. This means that the patient and patient's family must remain central to all planning. Including the patient and his or her family in planning takes time initially but is very valuable. The patient and his or her family can provide information that facilitates planning and the expenditure of resources. Including the patient and family in planning can save money in the long run. Families, and even young children, often want to participate in care and planning and feel validated. This creates a more positive attitude toward the medical system.

Motivational Interviewing

Motivational interviewing (Miller, 1983) aims to help people identify and resolve issues regarding ambivalence toward therapy and focuses on the role of motivation to bring about change. MI is a collaborative approach in which the interviewer assesses the patient's readiness to accept change and identifies strategies that may be effective with the individual patient.

- **Elements of MI**
    - *Collaboration* rather than confrontation in resolving issues
    - *Evocation* (drawing out) of the patient's ideas about change, rather than imposition of the interviewer's ideas;
    - *Autonomy* of the patient in making changes
- **Principles of MI**
    - *Expression of empathy*: showing understanding of patient's perceptions.
    - *Support of self-efficacy*: helping patients realize they are capable of change.
    - *Acceptance of resistance*: avoiding struggles/conflicts with patient;
    - *Examination of discrepancies*: helping patients see discrepancy between their behavior and goals
- **Strategies**
    - *Avoiding yes/no questions*: asking informational questions
    - *Providing affirmations*: indicating areas of strength
    - Providing reflective listening: responding to statements
    - *Providing summaries*: recapping important points of discussion
    - *Encouraging change talk*: including desire, ability, reason, and need

Palliative and End-of-Life Care

GRIEF AND LOSS

Older adults must cope with almost continuous **grief and loss**, including primary losses (spouse, friends, and family) and secondary losses (such as companionship and assistance). As losses accumulate, the older adult may become overwhelmed with grief and unable to cope. Patients may grieve the following losses:

- Body image (physical and psychological as physical condition deteriorates)
- Spouse/partner/friends (through death or distance)
- Self-identity and self-esteem (as roles change)
- Possessions (if people move from a home to an assisted living or other long-term care facility)
- Financial stability (as income decreases and expenses increase)
- Dignity (as others care for the person)
- Independence (as the person is forced to rely on others for assistance)
- Mental acuity
- Life itself (including that of significant others)

The older adult's ability to cope with grief and loss and find hope depends upon his or her support system, health status, mental status, and belief system.

LOSS OF A SPOUSE

The **loss of a spouse** can be devastating to the survivor, who often responds with severe depression and sometimes becomes suicidal. The response may depend on the quality of the relationship. If the partners had a poor or abusive relationship, the surviving spouse may feel some relief but also anger and guilt and may have difficulty assuming more independence. Because women tend to live longer than men, there are more widows than widowers. As some retirement benefits decrease when a spouse dies, women often lose a significant amount of their income when the spouse dies. Women often grieve more openly than men because men feel constrained by societal expectations. However, men may feel great loss. Men are often better able to afford to pay for assistance with chores previously done by a spouse, such as cooking and cleaning. Divorce, which is becoming more common with older adults, can result in similar effects.

DEPRESSION AND ANGER IN OLDER ADULTS

Older adults may exhibit a number of different psychological responses to loss. These responses may interfere with their ability to function and can interfere with medical care.

Depression is the most common response of older adults to loss. Patients may become increasingly withdrawn and sad. This response puts them at risk for suicide. They may feel that life is futile and refuse medical care.

Anger is also a response to loss. Some older adults focus on the unfairness of their situation and become mired in anger, often antagonizing friends and family and behaving belligerently. They may refuse to cooperate or actively resist care. These individuals may blame the doctors, nurses, and family for their circumstances and find fault with almost everything and everyone. Their relationships often suffer as a result of this behavior.

Acute Grief, Anticipatory Grief, and Chronic Grief

Grief is a normal response to loss. Patients may have to face the loss of their spouse, family, income, status, health, mobility, home, and independence. Mourning is the public expression of grief, and bereavement is the time period of mourning. There are three primary types of grief: acute, anticipatory, and chronic.

- **Acute grief** is immediate and occurs in response to some type of loss. It may be expressed as sadness, anger, fear, and anxiety.
- **Anticipatory grief** occurs when a loss is feared. For example, anticipatory grief may occur when the death of a spouse is impending.
- **Chronic grief** occurs when people are not able to come to terms with a loss so that grieving and mourning are prolonged, sometimes for years. People experiencing chronic grief may develop anorexia, insomnia, panic attacks, and self-destructive behaviors (alcohol and substance abuse). They may even contemplate or commit suicide. Chronic grief poses a serious risk to people and should be treated in the same way as depression with antidepressants, psychological evaluation, and counseling.

Elisabeth Kübler-Ross's Five Stages of Grief

Elisabeth Kübler-Ross developed a model of grieving. Her model is commonly referred to as the **five stages of grief**. She describes five distinct stages in the grieving process. Kübler-Ross postulated that people go through these stages in dealing with a tragedy, such as a terminal illness or death of a loved one. Kübler-Ross raised awareness of the need to treat individuals dealing with a terminal illness with compassion. The five stages of grief outlined by Kübler-Ross are denial, anger, bargaining, depression, and acceptance. A person may not go through every stage. The model has been criticized as having several flaws. There is little empirical research to support it. In addition, the model does not take into account how the patient's situation can affect the stages.

The following are the stages of grief in the Kübler-Ross model:

1. **Denial**: Denial is a defense. Patients and their families may be resistive to information and unable to accept the fact of dying or impairment. They may be stunned, immobile, or detached. Patients may be unable to respond appropriately. They may not remember what is said to them and repeatedly ask the same questions.
2. **Anger**: As reality becomes clear, patient and their families may react with pronounced anger directed inward or outward. Patients, especially women, may blame themselves, and self-anger may lead to severe depression and guilt. They may assume that they are to blame because of some personal action. Outward anger, more common in men, may be expressed as overt hostility.
3. **Bargaining**: Bargaining involves if-then thinking (often directed at a deity). For example, a patient may think "If I go to church every day, then God will prevent this." The patient or family may change doctors, trying to change the outcome.
4. **Depression**: As the patient and family begin to accept the loss, they may become depressed and overwhelmed with sadness. They may feel that no one understands. They may be tearful or cry and may withdraw or ask to be left alone.
5. **Acceptance**: This final stage represents a form of resolution and often occurs outside of the medical environment months after the diagnosis. Patients are able to accept death, dying, or incapacity. Families are able to resume their normal activities and lose the constant preoccupation with their loved one. They are able to think of the person without severe pain.

Hospice Care

Hospice care is designed to care for terminally ill individuals within the last six months of life. This period may be extended by physician authorization every 60 days. Medicare patients are covered for hospice care. The patient must be eligible for Medicare Part A, and a physician must certify that the patient is terminal with a life expectancy of six months or less. The patient (or responsible relative) must agree that the patient will receive hospice care rather than regular Medicare. The goal of hospice care is to maintain the person in the home environment. The patient is provided with home health aides and homemakers; durable goods (such as dressings, adult diapers, and underpads); counseling; and social worker assistance. Hospice care aims to manage the patient's pain and keep him or her comfortable. Routine home care is intermittent and must comprise 80 percent of total care. In-home continuous care is available for short periods of time in crisis. Inpatient hospice may be used for four to five days for symptom management and/or a five-day respite period for caregivers.

Palliative and End-of-Life Care

The World Health Organization (WHO) defines **end-of-life and palliative care** as active total care of patient whose disease is no longer responsive to treatment. Palliative care, especially pain management, is often delayed or inadequate. The dying patient and family must be considered a unit when planning for care, and a multidisciplinary approach that includes physicians, nurses, social workers, and chaplains or spiritual guides can help the family through this difficult period. Family may equate pain medication with euthanasia or assisted suicide. Additionally, family may feel that the patient's increased sedation robs them of time with the patient or may fear addiction. These concerns must be respected, but providing adequate information and support while allowing the patient and/or family to express their feelings can often allay many of these fears and facilitate decision-making.

Palliative Care

The purpose of **palliative care** is to make the patient comfortable during a chronic or terminal illness. It does not provide curative treatment. Palliative care is meant to improve the quality of life and relieve suffering. It neither prolongs life nor hastens death. The goals of palliative care include the relief of pain and the relief of symptoms (such as nausea or shortness of breath). In addition, palliative care provides support for the patient, caregivers, and/or family. It ensures that patients and their families receive psychosocial and spiritual support. Palliative care may provide bereavement services. While palliative care is often given in conjunction with hospice care, palliative care should begin prior to hospice care, because many issues, such as pain management, must be addressed prior to the last six months of the patient's life.

Supporting the Family of the Dying Patient

Families of dying patients often do not receive adequate support from nursing staff members, who feel unprepared for dealing with their grief and unsure of how to provide comfort. However, families may be in desperate need of this support. Before death the nurse should stay with the family and sit quietly, allowing them to talk, cry, or interact if they desire. The nurse should avoid platitudes such as "His suffering will be over soon."

The nurse should avoid judgmental reactions to what family members say or do and realize that anger, fear, guilt, and irrational behavior are normal responses to acute grief and stress. The nurse should display a caring attitude by touching the patient and encouraging family members to do the same. Touching the hands, arms, or shoulders of family members can provide comfort, but follow the cues of the family. Finally, the nurse should provide referrals to support groups if needed.

Support the Family During the Death of a Patient

At the time of death, the nurse should reassure the family that all measures have been taken to ensure the patient's comfort. The nurse should express personal feelings of loss. The nurse should provide information about what is happening during the dying process, explaining death rales and Cheyne-Stokes respirations, for example. The family members should be alerted to the patient's imminent death if they are not present. The family should be assisted in contacting clergy or spiritual advisors. The nurse should respect the feelings and needs of the spouse, children, and other family. After death, the nurse should encourage family members to stay with the patient as long as they wish to say goodbye. The nurse should assist the family to make arrangements, such as contacting the funeral home. If an autopsy is required, the nurse should discuss it with the family and explain when it will take place. If the patient's organs are being donated, the nurse should assist the family to make arrangements. The family members should be encouraged to grieve and express emotions.

End of Life

Physical Changes

There are a number of **physical changes** associated with the end of life. These changes are sensory, circulatory, respiratory, muscular, urinary, and integumentary.

- *Sensory*: Patients have reduced sensation of touch and pain, blurring of vision, and loss of blink reflex. Hearing is usually the last of the senses to fail, so the patient should be communicated with in a way he or she will understand during the dying process.
- *Circulatory*: Tachycardia is followed by bradycardia and weakening of the pulse with irregular rhythm. Blood pressure decreases.
- *Respiratory*: Tachypnea progresses to Cheyne-Stokes respirations. The patient is unable to cough or clear secretions, so rattling may be heard. Breathing becomes increasingly irregular with terminal gasping.
- *Muscular*: The patient loses the ability to move, talk, and swallow. The gag reflex is lost. The jaw begins to sag, and occasional jerking may be seen if the patient is receiving narcotics.
- *Urinary*: Urinary output decreases. The patient is incontinent and then unable to urinate.
- *Integumentary*: The skin becomes cold and clammy. Mottling and cyanosis may appear. The skin takes on a waxy appearance.

Individual Beliefs and Traditions

Individual beliefs and traditions regarding death vary widely, and these affect how the patient and his or her family deal with the end of life. The nurse should discuss these issues with the patient and/or family members in order to ensure that their needs are met. Those with strong spiritual beliefs may want spiritual advisors (such as priests, shamans, ministers, or monks) present to provide support or perform rituals. People who have no belief in an afterlife may face death with resolution or may be frightened at the thought of the total end of their existence. Individuals who believe in reincarnation may find comfort in the thought of their rebirth but may also fear karma for the mistakes they made in this life. Some people believe in a loving God, while others believe in a vengeful God. Some individuals may feel that they will be in a loving place after death, while others fear they will suffer torment for their sins. The nurse should remain supportive and allow patients and families to express their feelings, fears, and concerns.

End-of-Life Care Plan

The **end-of-life care plan** must consider advance directives, such as DNR, and the needs and desires of the patient and family.

End-of-life care plan	
Pain management	Although addiction is not a concern, patients may develop tolerance to pain medications, so careful pain assessment must be ongoing with adequate analgesia provided.
Oral care	Mouth care includes oral swabs to mucous membranes and petroleum jelly to lips. Dentures may cause discomfort or loosen and are usually removed.
Eye care	Eyelids may not close, so artificial tears or ophthalmic saline may relieve discomfort.
Anorexia Dehydration	Anorexia and dehydration are normal and may reduce pulmonary edema and the need to urinate.
Bowel/bladder control	Stool softeners may relieve constipation. Incontinence is common, so protective pads and briefs are used. Skin barrier ointments should be applied to perineal area.
Skin integrity	Frequent turning and application of lotion to skin and decreased frequency of bathing (to reduce drying) are indicated.
Anxiety reduction	Drugs to reduce anxiety have side effects, so comfort measures are most effective.

Care Transition and Coordination

Care Map

A **care map** is a concept map that provides an easily accessible visual representation of patient diagnoses, interventions, care, and outcomes. Care maps may be done in a variety of formats, from graphic flowcharts to tables. Care maps are useful in presenting the overall picture of patient needs and care.

- A simple care map may show progress through the medical care process, starting with admission and ending with discharge.
- A more complex care map may begin with the patient's name, diagnosis, and important identifying information as the core, with arrows linking to nursing diagnosis and interventions. For example, a diagnosis of impaired physical mobility may contain information about the impairment, interventions, and expected outcomes and may show a link to laboratory and radiographic studies to determine the cause, or to PT for therapy.
- An alternate form begins with the core information and provides categories in which details are provided. Categories may include nutrition, hydration, oxygen needs, neurological status, anxiety, skin integrity, mobility, sexuality, activity, body image, and elimination.

Discharge Plans

The **discharge plan** should begin on admission. Older adults do not always comply with the discharge plan, so including the patient and family in the planning process and establishing realistic goals are critical. If a patient is transferring to a long-term care facility or a home health-care program, the plan of care should be completely outlined and delivered along with copies of medical records. If a patient has had invasive procedures that increase risk for infection, the signs and symptoms of potential infection should be listed. Follow-up appointment dates with physicians, physical therapists, or other services should be included. Specific directions should be provided for all medications and treatments that are to be continued after discharge, with appropriate instruction completed prior to discharge. Contact information should be obtained from the patient so that post discharge follow-up can be conducted, and contact information should be provided to the patient or the transfer facility.

Assisting with Finding Financial Resources for Healthcare Costs

Not all patients have the financial means to pay for **healthcare costs**. Nurses should be aware of available resources for helping patients to pay for costs and provide patients with information that will assist with financial coverage. While it is not the nurse's duty to discuss personal finances in most situations, the nurse should have an understanding of available options to assist with payment of fees for healthcare. This involves having a basic knowledge of insurance coverage, co-payments, and benefits, as well as an understanding of Medicare and Medicaid services, and being able to guide patients to find answers to questions about these topics when they are outside of the nurse's expertise. The nurse should also be aware of state and local resources, as well as their qualifying conditions, to be able to guide the patient toward signing up for assistance, such as through state children's health insurance plans, non-profit organizations, healthcare payment plans, and financial aid available from local clinics or offices. Finally, the nurse should know whom to call within her organization or a local advocate who can help the patient if the situation falls outside of the nurse's scope of practice.

Change of Residence

Change of residence for an older adult may involve a move to an apartment, assisted living facility, or nursing home. These changes can be very disorienting for the older adult who must cope with a new environment and new people. The older adult must also cope with the grief of losing former associations and personal belongings. If at all possible, the older adult should be included in plans prior to a move. The move is made easier if the older adult is taken to visit the facility and allowed to meet some of the staff or people there. Even in very restricted environments, such as nursing homes, patients are usually allowed a few personal belongings, such as family pictures and a few items of clothing. Personal items can provide some comfort to older adults in new surroundings. Patients whose family and friends visit may cope better than those with no support system.

Home Meal Delivery Programs

Home meal delivery programs (such as Meals-on-Wheels) provide nutritious meals for homebound adults (often restricted to older adults). The programs usually serve meals 5-7 days a week with home delivery, often by volunteers. Meals are usually low cost ($2-4 per meal) but this varies with the program. Most programs deliver one hot meal a day and may provide food for one or two other meals (such as a sandwich for dinner and cold cereal for breakfast the next day). Requirements and age restrictions vary with some programs serving those over the age of 60 and others serving individuals over 65. People with temporary disabilities may be restricted in length of service. Some programs are intended for those with low incomes but others do not have income restrictions. Most programs provide little choice in menu but may offer low fat, low salt, or low carbohydrate diets. Many home meal delivery programs have waiting lists because the need outpaces the number of programs.

Assisted Living Facilities

There is a wide range of options in **assisted living facilities**. There are choices ranging from residential care facilities that house two to three patients in a home setting to large facilities with dozens or even hundreds of patients. Typically, nurses are not on duty. Therefore, medical assistance is limited. Services usually offered include staff on duty 24 hours a day to provide assistance if needed, provision of meals (two to three meals daily), cleaning, activities, and transportation. Costs vary widely from $500 per month to $10,000 per month. The goal of assisted living is to allow the patient to remain as independent as his or her physical and cognitive abilities allow. Residents often have individual apartments. Assisted living is usually limited to individuals with mild to moderate functional impairment, but licensure varies somewhat from state to state. Facilities focusing on patients with Alzheimer's disease may face further requirements, such as provision of a safe environment that prevents patients from wandering away from the facility.

RESIDENTIAL CARE FACILITIES

A **residential care facility** is a type of assisted living/group home. A typical residential care facility is a large home with two or more patients cared for by a person (often nonmedical) licensed by the state. Depending on the number of patients, nursing aides may be available to assist patients. Residents are assisted with activities of daily living, such as bathing and dressing, as required. Meals are cooked for the residents. The facilities have supervised activities for the residents. It is usually required that the residents be ambulatory, but this may vary according to the facility and state regulations. Residential care facilities do not usually provide medical care, so patients needing treatments (other than assistance with taking medications or minor treatments) are seen by home health agency nurses. Medicaid may provide funds to house older adults in residential care facilities, but the reimbursement rate is low. For this reason, finding a residential care facility that accepts Medicaid patients can be difficult. The cost for residential care ranges from $500 a month to thousands of dollars per month for luxury facilities.

SENIOR CENTERS

Senior centers provide services and recreational activities for older adults. Some senior centers offer day care programs, but services are generally intended for individuals who do not require supervision or assistance. Programs vary in the services they provide. Some senior centers are open a few hours a week for meetings and recreational activities (Bingo, cards, or dancing, for example). Other centers are open daily and offer programs (such as educational classes), meals (often at low cost), and recreational activities. Some senior centers provide transportation to and from the center, and some sponsor low-cost bus tours and vacation packages. Many communities have senior centers, and retirement communities often revolve around the activities provided by these centers. Senior centers sometimes provide low-cost legal assistance and help in filling out tax forms. Most centers provide information about senior services available in the community and may assist people in getting help they need.

REHABILITATIVE CARE

Rehabilitative care comprises a number of different services:

- *Physical therapy:* Exercises to strengthen muscles and increase or maintain mobility may involve active and passive exercises as well as computer/machine-mediated exercises, such as using a stationary bicycle. Physical therapy is often needed after injury to bones/muscles and strokes.
- *Occupational therapy:* Patients are taught modifications that allow them to be as independent as possible with activities of daily living. Patients might be taught, for example, safe methods of bathing or cooking. They may be provided assistive devices. Patients with strokes often receive occupational therapy.
- *Speech therapy:* Patients are helped to improve production and patterns of speech and to improve swallowing. Speech therapy is often used for stroke patients and those with neuromuscular diseases.

- *Respiratory therapy:* Patients are taught to manage respiratory limitations through paced-breathing/walking exercises and diaphragmatic breathing to increase their ability to function with lung disease.

Home Health Agencies

Home health agencies provide intermittent care in the home environment or assisted-living facilities. Home health care can include nursing care (assessment, medications, and treatment), social workers, speech pathologists, physical and occupational therapists, and certified nurse aides (personal care). Home health agencies may provide professionals to draw blood for lab tests and administer intravenous fluids. Home health care allows patients to be sent home earlier from acute hospitals and skilled nursing facilities and is more cost effective than in-patient care. Some insurance companies pay for home health care, and Medicare pays for care with requirements: Patients must be homebound, in need of skilled care more than 7 days/week or more than 8 hours each day over a period of 21 days or less. Those eligible may receive home health aide services but total hours of care may not exceed 28-35 hours/week (depending on need). Medicare pays a set amount for each "episode of care" (60-day period), depending on the health care condition.

Restorative Care/Supportive Care

Restorative care, usually provided after an injury (fractured hip) or illness (stroke), aims to restore the patient to optimal functioning and prevent complications. While restorative care often includes physical and occupational therapy, it is more comprehensive and includes encouraging the patient to be as independent in care as possible and to improve to his/her fullest potential. Restorative care includes activities to improve psychosocial adjustment and the patient's self-image. The patient is given short achievable goals (lift leg, hold a cup) to focus on so that he/she can see progress and gain confidence. As a goal is achieved, new goals are set.

Supportive care aims to reduce problems, complications, and symptoms associated with treatment or disease. For example, a patient receiving chemotherapy may receive supportive care to relieve nausea and vomiting, psychosocial support to deal with personal/financial issues, and spiritual support to provide comfort.

Skilled Nursing Facilities

Skilled nursing facilities (SNF, nursing homes) are licensed by states to provide both medical care (medications and treatment) and personal care (such as bathing, dressing, meals, and activities). Patients with insurance or Medicare may be transferred to an SNF after acute care in hospital. The length of stay at an SNF usually ranges from a few days to six weeks, depending on the patient's condition and progress. SNFs usually provide physical therapy and occupational therapy. They may also provide respiratory therapy. The purpose of SNF care is to provide transitional care between the hospital and the home environment. In some cases, patients who require medical care and cannot be cared for at home may remain in the SNF until death. Although Medicare will not pay for this, long-term insurance will cover the cost. State Medicaid programs may pay if certain restrictions (income, condition, and age) are met. Some patients pay privately. Costs range from about $4,000 to $10,000 per month.

Acute and Subacute Care

Patients requiring **acute care** are usually treated in hospital where diagnostic procedures (such as magnetic resonance imaging [MRI], computed tomography [CT] scan, lab tests, and x-ray) can be readily performed. Hospitals also have the sophisticated equipment necessary to monitor patients. Patients admitted to acute care facilities are usually extremely ill, requiring eight to nine hours of skilled nursing care daily. Physicians and highly skilled nursing staff are available for patients around the clock.

Subacute care provides a level of care between that of an acute hospital and a skilled nursing facility, although skilled nurses are available around the clock. Subacute care patients usually require four to six hours of skilled nursing care daily but may receive intensive therapy. Subacute care units may be contained within an acute hospital, but they may also exist as completely separate facilities. Most subacute care units do not offer monitoring or sophisticated diagnostic equipment, so patients treated in subacute units often have chronic (rather than acute) disorders, such as acquired immune deficiency syndrome (AIDS), head trauma, and neuromuscular diseases.

Information Technology

CPOE

Computerized physician/provider order entry (CPOE) is a set of clinical software applications that automate medication/treatment ordering, requiring that orders be typed in a standard format to avoid mistakes in ordering or interpreting orders. CPOE is promoted by Leapfrog as a means to reduce medication errors. About 50% of medication errors occur during ordering, so reducing this number can have a large impact on patient safety. Most CPOE systems contain a clinical decision support system (CDDS) as well so that the system can provide an immediate alert related to patient allergies, drug interactions, duplicate orders, or incorrect dosing at the time of data entry. Some systems can also provide suggestions for alternative medications, treatments, and diagnostic procedures. The CPOE system may be integrated into the information system of the organization for easier tracking of information and data collection. This system is cost-effective, replaces handwritten orders, and allows easy access to patient records.

BCMA

Barcode medication administration (BCMA) utilizes wireless mobile units at the point of care to scan the barcode on each unit of medication or blood component before it is dispensed. Scanning ensures the correct medication and dosage is given to the correct patient, eliminating most point of administration medication errors. The BCMA system can also be utilized for specimen collection. This system requires monitoring and input from the pharmacy, as each new barcode must be entered into the system. Additionally, some medications are received in bulk, so when they are dispensed in unit doses, barcodes must be individually attached. Staff must be trained to ensure that BCMA is utilized properly and consistently. The FDA has required that drug supplies provide barcodes on the labels of medications and other biological products. BCMA increases safety for patients. It integrates with the medication administration record and the information system of the organization, providing data for assessment of performance and performance improvement measures.

Computerized Notification System

The **computerized notification system** can be used to provide alerts to physicians related to abnormal laboratory or imaging results. This system has proven to be more effective in ensuring that alerts are communicated, although studies show that some results are still lost and follow-up is not always completed, especially in ambulatory care where the physician may not see the patient on a regular basis. There are steps in the design of the notification system that can improve safety and follow-up:

- Physician training with clear explanations of the goals in patient safety and the need and responsibility to check for computerized notices daily.
- Automatic notification to sender when the receiver opens the alert message.
- Automatic second notification to receiver if the alert message is not opened within a preset period of time.
- Automatic notification to sender to contact the physician by other means if the second notification is not opened within a preset period of time.
- Monitoring and evaluation for compliance.

EMR

The **Electronic medical record (EMR)** is a digital computerized patient record, which may be integrated with CPOE and CDSS to improve patient care and reduce medical error. Software applications vary considerably and standardization has not yet been implemented; therefore, the organization must carefully review current and future anticipated needs as well as the ability of applications to interface with each other to provide for adequate measurements, data collection, reports, retrieval of data, analysis, and confidentiality. Increasingly, physicians in private practice, especially those in large groups, are employing EMRs, and these systems might be different than those used in hospitals. Systems can be customized to meet the needs of the organization, but cost and lack of standardization remain barriers for implementation. However, studies indicate that there is a positive correlation between comprehensive EMR systems and patient outcomes. Quantifiable data about cost-effectiveness can be difficult to calculate because savings are often terms of saved time, fewer interventions, and reduced error.

RFI

Radio frequency identification (RFI) is an automatic system for identification that employs embedded digital memory chips, with unique codes, to track patients, medical devices, medications, and staff. A chip can carry multiple types of data, such as expiration dates, patient's allergies, and blood types. A chip/tag may, for example, be embedded in the identification bracelet of the patient and all medications for the patient tagged with the same chip. Chips have the ability to both read and write data, so they are more flexible than bar coding. The data on the chips can be read by sensors from a distance or through materials, such as clothes, although tags don't apply or read well on metal or in fluids. There are two types of RFI:

- *Active:* Continuous signals are transmitted between the chips and sensors.
- *Passive:* Signals are transmitted when in close proximity to a sensor. Thus, a passive system may be adequate for administration of medications, but an active system would be needed to track movements of staff, equipment, or patients.

Webinars and Internet Applications for Communication

Internet applications can make communicating with co-workers, peers, and other professionals simple and straightforward, at times requiring only an Internet connection.

- *Webinars* are online seminars that can reach large groups of people who all arrive at the same site online. Those attending the webinar can read information presented on the screen and listen to the speaker as if they were attending a seminar in person. Webinars are good tools for communication in that they can convey messages to large groups through relatively easy means. They also allow participants to ask questions or comment on the discussion by sending emails or instant messages during the session.
- *Online meetings* are another Internet application that allows users to communicate by presenting information through certain types of software. Online meetings are often geared toward smaller groups of people; those attending the meeting view the same screen and can discuss information through web conferencing. Both webinars and online meetings allow for gatherings and presentation of data without the expense or time of travel to meet together in person.

Healthcare Delivery Models and Settings

Telehealth

Telehealth is providing health care and monitoring to individuals at a distance utilizing **telecommunications and information technologies**. Telehealth may include two-way video conferencing for interviewing, diagnosing, monitoring and treating. Store-and-forward telehealth technology stores data (such as BP and heart rate) and transmits it electronically at specified times or under specified conditions (such as sending an ECG when tachycardia occurs). The aging population is a reason for the increasing trend of utilizing telehealth technologies as a **preventive measure** (monitoring patient's conditions) and to **reduce the need for hospitalization**. Other reasons include the increasing cost of healthcare and hospitalization, a more educated populace that wants to be involved in its own healthcare, the shortage of nursing and other healthcare personnel, and the increase (tied to the aging population) of chronic illnesses. If an outpatient facility plans to establish a telehealth program to provide medical consultation and services to multiple states, the first consideration is state laws and regulations, as these may vary considerably.

Ehealth

Ehealth (electronic health) is an emerging specialty that refers to the use of **information technology** in the care and treatment of patients. Ehealth is usually associated with the use of the Internet but in some cases may only refer to the use of computers and computer systems as definitions vary somewhat. Ehealth includes the use of:

- Electronic health records.
- CPOE and CDSS systems.
- Mobile health applications.
- Telemonitoring.
- Telehealth services.
- Virtual health care.
- Integrated networks.
- Mobile devices, such as tablets and smart phones.

CMS has an ehealth initiative that aligns health IT with industry electronic standards as part of the plan to promote the use of **electronic health records** throughout the healthcare industry. Health information exchanges (HIEs) are utilized to facilitate the secure exchange of information, always a concern in ehealth. Ehealth has shown a rapid growth but is impacted by shortage of trained personnel, high maintenance costs, and budgetary constraints.

Nursing Informatics

Informatics is basically the study of information and how it is managed. According the American Nurse Association scope and standards, nursing informatics is the integration of nursing, computer, and information sciences in the management of data and information. Much of nursing time is involved in documenting data and managing information, so informatics seeks methods to streamline and improve these processes. This involves research into the best systems and evaluation of existing systems. Credentialing is available for nurse informatics specialists, requiring specific coursework, although requirements may vary from one state to another. Nurse informatics specialists are involved in system design and often have a pivotal role in improving patient safety and facilitating user education. They facilitate the use of smart technology as well as wireless record keeping and remote monitoring. The role of the nurse informatics specialist will expand as more hospitals and institutions convert from traditional handwritten documentation to electronic record keeping, especially with incentives provided by the American Reinvestment and Recovery Act (2009).

Change Management

Communication Skills

Collaboration requires a number of **communication skills** that differ from those involved in communication between nurse and patient. These skills include the following:

- *Using an assertive approach:* It's important for the nurse to honestly express opinions and to state them clearly and with confidence, but the nurse must do so in a calm non-threatening manner.
- *Making casual conversation:* It's easier to communicate with people with whom one has a personal connection. Asking open-ended questions, asking about other's work, or commenting on someone's contributions helps to establish a relationship. The time before meetings, during breaks, and after meetings presents an opportunity for this type of conversation.
- *Being competent in public speaking:* Collaboration requires that a nurse be comfortable speaking and presenting ideas to groups of people, and doing so helps the person to gain credibility. This is a skill that must be practiced.
- *Communicating in writing:* The written word remains a critical component of communication, and the nurse should be able to communicate clearly and grammatically.

Intradisciplinary and Interdisciplinary Communication

There are a number of **skills** that are needed to lead and facilitate communication with **intra- and interdisciplinary teams**:

- *Communicating openly* is essential, and all members should be encouraged to participate as valued members of a cooperative team. To facilitate the flow of information, interrupting or interpreting the point of another is discouraged. Jumping to conclusions can effectively stop communication and should be avoided.
- *Active listening* requires paying attention and asking questions for clarification. Challenging the ideas of other team members is not appropriate.

- It is essential to *show respect* for the ideas of others. Care should be taken to react and respond to facts rather than feelings. This helps prevent angry confrontations and to diffuse anger.
- *Clarification* of information or opinions stated can help avoid misunderstandings. Unsolicited advice should not be offered, because it shows disrespect. Team members should feel comfortable about asking others for advice.

THERAPEUTIC COMMUNICATION

INTRODUCTIONS, ENCOURAGEMENT, AND EMPATHY

Therapeutic communication begins with respect for the patient/family and the assumption that all communication, verbal and non-verbal, has meaning. Listening must be done empathetically. Techniques that facilitate communication include the following:

- *Introduction:* Make a personal introduction and use the patient's name: "Mrs. Brown, I am Susan Williams, your nurse."
- *Encouragement:* Use an open-ended opening statement: "Is there anything you'd like to discuss?"
- *Acknowledge comments*: "Yes," and "I understand."
- Allow silence and observe non-verbal behavior rather than trying to force conversation. Ask for clarification if statements are unclear.
- Reflect statements back (use sparingly):
    - Patient: "I hate this hospital."
    - Nurse: "You hate this hospital?"
- *Empathy:* Make observations: "You are shaking," and "You seem worried."
- Recognize feelings:
    - Patient: "I want to go home."
    - Nurse: "It must be hard to be away from your home and family."
- Provide information as honestly and completely as possible about condition, treatment, and procedures and respond to the patient's questions and concerns.

EXPLORATION, ORIENTATION, COLLABORATION, AND VALIDATION

Methods to promote a caring and supportive environment with **therapeutic communication** include:

Exploration	Verbally express implied messages: Patient: "This treatment is too much trouble." Nurse: "You think the treatment isn't helping you?" Explore a topic but allow the patient to terminate the discussion without further probing: "I'd like to hear how you feel about that."
Orientation	Indicate reality: Patient: "Someone is screaming." Nurse: "That sound was an ambulance siren." Comment on distortions without directly agreeing or disagreeing: Patient: "That nurse promised I didn't have to walk again." Nurse: "Really? That's surprising because the doctor ordered physical therapy twice a day."

Collaboration	Work together to achieve better results: "Maybe if we talk about this, we can figure out a way to make the treatment easier for you."
Validation	Seek validation: "Do you feel better now?" or "Did the medication help you breathe better."

NON-VERBAL COMMUNICATION

EYE CONTACT AND TONE

Non-verbal communication can convey as much information as verbal communication, both on the nurse's part and the patient's. Non-verbal communication is used for a number of purposes, such as expressing feelings and attitudes, and may be a barrier to communication or a facilitator. While there are cultural differences, interpretation of non-verbal communication can help the nurse to better understand and promote communication:

- *Eye contact:* Making eye contact provides a connection and shows caring and involvement in the communication. Avoiding contact may indicate someone is not telling the truth or is uncomfortable, fearful, ashamed, or hiding something.
- *Tone*: The manner in which words are spoken (patiently, cheerfully, somberly) affects the listener, and when the message and tone don't match, it can interfere with communication. A high-pitched tone of voice may indicate nervousness or stress.

TOUCH, GESTURES, AND POSTURE

Additional elements of **non-verbal communication** include the following:

- *Touch*: Reaching out to touch an older adult's hand or pat a shoulder during communication is reassuring but hugging or excessive touching can make people feel uncomfortable. People may touch themselves (lick lips, pick at skin, scratch) if they are anxious.
- *Gestures*: Using the hands to emphasize meaning is common and may be particularly helpful during explanations, but excessive gesturing can be distracting. Some gestures alone convey message, such as a wave goodbye or pointing. Tapping of the foot, moving the legs, or fidgeting may indicate nervousness. Rubbing the hands together is sometimes a self-comforting measure. Some gestures, such as handshakes, are part of social ritual. Mixed messages, such as fidgeting but speaking with a calm voice may indicate uncertainty or anxiety.
- *Posture*: Slumping can indicate lack of interest or withdrawal. Leaning toward the opposite person while talking indicates interest and facilitates interaction.

NON-THERAPEUTIC COMMUNICATION

While using therapeutic communication is important, it is equally important to avoid interjecting **non-therapeutic communication**, which can effectively block effective communication. ***Avoid the following:***

Stating meaningless clichés	"Don't worry. Everything will be fine." "Isn't it a nice day?"
Providing advice	"You should..." or "The best thing to do is...." It's better when patients ask for advice to provide facts and encourage patients to make their own decisions.

Providing inappropriate approval	This can prevent the patient from expressing true feelings or concerns. Patient: "I shouldn't cry about this." Nurse: "That's right. You're an adult."
Asking for explanations of behavior not directly related to patient care	Asking for explanations such as "Why are you upset?" may require analysis and explanation of feelings on the patient's part.
Agreeing rather than accepting and responding	Agreeing with patient's statements "I agree with you" or "You are right" can make it difficult for the patient to change his/her statement or opinion later.
Making negative judgments	"You should stop arguing with the nurses."
Devaluing patient's feelings	"Everyone gets upset at times."
Disagreeing directly	"That can't be true" or "I think you are wrong."
Defending against criticism	"The doctor was not being rude; he's just very busy today."
Changing the subject	This avoids dealing with uncomfortable subjects: Patient: "I'm never going to get well." Nurse: "Your family will be here in a few minutes."
Making inappropriate literal responses	Even as a joke, this is not appropriate, especially if the patient is confused or having difficulty expressing ideas: Patient: "There are bugs crawling under my skin." Nurse: "I'll get some bug spray."
Challenging to establish reality	This often increases confusion and frustration: Patient: "I'm dying!" Nurse: If you were dying, you wouldn't be able to yell and kick."

Cultural Competence

Health professionals must be aware of issues related to cultural competence in dealing with patients and their families. **Cultural competence** is the ability to interact in an effective manner with people from different cultural groups. There are four different aspects of cultural competence:

- An individual's awareness of his or her own cultural view.
- An individual's attitudes toward the practices of other cultural groups.
- Knowledge of the practices of other cultural groups.
- The ability to interact effectively with other cultural groups.

Members of different cultural groups have different customs regarding eye contact, distance, and time. Some cultures avoid making eye contact, considering it rude. Individuals from these cultures may look down as a sign of respect. The space maintained between individuals varies among cultures. Members of some cultural groups stand close and some maintain a greater distance. While Americans tend to be concerned with being on time, other cultures have a more flexible view of time. It is important for health-care professionals to be sensitive to the needs of other cultural groups.

CHANGE THEORY/MANAGEMENT

LEWIN/SCHEIN

Change theory was developed by Kurt Lewin and modified by Edgar Schein. This management theory is based on 3 stages:

1. *Motivation to change (unfreezing):* Dissatisfaction occurs when goals are not met, but as previous beliefs are brought into question, survival anxiety occurs; however, sometimes learning anxiety about having to learn different strategies causes resistance that can lead to denial, blaming others, and trying to maneuver or bargain without real change.
2. *Desire to change (unfrozen):* Dissatisfaction is strong enough to override defensive actions and the desire to change is strong, but must be coupled with identification of needed changes.
3. *Development of permanent change (refreezing):* The new behavior that has developed becomes habitual often requiring a change in perceptions of self and the establishment of new relationships.

TRANSTHEORETICAL MODEL

The **Transtheoretical Model** focuses on changes in behavior based on the individual's (not society's or other's) decisions and is used to develop strategies to promote changes in health behavior. This model outlines stages people go through changing problem behavior and having a positive attitude about change.

The stages of change are as follows:

1. *Precontemplation:* The person is either unaware or under-informed about the consequences of a problem behavior and has no intention of changing behavior in the next 6 months.
2. *Contemplation*: The person is aware of the costs and benefits of changing behavior and intends to change in the next 6 months but is procrastinating and is not ready for action.
3. *Preparation*: The person has a plan and intends to instigate change in the near future (≤1 month) and is ready for action plans.
4. *Action*: The person will modify his/her behavior only if the behavior meets a set criterion (such as complete abstinence from drinking).
5. *Maintenance*: The person works to maintain changes and gains confidence that he/she will not relapse.

TEMPORAL DIMENSIONS AND INTERVENING VARIABLES

The **Transtheoretical Model** describes stages of change (precontemplation, contemplation, preparation, action and maintenance). These stages are a process that the individual goes through in order to change behavior and attitudes, but there are other aspects to be considered. There are two **temporal dimensions** to this process:

- *Distance* of the behavior (from the time the process begins to the time change is made) is an important consideration.
- *Duration* of the behavior (the time from change to relapse) is also important. Duration should become longer with a goal of no relapse.

Additionally, the model recognizes that there are **intervening variables:** decisional balance (the costs and benefits of change), self-efficacy (confidence in being able to change), and any other variables, such as social, environmental, psychological, or medical, which may affect behavior and change.

Juran's Quality Improvement Process

Joseph **Juran's quality improvement process (QIP)** is a 4-step method of change (focusing on quality control) which is based on a trilogy of concepts that includes quality planning, control, and improvement. The steps to the QIP process include the following:

1. *Defining* the project and organizing includes listing and prioritizing problems and identifying a team.
2. *Diagnosing* includes analyzing problems and then formulating theories related to cause by root cause analysis and test theories.
3. *Remediating* includes considering various alternative solutions and then designing and implementing specific solutions and controls while addressing institutional resistance to change. As causes of problems are identified and remediation instituted to remove the problems, the processes should improve.
4. *Holding* involves evaluating performance and monitoring the control system in order to maintain gains.

FOCUS

Find, organize, clarify, uncover, start (FOCUS) is a performance improvement model used to facilitate change:

1. *Find*: Identify a problem by looking at the organization and attempting to determine what isn't working well or what is wrong.
2. *Organize*: Identifying those people who have an understanding of the problem or process and creating a team to work on improving performance.
3. *Clarify*: Determining what is involved in solving the problem by utilizing brainstorming techniques, such as the Ishikawa diagram.
4. *Uncover*: Analyzing the situation to determine the reason the problem has arisen or that a process is unsuccessful.
5. *Start*: Determining where to begin in the change process.

FOCUS, by itself, is an incomplete process and is primarily used as a means to identify a problem rather than a means to find the solution. FOCUS is usually combined with PDCA (FOCUS-PDCA), so it becomes a 9-step process; however, beginning with FOCUS helps to narrow the focus, resulting in better outcomes.

Changes in Regulations/Standards

Communication of **changes in regulations and standards** must be made in a timely manner and disseminated widely, especially if the changes result in differences in processes or procedures. The CNS is often the first person to receive information about pending changes and should begin early to make plans to communicate to others. There are a number of ways to communicate changes:

- *Strategic Plan* should be updated on an annual basis to include all information related to changes in regulations and standards.
- *Consulting with administration* about impending changes and courses of action should be the practice.
- *Staff meetings* with department heads and staff who are directly impacted by changes should be held to outline changes.
- *Print materials*, such as documents, fliers, and posters should be prepared to provide the necessary information.

- *Email* communications can quickly alert staff to changes.
- *Training classes* that cover new standards should be provided as quickly as possible.

Interventions, Outcomes, and Changes in Practice

Interventions and outcomes should be tied to each other. After an initial cost-benefit analysis and institution of an intervention, outcomes need to be assessed carefully to determine if the intervention is meeting the goal set for it and if it is cost-effective. If, for example, a hospital is investing $93,000 additionally each year to control infections, expecting a savings of 5 infections at $135,000 ($43,000 net), but in fact the savings amount to only 2 infections at $34,000, then the added cost to the hospital is $59,000.

Changes in practice, however, cannot be made only on the basis of monetary figures. Further analysis must be done to determine if other variables affected the outcomes. If the hospital opened a transplant unit with additional surgical patients, then the reduction in 2 infections might be impressive. If there is a *staphylococcus* carrier among the staff, then this might account for additional infections. In some cases, a change of practice is required.

Resistance to Organizational Change

Performance improvement processes cannot occur without organizational change, and **resistance to change** is common for many people, so coordinating requires anticipating resistance and taking steps to achieve cooperation. Resistance often relates to concerns about job loss, increased responsibilities, and general denial or lack of understanding and frustration. Leaders can prepare others involved in the process of change by taking these steps:

1. Be honest, informative, and tactful, giving people thorough information about anticipated changes and how the changes will affect them, including positives.
2. Be patient in allowing people the time they need to contemplate changes and express anger or disagreement.
3. Be empathetic in listening carefully to the concerns of others.
4. Encourage participation, allowing staff to propose methods of implementing change, so they feel some sense of ownership.
5. Establish a climate in which all staff members are encouraged to identify the need for change on an ongoing basis.
6. Present further ideas for change to management.

Educational Initiatives

Patient Education

Patient education is a primary concern of nursing. Written materials for older adults should be age appropriate, clearly written with a large font, and illustrated. There are commercially prepared general health materials available, but educational materials are often prepared by staff for the population served by an institution. Materials should be written and then assessed to determine if they help to meet established goals for patient understanding and compliance. All aspects of patient and family education should be documented, including the date and time of the education, the type of presentation, the handouts or material provided to the patient and/or family, and the patient's response. Older adults may be overwhelmed by packets of information and may not be able to process the information. This is especially true of adults who are weak or cognitively impaired. Therefore, the nurse should be available to review the material with the patient and demonstrate any techniques. The material should be taught in small increments, as the patient may not be able to take in too much information at one time.

Methods for Learning Needs Assessment

There are a number of **methods** used to assess the educational needs of patients/families. Using multiple strategies provides the most accurate results:

- *Consult with the public health department* about community issues, such as rates of HBV, HIV, and TB, to determine shared educational needs.
- *Conduct mail surveys* either of the general populace or targeted surveys of former patients and families. Mail survey return rates are often low, so a large number of surveys must be prepared.
- *Conduct telephone surveys* of the same groups. This method usually has a better response rate and is less expensive, but is time-consuming and may require hiring temporary staff.
- *Conduct onsite surveys* for both inpatients and clinic patients, including both patients and family members. When surveys are requested by staff directly, return rates are good.
- *Conduct Interviews* for inpatients, clinic patients, and families. This method gives people the chance to elaborate but requires much staff time.

Readiness to Learn

The patient and family's **readiness to learn** should be assessed because if they are not ready, instruction is of little value. Often readiness is indicated when the patient/family asks questions or shows an interest in procedures. There are a number of factors related to readiness to learn:

- *Physical factors:* There are a number of physical factors that can affect ability. Manual dexterity may be required to complete a task, and this varies by age and condition. Hearing or vision deficits may impact ability. Complex tasks may be too difficult for some because of weakness or cognitive impairment, and modifications of the environment may be needed. Health status, age, and gender may all impact the ability to learn.
- *Experience*: People's experience with learning can vary widely and is affected by their ability to cope with changes, their personal goals, motivation to learn, and cultural background. People may have widely divergent ideas about what constitutes illness and/or treatment. Lack of English skills may make learning difficult and prevent people from asking questions.
- *Mental/emotional status:* The patient's support system and motivation may impact readiness. Anxiety, fear, or depression about condition can make learning very difficult because the patient and family cannot focus on learning, so the nurse must spend time to reassure them and wait until they are emotionally more receptive.
- *Knowledge/education:* The knowledge base of the patient and family, their cognitive ability, and their learning styles all affect their readiness to learn. The nurse should always begin by assessing what knowledge the patient and family already have about the patient's disease, condition, or treatment and then build from that base. People with little medical experience may lack knowledge of basic medical terminology, interfering with their ability and readiness to learn.

Variables

Methods used to instruct patients and families depend on many **variables**, which may include the following:

- *Goal:* instruction should be provided keeping the purpose in mind, whether it is to increase handwashing or promote vaccinations.
- *Necessity*: If the patient has a wound or invasive device that requires home care, then intensive one-on-one demonstration and observation is required, but if the need is more general, then fliers or handouts might be sufficient.

- *Educational background*: If most of the hospital population is from an affluent well-educated group, then detailed print information may be indicated. If there is a large illiterate or poorly educated population, then posters or handouts with pictures and little text might be more appropriate.
- *Language:* If there are sufficient populations of non-English speakers, then it may be necessary to produce instructive materials in Spanish, Russian, Chinese, or other languages or with primarily pictures/drawings.

LEARNING STYLES

Not all people are aware of their preferred **learning style.** A range of teaching materials/methods that relates to all 3 learning preferences—visual, auditory, kinesthetic—(and age-appropriate) should be available. Part of assessment for teaching involves choosing the right approach based on observation and feedback. Often, presenting learners with different options gives a clue to their preferred learning style. Some people have a combined learning style:

- **Visual learners**
  - Learn best by seeing and reading:
  - Provide written directions, picture guides, or demonstrate procedures. Use charts and diagrams.
  - Provide photos, videos.
- **Auditory learners**
  - Learn best by listening and talking:
  - Explain procedures while demonstrating and have the learner repeat. Plan extra time to discuss and answer questions. Provide audiotapes.
- **Kinesthetic learners**
  - Learn best by handling, doing, and practicing:
  - Provide hands-on experience throughout the teaching process. Encourage the handling of supplies/equipment. Allow the learner to demonstrate. Minimize instructions and allow the person to explore equipment and procedures.

DEALING WITH LEARNING STYLES

Recognizing and applying teaching methods to learning styles can improve learning markedly, but the instructor should keep a number of **principles of dealing with learning styles** in mind:

- Learning styles can and should be assessed for both the instructor and the patient family. People often can state a preference when asked how they best learn. If the nurse understands his/her own learning style, it can help the nurse understand its importance in teaching and learning.
- The nurse must use care not to prepare most educational materials to match his/her own learning style but to remember that other types of material must also be prepared.
- Helping the patient/family to understand their learning styles can make them more efficient learners.
- Materials that address more than one learning style (audio plus visual, for example) can help learners adapt learning to various types of presentations.
- Educational materials can be adapted to appeal to different learning styles.

LEARNER OUTCOMES

When the professional nurse plans an educational offering, be it a class, an online module, a workshop, or educational materials, the nurse should identify **learner outcomes,** which should be conveyed to the learners from the very beginning so that they are aware of the expectations. The subject matter of the educational material and the learner outcomes should be directly related. For example, if the nurse is instructing a patient on preparing and giving insulin injections, then a learner outcome might be as follows: "Accurately fill syringe with correct insulin dose." There may be one or multiple learner outcomes, but part of the assessment at the end of the learning experience should be to determine if, in fact, the learner outcomes have been achieved. A survey of whether or not the learners felt that they had achieved the learner outcomes can give valuable feedback and guidance to the quality professional.

Approaches to Teaching

There are many **approaches to teaching**, and the CNS must prepare, present, and coordinate a wide range of educational workshops, lectures, discussions, and one-on-one instructions on a variety of topics. Planning the amount of time for classes should be made part of the plan, but the CNS should allow for flexibility to contend with unexpected needs. All types of classes can be utilized, depending upon the purpose and material:

- *Educational workshops* are usually conducted with small groups. They allow for maximal participation and are especially good for demonstrations and practice sessions.
- *Lectures* are often used for more academic or detailed information. This format may include questions and answers but limits discussion. An effective lecture should include some audiovisual support.
- *Discussions* are best with small groups so that people can actively participate. This is a good format for problem solving.
- *One-on-one instruction* is especially helpful for targeted instruction in procedures for individuals.
- *Computer/Internet modules* are good for independent learners.

Facilitation of Learning

According to the synergy model, **facilitation of learning** is the ability to make learning easier. Facilitation of learning requires needs assessment. In addition, the material should be structured to suit the receiver in terms of delivery and content. There are a number of levels of facilitation of learning:

- At **level 1,** the nurse is able to deliver planned educational content that is disease specific but does not have the ability to assess patient readiness to learn or abilities. The patient and his or her family are considered to be passive recipients of knowledge.
- At **level 3,** the nurse is able to individualize treatment according to the patient's and family's needs and has an understanding of different methods of teaching and learning styles. The patient's needs are considered in planning.
- At **level 5,** the nurse has excellent understanding of teaching methods, learning styles, and assessment for learning readiness and develops an educational plan in cooperation and collaboration with others, including patients, families, and other health and allied professionals.

Health Literacy

Health literacy is the ability to obtain, understand, and consent to medical care and make informed healthcare decisions. Health literacy includes:

- Reading with comprehension and applying reason to context.
- Understanding graphs and other visual representations of information.

- Using the computer to obtain information.
- Understanding the results of laboratory and radiographic studies.
- Understanding and using basic mathematical computations.
- Articulating concerns and questions.
- Understanding basic anatomy and physiology.
- Having basic knowledge of disease.
- Understanding preventive health measures.
- Knowing how to access health care and health information.
- Health literacy may be affected by a number of factors, including lack of adequate education, low literacy or illiteracy, dementia, or learning disabilities. The most vulnerable include the elderly, ethnic minorities, immigrants, and those with low income and/or chronic mental or physical health problems.

Readability

Studies have indicated that learning is more effective if oral presentations and/or demonstrations are supplemented with reading materials, such as handouts. **Readability** (the grade level of material) is a concern because many patients and families may have limited English skills or low literacy level, and it can be difficult for the nurse to assess people's reading level. The average American reads effectively at the 6th to 8th grade level (regardless of education achieved), but many health education materials have a much higher readability level. Additionally, research indicates that even people with much higher reading skills learn medical and health information most effectively when the material is presented at the 6th to 8th grade readability level. Therefore, patient education materials (and consent forms) should not be written at higher than 6th to 8th grade level. Readability index calculators are available on the Internet to give an approximation of grade level and difficulty for those preparing materials without expertise in teaching reading.

Important Elements of Physical Environment Regarding Audiovisual Materials

There are a number of issues that must be considered when teaching a course and determining the appropriate audiovisuals and handout materials. The **physical environment** is a major consideration, especially when using **audiovisual materials**:

First, everyone in the room must be *able to hear and see*. In a small room, a television screen may suffice, but in a large space, a projection screen must be used.

Another issue is *lighting*. Some projectors have low resolution and the lights need to be turned off /dimmed or windows covered. Turning lights on and off a dozen times during a presentation can be very distracting. A small portable light at a speaker podium or an alternate presentation can be used.

Text size for presentations is another issue. PowerPoint or other presentations that include text must be of sufficient font size to be read from the back of the room.

Videos

Videos are a useful adjunct to teaching as they reduce the time needed for one-on-one instruction (increasing cost-effectiveness). Passive presentation of videos, such as in the waiting area, has little value, but focused viewing in which the nurse discusses the purpose of the video presentation prior to viewing and then is available for discussion after viewing can be very effective. Patients and/or families are often nervous about learning patient care and are unsure of their abilities, so they may not focus completely when the nurse is presenting information. Allowing the patients/families to watch a video demonstration or explanation first and allowing them to stop or review the video presentation can help them to grasp the fundamentals before they have to apply them, relieving some of the anxiety they may be experiencing. Videos are much more effective than written materials for those with low literacy or poor English skills. The nurse should always be available to answer questions and discuss the material after the patients/families finish viewing.

One-on-One Instruction Versus Group Instruction for Patient/Family Education

One-on-one instruction is the most costly type of instruction for an institution to conduct because it is time intensive. However, it allows the patient and family more time to interact with the nurse instructor and allows them to have more control over the process. The patient and family can ask questions or ask the instructor to repeat explanations or demonstrations. One-on-one instruction is especially valuable when patients and families must learn particular skills, such as managing dialysis. It is also a good method if confidentiality is important.

Group instruction is less costly than one-on-one instruction because the needs of a number of people can be met at the same time. Group presentations are more structured and are usually scheduled for a particular time-limited period (an hour, for example). Therefore, patients and families have less control over the instruction process. Questioning by patients is usually more limited and may be done only at the end of the session. Group instruction allows patients and families with similar health problems to interact. Group instruction is especially useful for general instruction, such as managing diet.

Coaching Patients and Families to Navigate the Healthcare System

Coaching patients and families to navigate the healthcare system to ensure safe passage includes the following:

Encouraging questions	Encouraging patient and/or family to ask questions is a beginning, but the nurse should suggest the types of questions to ask. A good starting point is: "What questions do you have about . . .?" and then respond with, "You might also want information about. . . ." The nurse should advise the patient to write down questions and refer to the list when speaking with the physician or others.
Educating	Providing information to the patient and/or family about treatments, changes, conditions, and other aspects of care helps them cope with the situations as they arise.
Avoiding medical errors	Patient and/or family should be advised to take steps to prevent medical errors: Provide all physicians a list of medicines. Ask healthcare personnel providing care to wash hands. Make sure healthcare personnel ask for two means of identification before administering any medication or treatment.

Teaching Older Adults

There are a number of strategies that facilitate **teaching older adults**:

- Spend a little time getting to know the patient so that he/she is more relaxed and receptive to learning.
- Determine what information is critical for the patient to learn and what is non-essential.
- Evaluate the patient's learning style and previous knowledge about the topic.

- Plan for ample time for each session of instruction and plan the probable number of sessions to determine how much instruction is needed for each session. Ensure that sessions are closely spaced to reinforce learning.
- Provide the patient ample time to practice.
- Allow the patient to guide the pace of the session as much as possible and encourage feedback.
- Prepare age-appropriate handouts at accessible reading level and with large-size font.
- Provide materials (pencil, paper) in case the patient wants to make notes.
- Be supportive, patient, and enthusiastic.

PEPLAU AND THE INTERPERSONAL RELATIONS MODEL OF NURSING

Hildegard Peplau developed the **interpersonal relations model of nursing** in 1952. This model focuses on the quality of nurse-client interaction. Peplau believed that patients deserve human care by educated nurses and should be treated with dignity and respect. She also believed that the environment (social, psychosocial, and physical) could affect health in a positive or negative manner. Peplau viewed the nurse as a person who could make a substantial difference for the patient and who acts as a "maturing force." The nurse can focus on the way in which patients react to their illness and can help patients to use illness as an opportunity for learning and maturing through the nurse-client interactions. The nurse helps the patient to understand the nature of his/her problem and to find solutions. Peplau's theory stresses the importance of collaboration between the patient and the nurse. The nurse-client relationship is viewed as a number of overlapping phases: orientation, identification of problem, explanation of potential solutions, and resolution of problem.

BENNER AND THE STAGES OF CLINICAL COMPETENCE

Benner developed the **stages of clinical competence** for nurses in 1984. These stages were based on the Dreyfus Model of Skill Acquisition. There are **5 stages of clinical competence** for nurses:

- *Novice*: The nurse has little experience and depends on rules and learned behavior and is not able to adapt easily.
- *Advanced beginner:* The nurse has some experience in coping with new situations and is able to formulate some principles of action.
- *Competent:* The nurse has 2 to 3 years of experience and has some mastery of new situations and goals and can cope well but may require time for planning and lack flexibility.
- *Proficient*: The nurse looks at situations holistically and relies on experience to determine goals and plans and can adapt plans to changing needs and make decisions based on understanding of maxims.
- *Expert*: The nurse has a wealth of experience to draw on and can provide care intuitively rather than relying on rules and maxims. The nurse is able to understand needs and determine quickly the most effective focus for providing care.

WATSON AND THE PHILOSOPHY OF HUMAN CARING

Watson developed the **philosophy of human caring** in 1979. Watson focused on transpersonal caring, which views the individual holistically from the perspective of the interrelationship among health, sickness, and behavior with a nursing goal to promote health and prevent illness. Watson's theory encompasses 10 caritas (methods of caring) the nurse can employ during caring occasions (opportunities to provide care) and caring moments (actions). The **10 caritas** include the following:

1. Having loving kindness and equanimity.
2. Being present and sustaining the spiritual beliefs of patient and self.
3. Cultivating personal spiritual practice.
4. Developing and maintaining a caring relationship.
5. Supporting both negative and positive feelings of the patient.
6. Being creative in caring.
7. Providing teaching-learning experiences within the patient's frame of reference.
8. Creating a physical and spiritual healing environment.
9. Providing for basic human needs.
10. Being open to spiritual concepts related to life-death of self and the patient.

Bloom's Taxonomy and 3 Types of Learning

Bloom's taxonomy outlines behaviors that are necessary for learning, and this can apply to healthcare. The theory describes 3 types of learning:

- *Cognitive* (This involves learning and gaining intellectual skills to master 6 categories of effective learning.)
  - Knowledge, Comprehension, Application, Analysis, Synthesis, Evaluation
- *Affective* (This involves recognizing 5 categories of feelings and values from simple to complex. This is slower to achieve than cognitive learning.)
  - *Receiving phenomena:* Accepting need to learn.
  - *Responding to phenomena:* Taking active part in care.
  - *Valuing:* Understanding value of becoming independent in care.
  - *Organizing values:* Understanding how surgery/treatment has improved life.
  - *Internalizing values:* Accepting condition as part of life, being consistent and self-reliant.
- *Psychomotor* (This involves mastering 7 motor skills necessary for independence. This follows a progression from simple to complex.)
  - *Perception*: Uses sensory information to learn tasks.
  - *Set:* Shows willingness to perform tasks.
  - *Guided response:* Follows directions.
  - *Mechanism:* Does specific tasks.
  - *Complex overt response:* Displays competence in self-care.
  - *Adaptation:* Modifies procedures as needed.
  - *Origination:* Creatively deals with problems.

Knowles' Theory of Andragogy

Knowles developed the **theory of andragogy** in relation to adult learners, who are more interested in process than in information and content. Knowles outlined some principles of adult learning and typical characteristics of adult learners that an instructor should consider when planning strategies for teaching parents, families, or staff:

Practical and goal-oriented	Provide overviews or summaries and examples. Use collaborative discussions with problem-solving exercises. Remain organized with the goal in mind.
Self-directed	Provide active involvement, asking for input. Allow different options toward achieving the goal. Give them responsibilities.
Knowledgeable	Show respect for their life experiences/education. Validate their knowledge and ask for feedback. Relate new material to information with which they are familiar.
Relevancy-oriented	Explain how information will be applied. Clearly identify objectives.
Motivated	Provide certificates of achievement or some type of recognition for achievement

Bandura's Theory of Social Learning

In the 1970s, A. Bandura proposed the **theory of social learning,** in which learning develops from observing, organizing and rehearsing behavior that has been modeled. Bandura believed that people are more likely to adopt the behavior if they value the outcomes and the outcomes have functional value and if the person modeling the behavior is similar to the learner and is admired because of status. Behavior is the result of observation of behavioral, environmental, and cognitive interactions. There are **4 conditions required for modeling***:*

- *Attention*: The degree of attention paid to modeling can depend on many variables (physical, social, environmental).
- *Retention*: People's ability to retain models depends on symbolic coding, creating mental images, organizing thoughts, and rehearsing (mentally or physically).
- *Reproduction*: The ability to reproduce a model depends on physical and mental capabilities.
- *Motivation*: Motivation may derive from past performances, rewards, or vicarious modeling.

Cognitive Flexibility

The **theory of cognitive flexibility**, focusing on the use of interactive technology such as computerized programs, was developed by Spiro, Feltovich, and Coulson. The theory recognizes the complexity and flexibility of learning and suggests that information must be presented from a variety of perspectives, and that materials and presentations must be context specific. According to this theory, the primary factor in learning is the ability of the person to construct knowledge. Basic concepts include the following:

- Provide multiple and varying presentations of content. This can include technological presentations (computerized) as well as input from instructors/experts who can facilitate learning.
- Avoid oversimplification of content and ensure that information relates to context.
- Promote the building of knowledge rather than the transfer of information. The learner must interact with the material by such actions as responding to questions or formulating hypotheses based on information presented in order to construct his/her own conclusions.
- Interconnect instructional sources.

Problem-Based Learning

Problem-based learning was developed by McMaster University in the 1960s. It is learner-centered with the instructor serving as facilitator rather than lecturer. The learner is presented with a problem and must search for the solution. Problem-based learning focuses on promoting the learner's ability to use critical thinking and problem-solving skills, increasing motivation. This process of problem-solving is believed to enhance transfer so that information learned in one context is internalized and can be utilized in other contexts as well. While effective, this method requires more preparation time and may require an extended learning period while the learner identifies the problem and attempts to formulate a solution. The teacher/facilitator can guide the learners by helping them to ask questions that lead to solutions.

Attribution Theory

Bernard Weiner developed the cognitive theory known as **attribution theory,** which focuses on explaining behavior. Weiner suggested that people attempt to attribute cause to behavior, based on 3-stages:

- Observing behavior.
- Determining that the behavior is intentional.
- Attributing the behavior to internal or external causes.

According to this theory, there are *factors to which achievement can be attributed:*

- Individual effort.
- Ability.
- Difficulty of task.
- Good or bad luck.

People often view their own achievement as the result of effort and ability and the achievements of others as the result of luck. By the same token, people may view personal failures as the result of bad luck and failures of others as the result of lack of effort or ability. Attributions are classified according to 3 factors:

- Locus of control (internal/external).
- Stability of causes for behavior.
- Ability to control causes.

Gardner's Theory of Multiple Intelligences

H. Gardner developed the **theory of multiple intelligences,** which states that there are at least 7 categories of "intelligences" that people utilize to comprehend the world around them and to learn. Gardner proposed that teaching that engages multiple intelligences is more effective than those focused primarily on linguistic or logical/mathematical intelligences (those most commonly addressed in education). Learners should be assessed to determine their personal intelligence strengths, and teaching should address the learner's preferences:

- *Linguistic*: Ability to use and understand language, written or spoken
- *Logical/mathematical:* Ability to utilize deductive and inductive reasoning, numbers, and abstract thinking
- *Visuospatial:* Ability to visualize and comprehend spatial dimensions
- *Body/Kinesthetic:* Ability to control physical action
- *Musical/rhythmic:* Ability to create/appreciate musical forms

- *Interpersonal*: Ability to communicate and establish relationships with others
- *Intrapersonal*: Ability to utilize self-knowledge and to be self-aware

Designing Programs to Promote Establishment of Appropriate Therapeutic Relationships

Programs to promote the establishment of **appropriate therapeutic relationships** should address all boundary issues. The most effective method is to integrate this material into all programs, including orientation, staff training, and evaluations, rather than addressing appropriate therapeutic relationships as a separate issue, although sexual harassment is usually addressed separately because of regulations. The primary issues in a therapeutic relationship are respect for the patient and family and self-awareness on the part of the healthcare practitioner, so these issues must be continually explored. The nurse must have self-awareness of personal values, biases, motivating forces, beliefs, strengths, weaknesses, feelings, and attitudes. The nurse's personal beliefs about others may affect a patient evaluation when the nurse makes judgments based on personal feelings rather than clinical observations. A strong self-awareness based on honest exploration can be an asset when working with the patient, as it can guide the nurse's behavior and responses to promote a better therapeutic relationship.

Development of Goals, Measurable Objectives, and Lesson Plans

Once a topic for performance improvement education has been chosen, **the goals, measurable objectives with strategies, and lesson plans** must be developed. A class should stay focused on one area rather than trying to cover many things.

Goal	Increase compliance with hand hygiene standards in ICU.
Objectives	Develop a series of posters and fliers by June 1. Observe 100% compliance with hand hygiene standards at 2 weeks, 1-month, and 2-month intervals after training is completed.
Strategies	Conduct 4 classes at different times over a one-week period, May 25-31. Place posters in all nursing units, staff rooms, and utility rooms by January 3. Develop a PowerPoint presentation for class and Intranet/Internet for access by all staff by May 25. Utilize handwashing kits.
Lesson plans	Discussion period: Why do we need 100% compliance? PowerPoint: The case for hand hygiene. Discussion: What did you learn? Demonstration and activities to show effectiveness Handwashing technique.

ADDIE Model

The American Society for Training and Development developed the **ADDIE Model** for instructional systems development. It provides an outline for development of training programs in 5 steps:

- *Step 1 – Analysis:* During this phase, the needs of the organization, the current level of knowledge, and the specific types of training needs are assessed, including goals and outcomes. Information about needs should be obtained from those involved in targeted processes. The training facilities, resources, and any limitations should be identified. Learning objectives should be developed.

- *Step 2 – Design:* This includes planning for the training based on what the learners already know and need to know. The strategy for instruction and course format should be clarified and an instructional plan written.
- *Step 3 – Development:* During development, the course materials are developed based on the analysis and design plan. The course should be presented for review to ensure it is accurate and complete and then piloted and reviewed again.
- *Step 4 – Implementation:* Implementation alone requires a great many considerations. A timeline for training must be provided with a schedule of courses. Learners must be enrolled, and classrooms must be made available. Coordination must be done with supervisors to assure that staff can attend classes. If trainers are needed, they must be trained. Course materials must be printed, purchased, or prepared, including certificates or participation records. Technological needs, such as for computers or Internet access, must be arranged, and travel plans made if necessary. Once all these things are taken care of, the training can begin.
- *Step 5 – Evaluation:* Pre-and post-tests can indicate if course material was learned, and a satisfaction survey can provide immediate feedback about whether learners like the course or feel it meets their expectations or the stated goals. However, long-term outcomes related to actual performance improvement are more difficult to quantify and may take months.

Counseling Principles

Counseling must have an ethical basis, based on respect for the client. General **principles of counseling** include the following:

- *Respect others:* Clients, families, and colleagues should be treated with respect and consideration. Cultural and lifestyle differences must be acknowledged and respected as well.
- *Avoid causing harm:* The wellbeing of the client must take precedence. Clients should be provided information based on interaction with the client that helps to elicit the client's concerns and need. Counseling should be tailored to assist clients to manage their problems/concerns.
- *Respect confidentiality:* The client should be assured that information provided will be kept in confidence and given an explanation regarding the need for questioning.
- *Provide opportunities for choice:* If the client is to remain engaged in the counseling process, he/she should be presented with some choices.
- *Be honest:* A relationship of trust cannot be established without honesty.
- *Remain within the scope of practice:* One should never counsel outside one's area of competence but should make referrals when appropriate.

Counseling Skills

There are a number of **basic skills** related to counseling that can be used when working with patients/clients outside of formal counseling. They are especially valuable skills when providing education. Skills include the following:

- *Paying attention:* Provide non-verbal feedback to the client by nodding the head, leaning forward, making eye contact, and sitting across from the client.
- *Making observations:* Watch the client's reactions carefully to determine if words and behavior (non-verbal clues) match.
- *Listening actively:* Listen to the words, the tone, the inflection, and the body language.
- *Summarizing/reflecting information:* Reflect back what the client states in order to clarify understanding and meaning. Summarize to help make points clear.

- *Asking questions:* Avoid yes/no questions but ask information (who, what, when, where, why, how, how much) questions.
- *Maintaining silence:* Follow the client's cues and allow periods of silence without becoming anxious.
- *Allowing independence*: Encourage the client to make choices.
- *Providing concrete examples:* Provide concrete rather than abstract examples and encourage the client to do the same through questioning.

Counseling for a Patient with a New Medication

Part of **medication management with new drugs** and prescriptions is to provide counseling for the patient who will be taking the medication. The nurse must provide information about the medication, including its name and dosage, and explain why the patient is going to be taking it. If the patient is going to self-administer the medication or if the nurse will be administering it (such as during an inpatient hospitalization), the nurse should provide information about the drug's effects, as well as potential side effects, therapeutic effects, proposed outcomes and pertinent information about how to take the medication. Certain medications require that the patient take all of the medication as directed, rather than stopping if symptoms abate, and information such as this would need to be specifically addressed. The nurse must counsel the patient about appropriate ways of taking medication, specifically regarding taking it at the same time each day, continuing until all of the medication is gone, or contacting the physician if certain effects develop.

Coordination and Collaboration

Intra- and Interdisciplinary Teams

The complexity of patient care requires collaboration among **intra- and interdisciplinary teams**. Collaboration may begin between the nurse and patient or nurse and doctor, but often, the expertise of others in the healthcare community must be included. Often, the nurse is in the position to seek collaboration and to recognize when multiple perspectives can be helpful in solving conflicts or making decisions about healthcare. Collaboration requires open sharing of ideas and respect for the expertise of the individual. Collaboration requires more than just talking, however. In many cases it may be more formalized, with specialized committees formed in order to solve specific problems. Studies have indicated that patients benefit from collaborative efforts between nurse and physician, and this benefit extends to others as well. In a collaborative environment, all of the participants benefit from sharing ideas and discussion that can lead to innovative problem solving.

Team Building

Leading, facilitating, and participating in performance improvement teams requires a thorough understanding of the dynamics of **team building:**

- *Initial interactions:* This is the time when members begin to define their roles and develop relationships, determining if they are comfortable in the group.
- *Power issues:* The members observe the leader and determine who controls the meeting and how control is exercised and begin to form alliances.
- *Organizing:* Methods to achieve work are clarified and team members begin to work together, gaining respect for each other's contributions and working toward a common goal.
- *Team identification:* Interactions often become less formal as members develop rapport, and members are more willing to help and support each other to achieve goals.

- *Excellence:* This develops through a combination of good leadership, committed team members, clear goals, high standards, external recognition, spirit of collaboration, and a shared commitment to the process.

Conflict Resolution Teams

Conflict is an almost inevitable product of teamwork, and the leader must assume responsibility for **conflict resolution.** While conflicts can be disruptive, they can produce positive outcomes by forcing team members to listen to different perspectives and opening dialogue. The team should make a plan for dealing with conflict resolution. The best time for conflict resolution is when differences emerge but before open conflict and hardening of positions occur. The leader must pay close attention to the people and problems involved, listen carefully, and reassure those involved that their points of view are understood. Steps to conflict resolution include the following:

- Allow both sides to present their side of conflict without bias, maintaining a focus on opinions rather than individuals.
- Encourage cooperation through negotiation and compromise.
- Maintain the focus, providing guidance to keep the discussions on track and avoid arguments.
- Evaluate the need for renegotiation, formal resolution process, or third-party involvement.
- Utilize humor and empathy to diffuse escalating tensions.
- Summarize the issues, outlining key arguments.
- Avoid forcing resolution if possible.

Negotiation

Negotiating may be a formal process, as when negotiating with administration for increased benefits, or an informal process, as arriving at a team consensus, depending on the purpose and the parties involved.

Competition	In this approach, one party wins and the other loses, as when parties feel their positions are non-negotiable and are unwilling to compromise. To prevail, one party must remain firm, but this can result in conflict.
Accommodation	One party concedes to the other, but the losing side may gain little or nothing, so this approach should be used when there is clear benefit to one choice.
Avoidance	When both parties dislike conflict, they may put off negotiating and resolve nothing, so the problems remain.
Compromise	Both parties make concessions in order to reach consensus, but this can result in decisions that suit no one; therefore, compromise is not always the ideal solution.
Collaboration	Both parties receive what they want, often by finding creative solutions, but collaboration may not be an option with highly competitive parties.

Consultation Theory

Caplan

The clinical nurse specialist is often actively engaged in a wide range of consultation services. In 1970, Gerald Caplan developed a **theory of mental health consultation** that delineated 4 types of consultation that are applicable to advance practice nurses both within and outside of mental health:

- *Client-centered*: The consultant takes an active role in working with the client in order to make recommendations, such as through making an assessment. This is usually a one-time consultation.
- *Consultee-centered*: The consultant focuses on assisting the consultee to manage problems. This may require education of the consultee or recommendations for alternative actions.
- *Program-centered administrative*: The consultant focuses on assisting the administration to improve clinical services related to specific programs.
- *Consultee-centered administrative*: The consultant assists consultees to meet administrative goals.

Barron and White

Barron and White (1996) built upon theories of Caplan and Lipowski and arrived at a consultation theory based on the nursing process. This model focuses on the purpose and outcomes of consultation as the central point surrounded by the ecological field that includes a number of interrelated factors that must be viewed in context:

- *Process of consultation*: Based on the steps of the nursing process (Assessment, diagnosis, planning, implementation, evaluation).
- *Characteristics of the consultee*: Includes education, experience, motivation, concerns, and time constraints.
- *Characteristics of the consultant*: Includes education, experience, skills, consultative competence, and knowledge of the situation and system.
- *Situation*: Includes consideration of the dynamics (patient-staff concerns, staff-staff concerns), aspects of the system, political considerations, and availability of resources.
- *Characteristics of the client/family:* Includes degree of problem and psychosocial and medical history.

Principles of Consultation

There are a number of **principles of consultation** that have resulted from consultation theory:

- The consultee initiates the consultation in order to meet specific needs.
- The consultant and consultee operate in a horizontal rather than vertical relationship and collaborate to reach solutions to problems.
- The consultant looks at problems and challenges in context rather than in isolation.
- The consultant does not assume responsibility for management of patient care and does not have direct authority.
- The consultant makes recommendations only. Recommendations should be presented in an objective, non-judgmental manner.
- The consultee is not under obligation to follow the recommendations of the consultant. The consultee makes the decision as to whether to accept or reject the consultant's recommendations.
- Consultation must be well documented, explaining not only the recommendations but also the observations and rationale for the recommendations.

Steps in Consultation

The clinical nurse specialist should develop and follow a consistent pattern of **steps in consultation**, understanding that each situation is distinct and may require flexibility. Usual steps include the following:

1. *Assessment*: The consultant must first assess the appropriateness of the request for consultation and the nature of the request, determining whether it is client-centered, consultant centered, or program-centered. The consultant must obtain data in order to identify the exact nature of the problem.
2. *Recommendations*: Based on data and observation, the consultant recommends interventions, such as further education or training for the consultee, clinical action, or changes in processes.
3. *Documentation*: The consultant documents findings and recommendations and establishes a method of evaluation (e.g., survey, data, observation, or outcomes).
4. *Evaluation*: The consultant uses appropriate feedback from evaluation to determine the effectiveness of the consultation.

Review Video: Steps in Consultation
Visit mometrix.com/academy and enter code: 566019

Internal and External Consulting

Internal consulting occurs within an institution or facility by a consultant who is a direct employee. Advantages to internal consultants include cost-effectiveness, especially if consultation is needed on an ongoing basis; familiarity with goals, mission, and needs of institution; ability to respond quickly; and maintenance of institutional privacy. However, internal consultants may have biases and may not represent best practices.

External consulting occurs when a consultant is contracted for a particular purpose, based on expertise. Advantages include the ability to find an expert in a specific area and cost-effectiveness if consultation is needed for only a prescribed period of time. The hourly wage may be higher, but benefit costs are lower. Additionally, the contract can more easily be terminated if results are unsatisfactory. Disadvantages include less control over institutional privacy, increased time needed for the consultant to become familiar with the institution, and less commitment to the institution's goals.

Promoting Collaboration

Promoting collaboration and assisting others to understand and use resources and the expertise of others requires a commitment in terms of time and effort:

- *Coaching others* on methods of collaboration can include providing information in the form of handouts about effective communication strategies and, in turn, modeling this type of communication with the staff being coached.
- *Team meetings* are commonly held on nursing units and provide an opportunity to model collaboration and suggest the need for outside expertise to help with planning patient care plans. The mentoring nurse can initiate discussions about resources that are available in the facility or the community.
- *Selecting a diverse group* for teams or inviting those with expertise in various areas to join the team when needed can help team members to appreciate and understand how to use the input of other resources.

Nursing Skills and Collaboration

Nurses must learn the **skill of collaboration** in order to advance the profession of nursing. Nurses must take an active role in gathering data for evidence-based practice to support the profession's role in health care. Nurses must share their knowledge with other nurses and health professionals in order to plan staffing levels and to provide optimal care to patients. Adequate staffing has consistently been shown to reduce adverse patient outcomes, but there is a well-documented shortage of nurses in the United States; more than half of current RNs work outside the hospital. Increased patient loads not only increase adverse outcomes but also increase job dissatisfaction and burnout. In order to manage the challenges facing nursing, nurses must develop skills needed for collaboration. Nurses must be willing to compromise. They must be able to communicate clearly. Nurses must be able to identify specific challenges and problems and must be able to focus on the task at hand. Finally, nurses must be able to work collaboratively as part of a team.

Interdisciplinary Collaboration

Interdisciplinary collaboration is absolutely critical to nursing practice if the needs and best interests of the patients and families are central. Interdisciplinary practice begins with the nurse and physician but extends to pharmacists, social workers, occupational and physical therapists, nutritionists, and a wide range of allied healthcare providers, all of whom cooperate in diagnosis and treatment, but state regulations determine to some degree how much autonomy a nurse can have in diagnosing and treating. While nurses have increasingly gained more legal rights, they have also become more dependent upon collaboration with others for their expertise and for referrals if the patient's needs extend beyond the nurse's ability to provide assistance. Additionally, the prescriptive ability of nurses varies from state to state, with some requiring direct supervision by other disciplines (such as physicians) while others require particular types of supervisory arrangements, depending upon the circumstances.

Content Expert

A **content expert** is a person who has knowledge of a certain area to the point of being an authority on the subject. Because of this knowledge and level of expertise, the content expert decides how the knowledge will be disseminated and taught to others. The content expert typically has an advanced degree and considerable experience working in the content area. The content expert passes on information to others, such as through a classroom or continuing education program. For example, a content expert may be a professor at a nursing school who teaches a specific course, such as mental health nursing for children and adolescents. In this example the content expert most likely has an advanced degree in nursing, and may have specialization or certification in the specific field of mental health nursing. Additionally, the content expert most likely has experience working in the field of mental health for children and adolescents, and can successfully pass the knowledge on to those who need to learn it for their own practices.

Expert Witnesses

The CNS may serve as an **expert witness** in his/her area of specialty. The nurse may be asked to interview witnesses, review documents, obtain experts, and act as liaison between lawyers and medical experts. The nurse should understand the Federal Rules of Evidence and his/her scope of competence. Nurses may serve as non-testifying consultants or testifying expert witnesses. States establish legal qualifications for expert witnesses, and this may vary somewhat. Responsibilities include the following:

- Providing objective opinions based on standards of nursing care rather than subjective opinions regarding morality or motivation
- Providing an opinion based on the information reviewed and the nurse's own educational expertise
- Providing an opinion based on reasonable nursing certainty related to the acts of negligence
- Educating the jury and helping them to understand nursing standards
- Being prepared and testifying truthfully, never guessing or offering information that is not a response to a direct question
- Maintaining composure and remaining calm under all circumstances

Case Management

Case management is used within acute, subacute, and skilled nursing facilities. The case manager chairs the interdisciplinary team responsible for the treatment of the patient and ensures that the needs of the patient are communicated to all members of the team. The case manager also ensures that all team members are focused on the same goal. As the patient moves back into the community, the case manager provides aid to the patient in securing any necessary social support services (such as home health care, transportation, and Meals on Wheels). The case manager supervises and manages all aspects of care to ensure continuity of care.

Models

There are a number of **models for case management** that can be utilized to integrate the outcome of utilization management assessment into the performance improvement process:

- *Type of provider care:* Provider care types include self-care (patient provides own care), primary care (patient and primary care physician), episodic care (patient, primary care physician, and specialist as well as the case manager), and brokered care (involves community, government, or private services).
- *Focus of care:* The focus may be on cost containment, common to managed care programs, where service depends upon the program's benefits and criteria for medical necessity and there is little or no direct contact with patient or family. The focus may also be on coordination of care, and this involves direct patient and family contact and individualized assessment and intervention.
- *Professional discipline:* Case management may be done by nursing, social workers, psychiatrists, or other specific disciplines, depending upon the goals of case management.

Health Promotion

Promoting Health and Preventing Illness

The goal of **health promotion** to assist people to maintain or achieve a high level of health and function is central to the nursing process. Health promotion involves teaching and encouraging people to make changes in their lifestyles, such as with diet and exercise. Health promotion activities can be done whenever the opportunity arises. **Preventing illness** involves more specific protection of people from illness or threats to their health or wellbeing. There are three types of prevention activities:

- *Primary*: Specific preventive interventions, such as immunizations, use of safety glasses, fluoridation of water, and changing habits (smoking, drinking, diet) to prevent disease
- *Secondary*: Screening to identify risks or disease (STDs, diabetes, hypertension) so preventive measures can be started to prevent progression of disease
- *Tertiary*: Interventions to promote recovery and prevent disabilities, such as turning patients to prevent pressure sores and enrolling patients in rehabilitation programs

American Diabetes Association Clinical Practice Recommendations for Preventing Complications

Preventing Neuropathic Complications of Diabetes

The American Diabetes Association Clinical Practice Recommendations for **preventing neuropathic complications** of diabetes include the following:

- *Screening*: Type 1 and type 2 diabetics should be screened for distal symmetric polyneuropathy at initial diagnosis and every year with pinprick, vibration sensation, and 10-g monofilament testing. Type 1 diabetics of more than 5 years and type 2 diabetics at diagnosis should be screened for autonomic neuropathy. Cardiovascular autonomic neuropathy is characterized by tachycardia (>100 at rest), and orthostatic hypotension. GI neuropathies, such as gastroparesis, esophageal enteropathy, may present as constipation alternating with diarrhea. Genitourinary neuropathy may cause erectile dysfunction. Comprehensive foot exam should include screening for PAD with ankle-brachial index.
- *Education*: All patients must be taught about foot care, including examination of feet and wearing of protective shoes.
- *Treatment*: Maintaining stable glucose levels and smoking cessation is critical. Drug treatments include tricyclic antidepressants (amitriptyline, nortriptyline, imipramine), anticonvulsants (gabapentin, carbamazepine, pregabalin), 5-hydroxytryptamine and norepinephrine uptake inhibitors (duloxetine), and substance P inhibitor (capsaicin cream). Other treatments specific to the neuropathy (such as penile implants) may also be employed.

Preventing Cardiovascular Complications of Diabetes

The American Diabetes Association Clinical Practice Recommendations for **preventing cardiovascular complications** (the most common cause of morbidity and mortality) include the following:

- Control of hypertension: The goal of screening, diagnosis, and treatment is to lower BP to <140/80 (preferably <130/80).
- Lipid management: Lifestyle modifications include diet and exercise. Statin therapy is indicated for overt CVD or for individuals over 40 without CVD but with other risk factors. Lower risk patients should have statin therapy if LDL is greater than 100 mg/dL or if there are multiple risk factors. Statin is optional with CVD if LDL is less than 70 mg/dL.
- Antiplatelet agents: ASA 75-162 mg daily (not recommended for those under 30 years of age). Combination therapy with clopidogrel if CVD is severe.
- Smoking cessation: No patient should smoke. Counseling and intervention should be provided.

- Coronary heart disease screening: A combination of ASA, statin, and ACE inhibitor may be used to reduce risk of acute cardiovascular events. Metformin and thiazolidinedione should not be used for those treated for congestive heart failure.

Preventing Renal Complications of Diabetes

The American Diabetes Association Clinical Practice Recommendations for **preventing renal complications of diabetes** are as follows:

- *Screening and diagnosis*: All individuals who have had type 1 diabetes for five or more years and all individuals with type 2 diabetes should have an annual urine albumin test. Serum creatinine should be assessed annually to estimate glomerular filtration rate (GFR) and determine degree of chronic kidney disease.
- *Treatment*: Treatment includes angiotensin-converting enzyme (ACE) inhibitors or angiotensin receptor blockers (ARBs) (with monitoring of serum creatinine and potassium) and reduction of protein intake to 0.8 to 1.0 g/kg/body weight per day in the early stages of chronic kidney disease and 0.8 g/kg/body weight per day in cases of advanced chronic kidney disease.
- *Glucose monitoring*: Maintaining normal steady glucose levels is critical to avoid renal disease. Twenty to forty percent of patients with persistent albuminuria (a marker for both type 1 and type 2 diabetes) develop diabetic nephropathy.

Preventing Retinal Complications of Diabetes

The American Diabetes Association Clinical Practice Recommendations for preventing retinal complications of diabetes include the following:

- *Screening*: Type 1 diabetics should be screened for diabetic retinopathy within 5 years of diagnosis and type 2 diabetics after initial diagnosis with subsequent yearly exams. This can be modified to every 2-3 years if 1 or more yearly exams are normal.
- *Treatment*: This includes prompt referral to ophthalmologist for laser photocoagulation therapy to prevent vision loss.

Diabetic retinopathy, a vascular complication, is the most common cause of new cases of blindness in adults 20-74. Initially, patients may have few symptoms, but as the condition progresses, they may begin to experience blurred vision, floaters, and decreased night vision. The condition is bilateral and can progress to blindness if untreated. Other eye disorders, such as cataracts, are also more common in those with diabetes.

Joint National Committee on Prevention, Detection, Evaluation, and Treatment of High Blood Pressure

The 8th Report of the Joint National Committee on Prevention, Detection, Evaluation, and Treatment of High Blood Pressure makes a number of specific **recommendations regarding evaluation**:

- *Follow-up:* Recheck in 2 years for normal, 1 year for prehypertension, 2 months for stage 1, and 1 month for stage 2 with immediate treatment for BP >180/110 mm Hg.
- *Ambulatory BP:* Done for suspected white-coat hypertension (reactive) hypertension if no target damage to organs (heart, brain, chronic kidney disease, peripheral artery disease, or retinopathy), drug resistance, hypotension related to antihypertensives, episodic hypertension, and autonomic dysfunction.
- *Diagnostic tests:* 12-lead EKG, urinalysis, blood glucose, Hct., K, creatinine (with estimated GFR), calcium, lipoprotein profile.

Classification and Methods in the 7th Report

The 8th Report of the Joint National Committee on Prevention, Detection, Evaluation, and Treatment of High Blood Pressure does not clearly delineate the stages of hypertension, and for that reason has sometimes been criticized for its scope. The 7th Report continues to be referred to for some of these specifics, and provides an evidence-based approach to the treatment and prevention of hypertension. The report concludes that systolic BP >140 mm Hg poses a greater risk for those over the age of 50 than increased diastolic BP. Increased diastolic pressure is more common in those under 50 years of age and is a cardiovascular risk factor until age 50. After this, increased systolic blood pressure is a risk factor as diastolic pressure tends to level off or decrease after age 50:

- Normal BP: <120/80
- Prehypertension: 120-130/80-89 mm Hg
- Stage 1 hypertension: 140-159/90-99 mm Hg
- Stage 2 hypertension: ≥160/100

BP should be checked with properly sized, inspected, and validated equipment using the auscultation method. Patients should be seated with feet on the floor for 5 minutes before the check. Patients should avoid caffeine, exercise and smoking for 30 minutes prior to the check. At least 2 measurements should be made to arrive at an average reading.

Risks for Cardiovascular Disease

The **8th Report of the Joint National Committee on Prevention, Detection, Evaluation, and Treatment of High Blood Pressure** identifies a number of risk factors for cardiovascular disease:

- Hypertension: >140/90 mmHg (>150/90 mmHg for adults over 60).
- ↑ Resting heart rate and ↓ variability of heart rate; ≥83 at rest increases risk.
- Age: >60.
- Diabetes mellitus: Associated with metabolic syndrome characterized by ↓HDL, ↑triglycerides, and abdominal obesity.
- Estimated glomerular filtration rate (eGFR) <60 ml/min: Chronic kidney disease.
- Family history of cardiovascular diseases: <55 years for men and <65 years for women.
- Microalbuminuria.
- Obesity: BMI ≥30 kg/m^2 for men at ≥55 years and women at ≥65 years.
- Physical inactivity.
- Use of tobacco: More cardiovascular disease caused by cigarettes than other types of tobacco use.

NIH, NHLBI Report of the National Cholesterol Education Program Expert Panel on Detection, Evaluation, and Treatment of High Blood Cholesterol in Adults

Lipid Classifications

The **NIH, NHLBI Report of the National Cholesterol Education Program Expert Panel on Detection, Evaluation, and Treatment of High Blood Cholesterol in Adults** classifies total cholesterol, LDL, HDL, and triglycerides to help to determine the need for treatment:

LDL cholesterol	<100: Optimal 100-129: Near optimal 130-159: Borderline high 160-189: High ≥190: Very high
Total cholesterol	<200: Optimal 200-239: Borderline high ≥240: High
HDL cholesterol	<40: Low ≥60: High
Triglycerides	<150: Normal 150-199: Borderline high 200-499: High ≥500: Very high

The optimal LDL goal for those with CHD or equivalent risk is < 100 mg/dL; 0-1 risk factors, <160 mg/dL; and more than 2 risk factors, <160 mg/dL. Those with coronary heart disease or equivalent risk factor have a risk of having major coronary events at the rate of >20% per 10 years.

Risk Assessment and Primary/Secondary Causes

The **NIH, NHLBI Report of the National Cholesterol Education Program Expert Panel on Detection, Evaluation, and Treatment of High Blood Cholesterol in Adults** stresses that LDL cholesterol is the major cause of coronary heart disease (CHD). Optimal LDL level is <100 mg/dL. **Management strategies include the following:**

- *Risk assessment:* A fasting lipoprotein profile should be obtained for adults over the age of 20 every 5 years. Major risk factors that modify LDL goals include smoking, hypertension, HDL < 40 mg/dL, family history of premature CHD (or risk equivalent, such as diabetes, peripheral arterial disease, abdominal aortic aneurysm, carotid arterial disease), and increasing age (≥45 for men and ≥55 for women).
- *Determining primary or secondary causes:* If LDL is elevated, causes of secondary dyslipidemia should be assessed prior to treatment. Secondary causes include diabetes, hypothyroidism, obstructive liver disease, chronic kidney failure, and drugs (progestins, anabolic steroids, corticosteroids).

Geriatrics Society Guideline for the Prevention of Falls in Older Persons

The **American Geriatrics Society Guideline for the Prevention of Falls in Older Persons** includes:

- All geriatric patients should be asked if they have had falls in the past year.
- If no falls have occurred, no intervention is needed.

- If one fall has occurred, the patient should be assessed for gait and balance, including the get-up-and-go test in which the patient stands up from a chair without using his or her arms, walks across the room, and returns. If the patient is steady, no further assessment is needed. If the patient demonstrates unsteadiness, further assessment to determine the cause is necessary.
- If multiple falls have occurred, a full assessment should be completed: history, vision, neurological status, muscle strength, joint function, mental status, reflexes, cardiovascular status (including rate and rhythm), postural pulse, and blood pressure. Referral to a geriatric specialist may be appropriate.

Interventions to Decrease Falls

The **American Geriatrics Society Guideline for the Prevention of Falls in Older Persons** recommends a number of interventions to decrease falls:

- Long-term exercise focusing on strength and balance training is recommended. Tai chi has been found to be helpful for some people.
- Modification of the home environment involves the removal throw rugs, installation of grab bars, and provision of easy access to the bathroom.
- A review of medications should be conducted to determine if the number can be reduced, especially if the patient is taking more than 4 medications or psychotropic medications as many medications or medication interactions can cause dizziness and instability.
- Assistive devices, such as walkers and crab canes are recommended to improve stability.
- Control of cardiovascular conditions, such as heart block or fibrillation, is essential. These conditions may cause dizziness/syncope and precipitate falls.
- Visual deficits should be addressed where possible (glasses).
- Footwear providing adequate support should be worn.

Helping Smokers Quit

The **US Department of Health and Human Services** guidelines for helping smokers quit includes:

- *Ask* about and record smoking status at every visit.
- *Advise* all smokers to quit and explain health reasons.
- *Assess* readiness to quit by questioning and if the patient is willing, provide resources. If patient is not willing, provide support and attempt to motivate the person to quit with information.
- *Assist* smokers with a plan that sets a date (within 2 weeks), removes cigarettes, enlists family and friends, reviews past attempts, and anticipates challenges during the withdrawal period. The CNS must give advice about the need for abstinence and discuss the association of smoking with drinking. Medications to help control the urge to smoke (patches, gum, lozenge, prescriptions) and resources should be provided.

Diabetic Foot Ulcers Screening

Most **diabetic ulcers** are on the foot, occurring from the toes to the heels. Ulcers may first appear as laceration, blisters, or punctures, and the wound is usually circular with well-defined edges. There is often callus in the periwound tissue.

The following are common sites:

- *Toes:* The toes are frequent sites for ulcers because of the potential for trauma. The interphalangeal joints often have limited flexibility that causes pressure and friction. The dorsal toes may have hammertoes from injuries or improperly fitted shoes that are easily injured. Distal toes may suffer injury from poor perfusion, heat, or short footwear.
- *Metatarsal heads* may have poor flexibility, increasing pressure.
- *Bunions* may erode because of deformities or narrow footwear.
- *Midfoot* may suffer injury from trauma or Charcot's fracture.
- *Heels* are susceptible to unrelieved pressure, often related to prolonged periods of bed rest.

Colorectal Screening

Colorectal screening recommendations include the following:

- Age ≥50—Average risk
- Asymptomatic without risk factors
- Age ≥40—Increased risk
- Family history of colorectal cancer in first or second-degree relatives
- Family history of genetic syndrome (FAP, HNLPCC)
- Adenomatous polyps in first-degree relatives before age 60
- History of polyps or colorectal cancer
- History of inflammatory bowel disease

Screening tests include:

- *Fecal occult blood—yearly:* This test checks for blood in the stool.
- *Flexible sigmoidoscopy—every 5 years*: This test uses a scope to check for polyps or signs of cancer in the rectum and lower third of the colon. It is often done with the fecal occult blood test.
- *Colonoscopy—every 10 years or as follow-up for abnormalities in other screening:* This test uses a longer flexible scope, usually with anesthesia, to check rectum and entire colon. It allows for removal of polyps, small cancerous lesions, and biopsies and provides surveillance of inflammatory bowel disease.
- *Double contrast barium enema—every 5 years*: This is an x-ray with contrast used to visualize intestinal abnormalities.

Prostate Cancer Screening

While **screening for prostate cancer** is generally recommended for men annually after age 50, there is not yet a specific screening recommendation or a consensus of medical opinion about screening. Men who have a close family member with prostate cancer (father, brother) or who are African American are at increased risk and may be advised to have screening earlier. Two tests are routinely done to screen for prostate cancer. One of these is the digital rectal exam (DRE) to palpate the size of the prostate and to note any abnormalities. The other test is the prostate specific antigen (PSA) test. The PSA level tends to increase with prostate problems, but many other factors can cause the PSA level to increase. Additionally, prostate cancers tend to grow slowly and may have little impact on a man's life while surgery can lead to impotence and/or incontinence. If screening indicates the possibility of cancer, further tests, such as a transrectal ultrasound and biopsy may be done.

Breast Cancer Screening

The National Cancer Institute recommends monthly breast self-exams for all women and **screening mammograms** every 1 to 2 years for all women ages over the age of 40. Women who are at increased risk for breast cancer may be advised to have mammograms prior to age 40, but breast tissue is denser and mammograms are less accurate. Risk factors include the following:

- Previous breast cancer
- Family history of breast cancer
- Genetic alterations (BRCA1, BRCA2)
- Early onset of periods (<12) or late menopause (>55)
- Long-term hormonal replacement therapy (HRT) of >5 years
- Hx of obesity, alcoholism, low activity
- Post-radiation therapy
- Hx of taking diethylstilbestrol (DES)
- Highly dense breasts

Both false positives and false negatives can occur. Any positive result should be verified by diagnostic mammogram, ultrasound, biopsy, MRI, or PET.

Cervical Cancer Screening

Screening for cervical cancer is recommended for all women beginning at age 21 or within 3 years of becoming sexually active. Because many teenagers engage in sexual activity at a young age, some may need screening by age 16 or 17. The most common screening test is the pelvic exam with a Papanicolaou (Pap) smear, which is examined for precancerous/cancerous cell changes. An additional test for women at age 30 or those with abnormal results on a Pap smear is the human papillomavirus (HPV) test to determine if the woman has antibodies to HPV, indicating a prior infection that increases risk of developing cervical cancer. A positive finding is verified by biopsy. If screening tests are negative by age 30, many physicians recommend screening only every 2 to 3 years. Additionally, women who are over age 65 or post-hysterectomy (with cervical removal) and have had normal Pap smears are usually advised that they do not need to continue regular screening as risks of developing cervical cancer are very low.

Vision/Glaucoma Screening

Glaucoma, usually associated with an increase in intraocular pressure, is a leading cause of blindness because of damage to the optic nerve. Onset may be gradual or abrupt, depending upon the type of glaucoma. Screening for glaucoma is essential because there may be no symptoms until irreversible damage has occurred. Routine screening tests include tonometry to measure pressure in the eye and an ophthalmoscopic exam to examine the optic nerve. If screening is positive for glaucoma, further tests include visual field testing (peripheral vision is usually affected) and gonioscopy to study the drainage system of the eye. **The American Academy of Ophthalmology has established a schedule for screening:**

Age	Recommendations
20-29	One screening during this period for most individuals Every 3-5 years for those of African descent or with family history of glaucoma
30-39	Two screenings during this period for most individuals Every 2-4 years for those of African descent or with family history of glaucoma
40-64	Every 2-4 years

Age	Recommendations
≥65	Every 1-2 years

Screening for macular degeneration (Amsler grid) and visual acuity should be done at the same time.

Osteoporosis Screening

The United States Preventive Task Force recommends all people, especially women over the age of 65, be screened for **osteoporosis**. In addition, those with increased risk factors should be screened from age 60. Risk factors include the following:

- **F: Fractures**: Risk factors include a family history of osteoporotic fractures or a personal history of vertebral or hip fractures.
- **R: Race**: Asians and Caucasians have the highest risk.
- **A: Age and gender**: Women over age 65 have the highest risk.
- **C: Chronic disease/medications**: Diabetes, Addison's disease, Cushing's disease, inflammatory bowel disease, eating disorders, and hyperparathyroidism are risk factors. Medications such as corticosteroids, thyroid medication in excess, and chemotherapy drugs may increase risk.
- **T: Thin bones, low weight**: Individuals who weigh less than 134 pounds are at higher risk.
- **U: Underactive**: Inadequate exercise puts an individual at higher risk.
- **R: Reduced estrogen**: Post-menopausal women are at higher risk.
- **E: Excessive alcohol intake and smoking**: Alcohol disrupts calcium balance and impairs vitamin D metabolism. Smoking has an anti-estrogen effect.
- **D: Diet**: A diet deficient in calcium and/or vitamin D is a risk factor.

Screening is per a bone density test, usually a DEXA scan. Results are expressed as a T-score with a -2.0 score the starting point for osteoporosis:

- 0-10: Normal -1.0: 10% below normal -2.0: 20% below normal

Influenza Vaccine

A different **influenza ("flu") vaccine** is formulated each year, and administration begins in September prior to flu season. There are two types of flu vaccines:

- *Trivalent inactivated influenza vaccine (TIV)* (injectable) is available for use in those over 6 months old, including older people who are healthy or have chronic medical conditions.
- *Live attenuated influenza vaccine* (LAIV) is a nasal spray for use in those 2 to 49 years of age. It is not for use in pregnant women and is not used for older adults.

Antibodies against the viruses used to formulate the vaccines develop in about 2 weeks. Vaccination is recommended for all people over six months of age.

The flu vaccine is **contraindicated** in individuals with an allergy to eggs, a history of reaction to flu vaccine, and a history of Guillain-Barré. The vaccine should not be administered 6 weeks or less after a previous flu vaccine. Adverse effects include infection with local inflammation, fever, and aching.

Hepatitis A Vaccine

Hepatitis A is the cause of a serious liver disease, which can result in morbidity and death. Hepatitis A is spread through the feces of a person who is infected and often causes contamination of food and water. Outbreaks have been traced to restaurants and kitchens in large facilities. This vaccine is now routinely given to children. Older adults may receive the two-injection series if they are considered at risk, depending upon lifestyle (males have sex with other males or illegal drug users) or medical condition (e.g., chronic liver disease and those receiving clotting factor concentrates). It is also recommended if traveling to endemic areas and if outbreaks occur. Adverse reactions are mild and include soreness, headache, anorexia, and malaise although severe allergic reactions can occur as with all vaccines.

Hepatitis B Vaccine

Hepatitis B can cause serious liver disease leading to liver cancer. Hepatitis B is transmitted through blood and body fluids: therefore, it is now recommended for all newborns, individuals under 18, individuals over 18 in high-risk groups (drug users, men having sex with men, individuals with multiple sex partners, partners of individuals with HBV, and healthcare workers). Older adults with end-stage renal disease (including those receiving hemodialysis), chronic liver disease, or HIV/AIDS should receive the vaccine. The vaccination is also recommended for international travelers to areas in which hepatitis B is endemic. Older adults in correctional facilities, drug-abuse treatment facilities, dialysis facilities, and non-residential daycare facilities for people with developmental disabilities should be vaccinated. Three injections of monovalent HepB are required to confer immunity. Adverse reactions include local irritation and fever. Severe allergic reactions can occur to those allergic to baker's yeast.

Herpes Zoster Vaccine

Adults who have had chicken pox as children or adults retain the varicella zoster virus in the nerve cells, and the virus can become reactivated and cause herpes zoster ("shingles"). Herpes zoster is most common in those over the age of 50 with chronic medical conditions and those who are immunocompromised. Since 2006, the **herpes zoster vaccine** has been recommended for those 60 years of age and older. A single dose of the vaccine is needed. Studies indicate that it prevents about 50% of herpes zoster cases and decreases pain and severity in those who still develop the disease. It is contraindicated in those with an allergy to gelatin or neomycin and those who are immunocompromised because of HIV/AIDS, chemotherapy, radiation, steroid use, history of leukemia or lymphoma, and active TB. Adverse reactions are rare and include allergic response, local inflammation, and headache.

Pneumococcal Polysaccharide-23 Vaccine

Pneumococcal polysaccharide-23 vaccine (PPV) (Pneumovax® and Pnu-Immune®) protects against 23 types of pneumococcal bacteria. Pneumococcal vaccine is now routinely given to children, and this has reduced the overall incidence of infection in both children and older adults. The vaccine is given to adults 65 years of age and over and to those at increased risk from chronic disease (sickle cell, asplenia, Hodgkin's, COPD, HIV/AIDS, cardiopulmonary and liver disease, diabetes).

Administration is explained below:

- One dose is usually all that is required, although a second dose may be advised with some conditions, such as cancer or organ/bone marrow transplantations.
- Revaccination is recommended for those over 65 if the first vaccination was administered 5 years or more previously and the patient was under 65 at the time.

Studies have indicated that this vaccine protects against pneumococcal bacteremia in older adults but is less successful in protecting against pneumonia, the primary form of pneumococcal infection.

Immunizations for International Travel

International travelers should check the CDC Traveler's Health page (http://www.cdc.gov/Travel/contentVaccinations.aspx) to determine which vaccinations are needed for different destinations. Vaccinations should be taken 4-6 weeks prior to travel to ensure effectiveness. The CDC recommends 3 categories of vaccinations for travelers:

- *Routine vaccinations* are advised for all adults.
- *Recommended vaccines* vary according to destination.
- *Required vaccines*: Only 2 vaccinations are currently required by international health regulations. Yellow fever vaccination is required for travel to some countries in sub-Saharan Africa and tropical areas of South America. Meningococcal vaccination is required for travel to Saudi Arabia during the annual Hajj pilgrimage.

Vaccinations may be contraindicated in those with immune deficits related to disease or treatment, so this should be discussed with a physician. In some cases, travel to some areas may not be advisable because of the inability to receive vaccinations.

Anticipatory Guidance for Adults

Routine Screening	Annually: height, weight, vital signs Every 5 years: fasting lipoproteins Age 50 and every 5 years thereafter: flexible sigmoidoscopy, and every 10 years, colonoscopy (colorectal screening) Annually (with risk factors): diabetic screening Females: annual mammogram to age 40 and then every 1 to 2 years; Pap tests every 2 years; osteoporosis screening (ages 60 to 64) Males: prostate screening as recommended
Vaccinations	DTaP X 1 and then TD every 10 years >Age 60: herpes zoster (shingles) Yearly: influenza. <Age 26 x 3 doses: HPV Age 0 to 49: MMRI (1 to 2 doses) Others according to risk factors
Assessment and Education	Substance abuse: alcohol, OTC, prescription drugs, or illicit drugs; Smoking assessment: smoking cessation; Diet and nutrition: vitamins, calcium needs; Obesity: BMI, waist-hip ratio Exercise; Contraception/at-risk sexual behaviors Dental care; Mental status: depression, anxiety

Nosocomial Infection

A **nosocomial infection** is defined by the National Nosocomial Infections Surveillance (NNIS) as a localized or systemic hospital-acquired infection that was not present or (incubating) in the patient at the time he or she entered the hospital. The infection may be caused by a toxin or pathogen. In some cases, infection may be evident within the first 24 to 48 hours, but other infections may not be evident until after discharge from the hospital. This is because incubation times and resistance vary. An infection that occurs after discharge but is hospital acquired is also nosocomial. A nosocomial infection is identified by laboratory analyses and clinical symptoms. A diagnosis of infection by an attending physical or surgeon is also considered acceptable identification. Colonization that is not causing an inflammatory response or evidence of infection is not considered nosocomial for reporting purposes. The most common nosocomial infections are *Staphylococcus aureus* and methicillin-resistant *Staphylococcus aureus* (MRSA).

Clostridium Difficile Infection

Clostridium difficile is an anaerobic gram-positive bacillus that produces endospores. It is commonly found in health-care facilities, such as hospitals. Intestinal flora (microorganisms) normally provide resistance to *C. difficile*, but if the flora are disrupted by antibiotic use (or sometimes chemotherapeutic agents) and the host is an asymptomatic carrier or has acquired the infection during or after treatment, then *C. difficile* can begin to overgrow. *C. difficile* produces a lethal cytotoxin called toxin B. It also produces an endotoxin with cytotoxic action (toxin A) that causes fluid to accumulate in the colon and causes severe damage to mucous membranes. *C. difficile* causes more cases of nosocomial diarrhea than any other microorganism. All antibiotics can cause *C. difficile* infections, but clindamycin and cephalosporins are most frequently implicated. Symptoms of *C. difficile* infection vary widely from mild diarrhea to lethal sepsis. *C. difficile* can cause diarrhea, colitis, pseudomembranous colitis, and megacolon. Infection may not be obvious for weeks after completion of treatment with antibiotics.

MRSA

***Methicillin-resistant Staphylococcus aureus* (MRSA)** is caused by a mutation in *S. aureus* that confers resistance to methicillin (amoxicillin), other beta lactamase-resistant penicillins, and cephalosporins. First identified in 1945, MRSA has become endemic in hospitals. It is the cause of surgical site and bloodstream infections and pneumonia. More than half of *S. aureus* infections are now classified as MRSA. The mortality rate of MRSA is 21 percent. MRSA often colonizes the skin, especially in the anterior nares, and can easily spread through contact with contaminated surfaces or contaminated hands. Community-acquired as well as hospital-acquired infections are of grave concern. Prompt diagnosis and treatment with vancomycin or other antibiotics are essential. Standard and contact precautions with use of gloves, gown, and masks should be instituted if deemed appropriate. Droplet precautions should be taken in cases of pneumonia. Patients with MRSA should be placed in a private room or cohort room. Routine surveillance of high-risk patients or those with a previous history of MRSA should be conducted.

VRE and MDRE

***Vancomycin-resistant enterococci* (VRE)** and ***multidrug-resistant enterococci* (MDRE)** create serious problems for health-care facilities. VRE was first identified in the United States in 1989. By 2004, VRE was the cause of one-third of all the infections acquired in intensive care units related to the use of vancomycin. There are several phenotypes, but two types are most common in the United States: VanA (resistant to vancomycin and teicoplanin) and VanB (resistant to just vancomycin). VRE infections are treatable by other antibiotics, but MDRE infections are increasingly resistant to two or more antibiotics, including vancomycin. Restriction of vancomycin use alone has not proven successful in controlling the development of VRE or MDRE because other antibiotics, such as clindamycin, cephalosporin, aztreonam, ciprofloxacin, aminoglycoside, and metronidazole are implicated. Prior antibiotic use is present in almost all patients with MDRE. Other risk factors include prolonged hospitalization and intraabdominal surgery.

The **incidence of VRE infections** has increased greatly in both intensive care units and medical/surgical units. Approximately 25 percent of enterococci infections are now classified as VRE. Patients who are immunocompromised or severely ill are at increased risk. Also, at increased risk are those admitted to intensive care units or hospitalized for lengthy periods. VRE is also associated with antibiotic use, including vancomycin, clindamycin, and ciprofloxacin. VRE can occur systemically or infect the urinary tract or surgical sites. Some people are colonized but have no symptoms. These individuals may pose a threat to others as the bacterium may survive on surfaces for up to six days. A number of precautions should be taken to prevent the spread of infection. Infected patients should be placed in isolation. All individuals entering the patient's room should use barrier precautions (gowns, gloves, and masks). All individuals must wash their hands thoroughly after contact with the patient. Dedicated equipment should be used to treat infected patients in order to reduce transmission. There should be a policy to limit vancomycin use. Isolation rooms should be cleaned thoroughly.

Management of Suicidal Patients

Approximately 50 percent of suicides involving older adults are associated with depression. For this reason, all depressed older patients should be assessed for suicide risk. Suicide has many possible causes, including severe depression, social isolation, situational crisis (move to nursing home), bereavement, and psychosis. The nurse should provide support without being judgmental because this may further harm the patient's self-esteem and increase the risk of another suicide attempt. **Suicidal patients** should be referred to a mental health professional for evaluation. Treatment for a suicide attempt depends on the type of suicide attempt. There are antidotes available for certain common drugs. For example, naloxone (Narcan) is given for opiate overdose and *N*-acetylcysteine is administered for acetaminophen overdose. Individuals at high risk for a further suicide attempt should be hospitalized. High-risk situations include violent suicide attempt (knives, gunshots); suicide attempt with low chance of rescue; ongoing psychosis; ongoing severe depression; repeated suicide attempts; and lack of a social support system.

Evidence-Based Practice

Critical Pathways

Types

Critical pathways are plans that involve diagnosis, procedure, or condition-specific care. Critical pathways involve the services of individuals from numerous disciplines. Critical pathways outline the steps in a patient's care and the expected outcomes. The pathways outline goals in patient care and the sequence and time of interventions taken to achieve those goals. Critical pathways may be developed for physician care or nursing care. Increasingly, critical pathways are being used as a method to improve and standardize care and decrease hospital stays. There are two basic types of pathways: guidelines and integrated care plan/pathways. *Guidelines* outline patient care. Documentation is not required to demonstrate that guidelines have been followed. The pathway may be in the form of a flow sheet, with different paths to follow depending on the patient's outcomes.

An **integrated care plan/pathway** must be followed. Documentation with dates and signatures is necessary to show that the steps have been carried out and to indicate specific outcomes. Pathways should be based on best practices. Their effectiveness should be monitored and evaluated to determine if modifications are needed.

Steps of Development

Clinical/critical pathway development is done by those involved in direct patient care. The pathway should require no additional staffing and cover the entire scope of an illness. Steps include the following:

1. Selection of patient group and diagnosis, procedures, or conditions based on analysis of data and observation of a wide variety of treatment approaches.
2. Creation of an interdisciplinary team of those involved in the process of care, including physicians to develop pathway.
3. Analysis of data including literature review and study of best practices to identify opportunities for quality improvement
4. Identification of all categories of care, such as nutrition, medications, nursing.
5. Discussion, reaching consensus.
6. Identifying the levels of care and number of days to be covered by the pathway.
7. Pilot testing and redesigning steps as indicated.
8. Educating staff about standards.
9. Monitoring and tracking variances in order to improve pathways.

Evidence-Based Practice

Cochrane Database

The **Cochrane Database** is a primary resource in the development of evidence-based practice. Cochrane provides a collection of different medical databases in the Cochrane Library for easy internet access. Cochrane databases include the following:

- Cochrane Database of Systemic Reviews
- Cochrane Methodology Register
- Health Technology Assessment Database (HTA)
- Database of Abstracts of Reviews of Effects (DARE)
- Cochrane Central Register of Controlled Trials (CENTRAL)
- NHS Economic Evaluation Database (NHS EED)

Cochrane also provides reviews of research and meta-analysis to synthesize the research findings of various research studies. Researchers for Cochrane conduct statistical analysis when comparing data from a variety of studies or trials. The Cochrane Database can be freely accessed in many countries, but requires a subscription for complete access to reports in all US states except Wyoming, although a two page summary of findings is available.

Evidence-Based Practice Guidelines

Evidence-based practice guidelines are commonly used for such things as standing medicine orders or antibiotic protocols. However, decisions are often made based on biased expert opinion or on studies that lack internal and/or external validity. Evidence-based practice guidelines should be established in a systematic way. It's important that decisions be based on solid evidence and not personal belief. The establishment of evidence-based practice guidelines does not ensure that they will be followed. Some individuals will resist changing their practices, so consideration must be given to implementation. A policy must be developed as to whether the use of the guidelines is mandatory or voluntary. In addition, it must be decided to what degree individual practitioners can choose other options. Rigid guidelines may be counterproductive. In some cases, establishing guidelines may affect cost reimbursement from third-party payers.

Developing Evidence-Based Practice Guidelines

Steps to developing **evidence-based practice guidelines** include the following:

- *Focus on the topic/methodology:* This includes outlining possible interventions/treatments for review, choosing patient populations and settings and determining significant outcomes. Search boundaries (such as types of journals, types of studies, dates of studies) should be determined.
- *Evidence review:* This includes review of literature, critical analysis of studies, and summarization of results, including pooled meta-analysis.
- *Expert judgment:* Recommendations based on personal experience from a number of experts may be utilized, especially if there is inadequate evidence based on review, but this subjective evidence should be explicitly acknowledged.
- *Policy considerations:* This includes cost-effectiveness, access to care, insurance coverage, availability of qualified staff, and legal implications.
- *Policy:* A written policy must be completed with recommendations. Common practice is to utilize letter guidelines with "A" the most highly recommended, usually based on the quality of supporting evidence.
- *Review:* The completed policy should be submitted to peers for review and comments before instituting the policy.

Using Evidence-Based Research to Provide Care

Evidence-based research is the use of current research and patient values in practice to establish a plan of care for each patient. Research may be the result of large studies of best practices or individual research from observations in practice about the effectiveness of treatment. Evidence-based practice requires a commitment to ongoing research and outcomes evaluations. Many resources are available:

- Guide to Clinical Preventive Services by the Agency for Healthcare Research and Quality of the U.S. Department of Health and Human Services (http://www.ahrq.gov/clinic/cps3dix.htm).
- Evidence-based practice requires a thorough understanding of research methods in order to evaluate the results and determine if they can be generalized. Results must also be evaluated in terms of cost-effectiveness.
- Steps to evidence-based practice include:
- Making a diagnosis
- Researching and analyzing results
- Applying research findings to plan of care
- Evaluating outcomes

Role of the AHRQ in Evidence-Based Practice

Surveys

One tool used to assess an organization's patient safety culture when establishing evidence-based practice is a survey. The **Agency for Healthcare Research and Quality (AHRQ)** has sponsored the development of surveys to assess patient safety for different healthcare organizations, including hospitals, nursing homes, and outpatient facilities. These surveys are available for download and can be used easily by all levels of staff within an organization. The surveys ask questions related to safety, error in medications/treatments, and incident reporting and typically take ≤15 minutes to complete, so they can be done as part of staff meetings or during clinical hours. Each survey consists of questions about a number of sections using a scale of 1 to 5, along with checklists and narrative for responses. Sections include work area/unit, supervisor/manager, communications, frequency of events reported, patient safety goals, hospital/facility, number of events reported, background information, and comments.

EVIDENCE-BASED PRACTICE CENTERS

The **Agency for Healthcare Research and Quality** (AHRQ) promotes evidence-based practice through funding of 14 Evidence-based Practice Centers (EPCs) in order to develop evidence-based practice guidelines to disseminate and use in developing patient care plans, establishing insurance coverage, and developing educational materials. These centers issue research reports, including meta-analysis of all relevant research on a wide range of topics, such as "Pain Management Interventions for Elderly Patients with Hip Fracture," which include morbidity/mortality rates and cost-effectiveness of different treatments and procedures. Research focuses on areas of significance to those receiving Medicaid and Medicare. For example, 5 EPCs are engaged in research on technology for CMS, focusing on topics related to the U.S. Preventive Services Task Force. Topics for review are proposed by partners, such as insurance companies, professional associations, patient advocacy groups, and employers. Guides are available for both consumers and clinicians.

LEVELS OF EVIDENCE IN EVIDENCE-BASED PRACTICE

Levels of evidence are categorized according to the scientific evidence available to support the recommendations, as well as existing state and federal laws. While recommendations are voluntary, they are often used as a basis for state and federal regulations.

- *Category IA* is well supported by evidence from experimental, clinical, or epidemiologic studies and is strongly recommended for implementation.
- *Category 1B* has supporting evidence from some studies, has a good theoretical basis, and is strongly recommended for implementation.
- *Category IC* is required by state or federal regulations or is an industry standard.
- *Category II* is supported by suggestive clinical or epidemiologic studies, has a theoretical basis, and is suggested for implementation.
- *Category III* is supported by descriptive studies, such as comparisons, correlations, and case studies, and may be useful.
- *Category IV* is obtained from expert opinion or authorities only.
- *Unresolved* means there is no recommendation because of a lack of consensus or evidence.

Nursing and Healthcare Advocacy

CNS PROMOTION

The CNS is in a unique position to serve as a **consultant and educator** for the community regarding health promotion and disease prevention, promoting the CNS role. There are many avenues that the CNS can explore:

- *Schools and universities* present many opportunities for education from demonstrating handwashing to small children in elementary school to speaking with students in medical fields to giving lectures on health care in university classes or public seminars.
- *Service organizations* often invite speakers to discuss topics of interest, and this presents an opportunity to discuss health issues and to enlist the aid of other organizations in spreading information.

- *News media* is especially interested in information during times of outbreaks or specific health concerns, but they may also be willing to interview or allow reports on a regular basis.
- *Job fairs* present an opportunity to speak to a wide range of people.
- *Unions* may be interested in field-related information.

SPHERES OF INFLUENCE

The CNS works in the three **spheres of influence** (patient/client, nurse and nurse practice, and organization/system), affecting outcomes through provision of care that includes expertise in diagnosis and treatment of disease as well as prevention and health promotion. These 3 spheres of influence are not mutually exclusive but are interrelated in almost all cases and are within the specialty area of the CNS. For example, a CNS may serve in all 3 spheres:

- *Patient/client sphere*: The CNS may provide assessment and direct care of the patient and family members related to a particular focus of health, such as diabetic care.
- *Nurse/nursing practice sphere*: The CNS may serve as a mentor, educator, or supervisor for other nursing staff. The goal of the CNS is to advance the practice of nursing.
- *Organization/system sphere*: The CNS may be actively involved in administrative committees and may participate in planning for the organization.

PROFESSIONAL INFORMATION DISSEMINATION AND NEWSLETTERS

Dissemination of pertinent information and literature should be an ongoing scheduled process, at least monthly. The easiest way to disseminate this type of information is through newsletters, either print or electronic.

- *Print newsletters* involve costs that must be considered as part of operating expenses. There is also staff time involved in preparing the document as well as copyright considerations. Most government publications are copyright exempt and can be reproduced, but articles of interest from journals require permission to reproduce, which may be difficult to obtain for new material. An alternative method is for someone to write a review of an article or articles, including a summary of the main points. Use of pictures adds expense, especially if they are in color.
- *Electronic newsletters* involve staff time but are considerably less expensive. Additionally, links to online articles and color pictures can be easily inserted into the newsletter.

PEER SUPPORT

Nursing is a high stress profession and almost all nurses benefit from informal **peer support** from others in the profession through discussion and networking. In addition, formal peer support groups are becoming more common as the profession recognizes that the nurse must often cope with psychologically traumatic experiences as part of their profession as well as in their personal lives. Formal peer support groups may comprise members from various levels of the organization, but when possible, the members should be chosen by staff rather than assigned. Peer support groups may provide ongoing support of staff through meetings and newsletters but are also used for debriefing and provision of emotional support to help nurses cope with traumatic events, such as a disaster with multiple victims. Peer support groups should receive training but do not take the place of psychologists or other counselors, so members must make referrals when appropriate.

PEER REVIEW

Peer review is an intensive process in which an individual practitioner is reviewed by like practitioners. It may be used for an individual practitioner and patient or a group of patients and often relates to data found as part of root cause analysis, infection control, or other surveillance measures. Peer review is usually conducted within the specified department by a committee. A ranking system is usually used to indicate compliance with standards:

- Care is based on standards and is typical of that provided by like practitioners.
- Variance may occur in care, but outcomes are satisfactory.
- Care is not consistent with that provided by like practitioners.
- Variance resulted in negative outcomes.

In some cases, this ranking system is not used and is replaced with a series of questions with affirmative answers indicating cause for concern.

Peer Review and Joint Commission Focus

The **Joint Commission** focuses on the process of **peer review** in both design and function. Peer review should be a review by a like practitioner with similar training, experience, and expertise. In some cases, the pool of practitioners may be too small within one organization; so external peer reviews may be required. Peer review is often triggered by root cause analysis that indicates the need to focus on an individual, sometimes related to utilization review:

- *The design* should include definitions of peer, methods in which peer review panels are selected, triggering events, and timeframes. It should also outline the participation of the person being reviewed.
- *The function* must be consistently applied to all individuals, balanced and fair, adherent to timelines, ongoing, and valuable to the organization, Decisions should be based on solid reason and literature review and must be defensible.

Fostering Healthy Work Environments

Nursing associations have taken an active role in stressing the importance a **healthy work environment** in terms of physical and emotional well-being. Standards include:

Effective Communication	Teaching communication skills and using them to improve outcomes, providing access to communication technologies, accountability, and policies regarding verbal or physical abuse, including consequences
Collaboration	Teaching collaboration skills and clearly outlining accountability and expectations
Decision-Making	Administration, team members, and patients included, with processes clearly outlined
Adequate Staffing	Assessment and input by all team members to ensure that the needs of the patients are adequately matched with nurse competencies
Recognition	Ensuring that staff members feel valued for their contributions
Effective Leadership	Leaders serving as models for attaining the goal of a healthy work environment with adequate time and resources to achieve goals

Workplace Regulations and Standards

Regarding Sexual Harassment

Sexual harassment regulations include these:

- The 1964 Civil Rights Act (Title VII) prohibited gender discrimination and sexual harassment by employers.
- The 1972 Education Amendments (Title IX) extended protection to education institutions.

- The 1980 Equal Employment Opportunity Commission (EEOC) defined sexual harassment as quid pro quo (expecting something in return for a favor) or hostile work environment (unwelcome advances or conduct).
- The 1991 Civil Rights Act allowed victims to obtain punitive/compensatory awards if subjected to sexual harassment.
- Additionally, many state laws have requirements regarding sexual harassment, and protection has been extended to same-gender harassment.

Sexual harassment includes unwelcome verbal advances (comments, asking for dates), personal comments (appearance, lifestyle, body), offensive behavior (bullying, leering), offensive materials (jokes, posters, videos, emails), and unwelcome physical contact (touching, hugging, kissing, molesting). Sexual harassment in the healthcare industry is high, with studies showing that offenders are most often physicians, but co-workers, supervisors, and patients also commit sexual harassment. Healthcare providers may be legally and financially liable for harassment.

Regarding Workplace Violence

While there are no specific federal laws requiring protection against **workplace violence,** including verbal and non-verbal threatening actions, OSHA provides preventive guidelines, and the Joint Commission (2009) has established leadership standards requiring a code of conduct and management procedures for inappropriate behavior. A number of states have also enacted laws requiring workplace violence prevention programs and specifying penalties for attacks on healthcare workers. The healthcare industry leads all others in the number of assaults, because of many factors, including increased prevalence of guns, placement of criminals in hospitals, release of mentally ill without adequate follow-up, increased substance abuse, inadequate staffing, inadequate training, and availability of drugs. Violence prevention policies should include:

- Establishment of zero-tolerance policy and dissemination of the policy to all staff, patients, and visitors
- Prevention of reprisals for reporting workplace violence
- Creation of a plan to reduce risk and increase safety
- Establishment of liaison with local law enforcement agencies

Regarding Equal Employment Opportunity

The **Equal Employment Opportunity Commission** enforces federal laws against discrimination in employment for employers with ≥15 employees and age-discrimination for employers with ≥20 employees. The EEOC investigates, provides guidance, and enforces a number of laws:

- Civil Rights Act (1964), Title VII, including Pregnancy Discrimination Act: Employers cannot discriminate based on race, color, gender, pregnancy, religion, and national origin.
- Civil Rights Act (1991), Sections 102 and 103: Amends previous laws to allow jury trials and punitive and compensatory damages.
- Equal Pay Act (1963): Males and females must receive equal pay for equal work.
- Age Discrimination in Employment Act (ADEA) (1967): Law provides protection against age discrimination for those ≥40.
- Americans with Disabilities Act (ADA) (1990): Law prevents discrimination in private sector and state and local levels against qualified individuals with disabilities and requires reasonable accommodations.

- Rehabilitation Act (1973), Sections 501 and 505: Law is similar to ADA but applies to discrimination against those with disabilities in the federal government.
- Genetic Information Nondiscrimination Act (GINA) (2008): Employers cannot discriminate based on genetic information.

Transtheoretical Model

During each stage of the process of the **Transtheoretical Model**, people go through 10 **processes of change** as they attempt to modify their behavior:

- *Consciousness raising*: Seeking information.
- *Counterconditioning:* Substituting alternative action for problem behavior, such as using relaxation techniques, positive statements, and desensitization.
- *Dramatic relief:* Expressing feelings (positive and negative) about change of problem behavior and solutions.
- *Environmental reevaluation:* Determining the effect the problem behavior has on others and developing empathy.
- *Helping relationships:* Accepting assistance from others to effectuate change.
- *Reinforcement management:* Accepting reward (from self or others) for changing problem behavior.
- *Self-liberation:* Believing change is possible and committing to change.
- *Self-reevaluation:* Reevaluating values in relation to problem behavior.
- *Social liberation:* Becoming aware (emotionally and cognitively) of positive lifestyles and feeling empowered.
- *Stimulus control:* Controlling situations in which problem behavior is triggered.

Evaluation

Scope and Standards

Standards of Care

The ANA has established standards of specialty nursing practice that represent the duties of the CNS and promote evidence-based care and development of individual care plans. **Standards of care,** which encompass the nursing process, include the following:

- **Core Practice Standards**
  - Assessment
  - Diagnosis
  - Outcomes identification
  - Planning
  - Implementation
  - Evaluation
- **Professional Practice Standards**
  - Ethics
  - Education
  - Evidence-based practice and research
  - Quality of practice
  - Communication
  - Leadership
  - Collaboration
  - Professional practice evaluation
  - Resource utilization
  - Environmental health

Core practice standards are required for the nurse to achieve a competent level of patient care, while professional practice standards relate to professional behavior. The CNS is responsible for competency in both areas of practice, should be actively involved in activities related to professional standards, such as evidence-based practice and research, and should serve as a resource person for other staff members, helping them to achieve adequate standards of care.

Joint Commission's Core Measures

The Joint Commission has established **core measures** to determine if healthcare institutions are in compliance with current standards. The core measures involve a series of questions that are answered either "yes" or "no" to indicate if an action was completed. Currently, the Joint Commission's core measures are as follows:

- Acute Myocardial Infarction (AMI)
- Children's Asthma Care
- Emergency Department
- Hospital Outpatient Department
- Hospital-Based Inpatient Psychiatric Services
- Immunization
- Perinatal Care

- Stroke
- Substance Use
- Tobacco Treatment
- Venous Thromboembolism

For each condition, questions relate to whether or not **standard care** was provided, such as giving an Aspirin for those patients with an acute MI. This data is public and provides useful information about these particular standards, but does not necessarily reflect the overall quality of care. Core measurements alone are not adequate performance measures, but must be considered along with other indicators.

Nurse Practice Act

Each state has its own **Nurse Practice Act,** which is administered by the state Board of Nursing. The Nurse Practice Act outlines requirements for licensure and certification and delineates the scope of practice of nurses, including duties and delegation. Typically, licensure is granted to those who complete an accredited LVN/LPN or RN program and pass the nursing exam (NCLEX) or receive endorsement because of licensure in another state. RN programs may be 3-year hospital-based programs, associate degree programs, or bachelor's degree programs. Foreign-trained nurses may need to meet special requirements that are determined by the state Board of Nursing and included in the Nurse Practice Act. The Nurse Practice Act of each state provides the requirement for advanced practice certification and the professional designation. Additionally, the Nurse Practice acts outline the requirements for relicensing or recertification, often including the need for continuing education. The Nurse Practice Act also includes provisions for disciplinary action.

CNS Scope of Practice

Each state has a nurse practice act that outline the **scope of practice** of advanced practice nurses, such as clinical nurse specialists. Additionally, the American Association of Clinical Nurse Specialists has established guidelines in relation to activities allowed under scope of practice. Primary responsibilities include activities aimed at health promotion and disease prevention:

- *Assessing* includes history, physical evaluation, screening tests, identifying risks, and ordering routine laboratory/radiographic tests.
- *Diagnosing* includes integrating information from assessment with specific laboratory tests to arrive at a clinical diagnosis.
- *Managing* includes establishing a plan of care, providing interventions and education, referring to other healthcare providers or agencies, and reassessing the care plan based on outcomes.

Clinical nurse specialists with a specific clinical focus may have added responsibilities.

NACNS Statement of Practice

The **clinical nurse specialist (CNS)** is one of 4 advanced practice nursing professionals recognized in the United States along with nurse practitioners, certified midwives, and certified nurse anesthetists. In 1998, the National Association of Clinical Nurse Specialists (NACNS) (founded in 1996) clarified the role of the CNS and identified 3 interrelated spheres of influence: Patient/client, nurse/nursing practice, and organization/system. In 2004, the NACNS expanded on its original statement and outlined core competencies and outcomes based on the spheres of influence and the CNS specialty focus with the Statement on CNS Practice. These core competencies have been further refined by specialty organizations, such as the American Association of Critical Care Nurses. In order to be a Medicare provider, the CNS must have a master's degree and obtain certification through an accredited credentialing agency even though state regulations vary in the use of the CNS designation, certification requirements, and prescriptive authority.

ANA's Scope and Standards of Gerontological Nursing Practice

The **American Nurses Association's Scope and Standards of Gerontological Nursing Practice** includes many skills, such as providing care, managing care, advocating for the patient, and researching ways to improve care. Education is an essential role of the gerontological nurse. Duties outlined by the Scope and Standards of Gerontological Nursing Practice include utilizing data, information, and knowledge to develop a patient care plan; assessing information for diagnosis; influencing health outcomes; planning care to provide appropriate treatment; implementing interventions and evaluating treatment progress; evaluating the quality of care; self-assessment of abilities and performance in relation to professional standards; keeping up to date in the field; providing care in an ethical manner; working collaboratively with patients, family, caregivers, and interdisciplinary team members; utilizing research to provide evidence-based care; and providing and promoting safe and cost-effective care to all patients.

ANA Social Policy Statement

The **American Nurse Association Social Policy Statement** was written in 1980, revised in 1995, and revised again in 2003. The ANA Social Policy Statement provides a description and definition of nursing practice and outlines the knowledge base required for nursing and the requirements and scope of practice for advance practice nurses, such as the CNS. The ANA Social Policy Statement recognizes the social contract that exists between nursing and society and the responsibilities that the social contract entails. Nursing requires a holistic approach rather than problem-focused approach to care, integrating objective data and knowledge and utilizing the scientific method. The ANA Social Policy Statement also describes the regulation of nursing, including self-regulation, professional, and legal, centering on the code of ethics and meeting of certification requirements. Nurses are accountable for their actions under the law but also must assume personal responsibility for maintaining their knowledge base.

Scope and Standards of Advance Practice

The clinical nurse specialist (CNS) must practice within the **standards of advance practice** and the individual's scope of practice, which is directly related to the individual's educational preparation and certification. A CNS must have two types of licenses/certificates: an RN and an advanced practice certificate. Advance practice nurses are those who have completed additional education in an accredited nursing program (usually at a Master's level) and have received certification with a national certifying organization, such as the American Nurse's Credentialing Center. The CNS must function legally under the Nurse Practice Act of the state in which the person resides. In some cases, a CNS license/certification in one state is automatically recognized in other states through the Compact agreement, but advance practice nurses are often excluded from these agreements. Educational experience and scope of practice must relate to patient population in terms of age, disease, diagnosis, and treatment.

Care Process, Establishing Priorities, and Collaboration

The nurse must adhere to the **standards of advance practice**. These standards provide the guidelines for practice and describe the responsibilities of the gerontological nurse. The standards outline the values and priorities of the profession.

In the *care process*, the nurse assesses, develops, and implements a plan of care and evaluates the patient's response; the nurse must use the scientific method and national standards as the basis for care. In *establishing priorities*, the nurse provides education and encourages the patient and his or her family to take an active role in self-care. The nurse must be sure that the patient is able to make informed decisions. The nurse must assist the patient through all aspects of health care to ensure patient safety and optimal care. *Collaboration* is essential. As a member of an interdisciplinary health team, the nurse must consult with other team members when appropriate.

Documentation, Patient Advocacy, Continuous Quality Improvement, Research and Education

Standards of advance practice specific responsibilities include the following:

- *Documentation*: The CNS keeps accurate, legal, legible records and maintains patient confidentiality. The CNS ensures that the patient signs a release before providing medical records to other parties.
- *Patient advocacy:* The CNS advocates for the individual patient in the process of care but also advocates for patients at the state and national level in order to facilitate patient access to care and improve the quality of care.
- *Continuous quality improvement:* The CNS recognizes the need for constant learning and evaluation and reevaluation. It participates in quality review and continuing education while maintaining certification and utilizing clinical guidelines and standards of care.
- *Research and education:* The CNS initiates, participates in, and utilizes the results of research in clinical practice.

Prescriptions and Diagnostic Tests

Both **prescribing** medications and treatment and ordering **diagnostic** tests are within the scope of practice of the clinical nurse specialist, but as with other aspects of practice, each state establishes how that will be carried out. Additionally, insurance reimbursement varies from one area to another and must be considered:

- *Prescription*: Terminology varies from state to state with clinical nurse specialists allowed to "furnish" or "prescribe" some types of medications. In some states they may do so independently; in others, they must be "supervised" by a physician under whose auspices they provide care to patients. The CNS should maintain a list of medications and consider cost-effectiveness when ordering medications.
- *Diagnostics:* The CNS can order laboratory, EKG, and radiographic tests for routine screening and health assessment. The CNS can also diagnose based on assessment. There are limitations, depending upon the individual state nursing practice act.

Consultation, Referral, and Coordination

As part of the **scope of practice**, the CNS is able to provide and augment primary care to adults through a number of different services:

- *Consultation* services may include a variety of services, such as assessment of growth risk factors, providing interventions (e.g., diet and exercise programs), and educating patients/families.
- *Referral services* include referring patients to physicians, such as orthopedic specialists, and to organizations or agencies, such as drug rehabilitation programs.
- *Coordination services*, with the nurse maintaining contact and receiving reports from referrals in order to provide an integrated plan of care, serves as a valuable service to patients who often must deal with many different healthcare providers who have little or no contact with each other. This type of service can prevent unnecessary duplications of service but also ensure that findings are not overlooked.

Care Process, Establishing Priorities, and Collaboration

The clinical nurse specialist is guided by the **standards of advance practice**, which provide the framework for practice and describes the CNS's responsibilities, related to the values and priorities of the profession:

- *Care process:* In assessing, diagnosing, developing, and implementing a plan of care, and evaluating the patient's response, the CNS must use the scientific method and national standards as the basis for care.
- *Establishing priorities:* Providing education and encouraging the patient/family to take an active role in self-care is of primary concern. The CNS must ensure that the patient can make informed decisions. The CNS must assist the patient through all aspects of health care to ensure patient safety and optimal care.
- *Collaboration*: The CNS is a member of the interdisciplinary health team and consults with others when appropriate and refers the patient to specialists as needed. When collaboration is mandated by law, the CNS complies with all requirements.

Delegation of Tasks

One major responsibility in the leadership and management of a performance improvement team is effective **delegation**. The purpose of forming a team is to share the workload. Leaders cannot perform effectively if they take on too much of the workload. Additionally, failure to delegate shows an inherent distrust in team members. The leader is ultimately responsible for the delegated work. Mentoring, monitoring, and providing feedback and intervention are necessary components of leadership. Delegation includes the following:

- Assessing the skills and availability of the team members, determining if a task is suitable for an individual
- Assigning tasks with a time line
- Ensuring that the tasks are completed properly and on time by monitoring progress but not micromanaging
- Reviewing the final results and recording outcomes.

5 Rights of Delegation

Prior to delegating tasks, the nurse should assess the needs of the patients and determine the task that needs to be completed and ensure that he/she can remain accountable and can supervise the task appropriately and evaluate effective completion. The **5 rights of delegation** include the following:

- *Right task:* The nurse should determine an appropriate task to delegate for a specific patient.
- *Right circumstance:* The nurse has considered the setting, resources, time factors, safety factors, and all other relevant information to determine the appropriateness of delegation.
- *Right person:* The nurse is in the right position to choose the right person (by virtue of education/skills) to perform a task for the right patient.
- *Right direction:* The nurse provides a clear description of the task, the purpose, any limits, and expected outcomes.
- *Right supervision:* The nurse is able to supervise, intervene as needed, and evaluate performance of the task.

Delegating Tasks to Unlicensed Assistive Personnel

The scope of nursing practice includes **delegation of tasks** to unlicensed assistive personnel, providing those personnel have adequate training and knowledge to carry out the tasks. Delegation should be used to manage the workload and to provide adequate and safe care. The nurse who delegates remains accountable for patient outcomes and for supervision of the person to whom the task was delegated, so the nurse must consider the following:

- Whether the knowledge, skills, and training of the unlicensed assistive personnel provides the ability to perform the delegated task
- Whether the patient's condition and needs have been properly evaluated and assessed
- Whether the nurse is able to provide ongoing supervision

Delegation should be done in a manner that reduces liability by providing adequate communication. This includes specific directions about the task, including what needs to be done, when, and for how long. Expectations related to consultation, reporting, and completion of tasks should be clearly defined. The nurse should be available to assist if necessary.

Documentation

Documentation is a form of communication that provides information about the healthcare patient and confirms that care was provided. Accurate, objective, and complete documentation of patient care is required by both accreditation and reimbursement agencies, including federal and state governments. Purposes of documentation include the following:

- Carrying out professional responsibility
- Establishing accountability
- Communicating among health professionals
- Educating staff
- Providing information for research
- Satisfying legal and practice standards
- Ensuring reimbursement

While documentation focuses on progress notes, there are many other aspects to charting. Doctor's orders must be noted, medication administration must be documented on medication sheets, and vital signs must be graphed. Flow sheets must be checked off, filled out, or initialed. Admission assessments may involve primarily checklists or may require extensive documentation. The primary issue in malpractice cases is inaccurate or incomplete documentation. It's better to over-document than under, but effective documentation does neither.

Importance of Accuracy

There are a number of requirements regarding **written communication/documentation.** Regardless of format, charting should always include any change in client's condition, treatments or other interventions, medications, client responses, and complaints of family or client. Nurses should avoid subjective descriptions (especially negative terms, which could be used to establish bias in court), such as tired, angry, confused, bored, rude, happy, and euphoric. Instead, more objective descriptions, such as "Yawning 2-3 times a minute," should be used. Clients can be quoted directly. "I shouldn't have to wait for pain medication when I need it!" If errors are made in charting, for example, charting another patient's information in the record, the error cannot be erased, whited-out, or otherwise made illegible. The error must be indicated by drawing a line through the text and writing "Error."

Importance of Legibility and Clarity

Written communication/documentation requirements include the following:

- *Legibility*: If hand entries are used, then writing should be done with a blue or black permanent ink pen, and writing should be neat and legible, in block printing if handwriting is illegible. Some facilities require black ink only, so if unsure, nurses should use black ink. No pen or pencil that can be erased can be used to document in a patient's record because this could facilitate falsification of records. For the same reason, a line must be drawn through empty spaces in the documentation.
- *Clarity*: A standardized vocabulary should be used for documenting, including lists of approved abbreviations and symbols. Abbreviations and symbols, especially, can pose serious problems in interpretation, so they should be used sparingly.

Timeliness

Nurses should chart every 1-2 hours for routine care (bathing, walking), but medications and other interventions or changes in condition should be charted immediately. Failure to chart medications, especially prn medications, in a timely manner may result in the client receiving the medication twice. Additionally, if one nurse is caring for a number of patients, it may be easy to forget and omit or confuse information. Nurses must never chart in advance because it is illegal and can lead to unforeseen errors. Guessing that a client will have no problems and care will be routine can result in having to make corrections. Nurses must chart the time of all interventions and notations. Time may be a critical element, for example, in deciding if a patient should receive more pain medication or be catheterized for failure to urinate. Military time is used in many healthcare institutions but if standard time is used, the nurse should always include "AM" or "PM" with time notations.

Methods

Different **methods of documentation** used for patient's medical records include the following:

- *Narrative*: This charting provides a chronological report of the patient's condition, treatment, and responses. It is an easy method of charting but may be disorganized and repetitive, and if different people are making notes, they may address different issues, making it difficult to get an overall picture of the patient's progress.
- *SOAP (subjective data, objective data, assessment, plan of action):* This problem-oriented form of charting includes establishing goals, expected outcomes, and needs and then compiling a numbered list of problems. A SOAP note is made for each separate problem.
    - ***Subjective***: Client's statement of problem
    - ***Objective***: Nurse's observation
    - ***Assessment***: Determination of possible causes
    - ***Plan***: Short- and long-range goals and immediate plan of care

If there are multiple problems (edema, pain, restricted activity, etc.), this charting can be very time-consuming as each element of SOAP must be addressed. SOAP notes may also be extended to ***SOAPIER*** (including ***intervention, evaluation, and revision***.)

PIE and Focus/DAR

Different **methods of documentation** for patients include the following:

- *PIE (problem, intervention, evaluation):* This problem-oriented form of charting is similar to SOAP but is less complex. It combines use of flow sheets with progress notes and a list of problems. Each problem is numbered sequentially, and a PIE note is made for each problem at least one time daily (or during treatment, depending on the frequency).
- *Focus/DAR (data, action, response):* This type of focused charting includes documentation about health problems, changes in condition, and concerns or events, focusing on data about the injury/illness, the action taken by the nurse, and the response. The written format is usually in 3 columns (D-A-R) rather than traditional narrative linear form. A DAR note is used for each focus item.

Charting by Exception and Computerized Charting

Different **methods of documentation** for patients include the following:

- *Charting by exception*: This form of charting was developed in response to problem-oriented charting in an attempt to simplify charting. It includes extensive use of flow sheets and intermittent charting to document unexpected findings and interventions. However, because this focuses on interventions, those problems that require no particular intervention (such as increased discomfort after ambulating) may be overlooked, and charting may not be adequate for legal challenge because lack of charting may be construed as lack of care of evaluation.
- *Computerized:* All record keeping is done electronically, usually at point of care. Computer terminals must be placed where others cannot read notes being written, and access must be password protected. These systems may include clinical decision support systems (CDSS), which provide diagnosis and treatment options based on symptoms. Computerized charting has some advantages: It is legible and tamper-proof and tends to reduce errors as many systems signal if a treatment is missed or the wrong treatment is given.

Flow Sheets and Critical Pathways

Different **methods of documentation** for patients include the following:

- *Flow sheets:* These are often a part of other methods of charting and are used to save time. They may be used to indicate completion of exercises or treatments. They usually contain areas for graphing data and may have columns or rows with information requiring checkmarks to indicate an action was done or observation made.
- *Critical pathways:* These are specific multi-disciplinary care plans that outline interventions and outcomes of diseases, conditions, and procedures. Critical pathways are based on data and literature and best practices. The expected outcomes are delineated as well as the sequence of interventions and the timeline needed to achieve the outcomes. There are many different types of forms that appear similar to flow sheets but are more complex and require more documentation. Any variance from the pathway or expected outcomes must be documented. Critical pathways are increasingly used to comply with insurance limitations to ensure cost-effective timely treatment.

Scope of Malpractice

Clinical nurse specialists, as all advance practice nurses, are usually insured for **malpractice** at a higher rate than registered nurses because their scope of practice is much wider. A CNS may be sued individually or as part of a medical group to which the CNS is associated. Because a suit is a civil matter, loss of judgment may not be reported to the state board of nursing. If a charge of negligence is brought to the attention of the board, the board may initiate an investigation and disciplinary action. Negligence may involve a number of failures, such as not referring a patient when needed, incorrect diagnosis, incorrect treatment, and not providing the patient/family with adequate or essential information. Once a CNS has established a duty to a patient—by direct examination or even casual or telephone conversation that involves professional advice—the CNS may be liable for malpractice if he/she does not follow up with adequate care.

Patient Outcomes

NDNQI

The National Database of Nursing Quality Indicators (NDNQI) is a database containing information collected at the level of the nursing unit. This database was initiated by the American Nurses Association (ANA) and began in 1997 when the ANA selected the Midwest Research Institute and the University of Kansas School of Nursing to take on the task to develop and maintain the NDNQI. From 1997 to 2000 the ANA funded several studies to test selected indicators. Since then the database has grown tremendously in the number of indicators evaluated and in the number of participating hospitals.

Benefits

One of the biggest benefits of the National Database of Nursing Quality Indicators (NDNQI) comes from the comparisons generated from participating hospitals. In 1998 the NDNQI started accepting data from participating hospitals and then began to charge for data submission and the creation of comparison reports in 2001. Comparison information is grouped based on the patient and unit type. Quarterly reports provide information including national comparisons along with performance trends of the specific unit over the last eight quarters. Many hospitals utilize this information to assist with quality improvement, nursing recruitment and retention, patient recruitment, research, and development of staff education topics. This information is also valuable to the participating hospital because it can be utilized to meet report requirements for different regulatory bodies or magnet designations.

HEDIS

HEDIS stands for Healthcare Effectiveness Data and Information Set, which are the accreditation standards by which managed health care plans are evaluated and judged. HEDIS looks at the quality of the systems, the process, the care, and the services that a managed care plan delivers to its members. The information provided by HEDIS helps the consumer and employers choose the plan that offers the highest quality of care at the best cost. The HEDIS standards look at the effectiveness of care, accessibility, consumer satisfaction, cost, the stability of the plan, and the credentials of the health care providers. A program evaluated through the use of HEDIS ensures quality for the consumer.

Nursing Sensitive Indicators

Nursing sensitive indicators are those structures, processes, and patient outcomes that are influenced (not necessarily controlled) by nursing. Nursing sensitive indicators are developed to determine the degree of influence that nursing provides; that is, they establish correlation between nursing interventions and patient outcomes. For example, indicators may be used to determine what effect increasing staffing levels has on patient outcomes:

- Structures include staffing levels, educational attainment of staff, skill levels, and certification levels.
- Processes include procedures, assessment, and implementation of care, and nursing satisfaction.
- Outcomes include patient outcomes (infection rates, pressure sores) that are directly influenced by nursing care.
- Nursing sensitive indicators currently in use include nursing hours/day, nurse-to-patient ratio, staff turnover, nosocomial infections, patient falls, patient injuries, rate of pressure sores, use of restraints, staff mix, pediatric peripheral IV infiltration, and RN education. The National Database of Nursing Quality Indicators (NDNQI) provides reports that measure the impact of nursing care.

Outcomes in the Patient/Client Sphere

The NACNS has outlined core competencies the CNS must master to achieve outcomes (clinical/economic) in each sphere of influence. **Outcomes associated with the patient/client sphere** include:

- Care is provided for specific patient populations.
- Areas requiring nursing intervention are identified.
- Nursing care targets specific causes of health disorders.
- Goals related to health promotion and prevention are met.
- Nursing care plan meets the needs of patients.
- Adverse events are prevented.
- Nursing outcomes are clarified.
- Effective interventions are included in evidence-based guidelines.
- Ineffective interventions are eliminated.
- Collaboration with the patient/family, physician, and other staff is utilized as appropriate.
- Educational programs are presented and evaluated.
- Smooth transitions occur.
- Results are published/shared.

Outcomes in the Nurse/Nurse Practice Sphere

The NACNS has outlined core competencies the CNS must master to achieve outcomes (clinical/economic) in each sphere of influence. **Outcomes associated with the nurse/nurse practice sphere** include the following:

- Needs for staff training and development are outlined.
- Practice reflects current best practices.
- Changes in practice result from accessible research.
- Nurses identify contributions specific to nurses and expected outcomes.
- Care providers develop solutions to patient problems.
- Collaborative efforts achieve target patient outcomes.
- Nurses have educational programs that are readily available to enhance their careers.
- Nursing staff gains confidence in providing patient care.
- Job satisfaction increases.
- Staff retention improves.

- Staff is engaged in the learning process.
- Programs developed for nursing education are implemented and evaluated for effectiveness.
- Care is cost-effective through the efficient use of resources.

Outcomes in the Organization/System Sphere

The NACNS has outlined core competencies the CNS must master to achieve outcomes (clinical/economic) in each sphere of influence. **Outcomes associated with the organization/system sphere** include the following:

- Continuous improvements in care benefit the organization/system.
- Evidence-based policies and care improve nurse/team practice.
- Innovations occur throughout the continuum of care.
- Innovative care provides cost-effective positive outcomes for patients.
- A common vision is shared by health professionals and management.
- Factors contributing to problems, costs, and outcomes are clear to those who make decisions.
- Nursing care programs reflect the strategic plan, mission, and vision of the organization/system.

Research Methodology

Fostering a Culture of Scientific Inquiry, Considering Barriers and Facilitators

Numerous factors influence development of **scientific inquiry across the spheres of influence**, with both drivers and barriers affecting decisions:

- **Drivers**
  - *Financial goals*: Cost is of primary importance with increasing costs of medical care and reduced reimbursement, so processes must demonstrate cost-effectiveness.
  - *Political support*: Buy-in of those in power is critical to success. This support should be used to encourage participation and acceptance.
  - *Regulations require changes*: Federal (CDC, FDA), state (State Department of Public Health), and local (County Department of Public Health) regulations may require practice improvement.
- **Barriers**
  - *Financial concerns*: Improved processes that increase costs may not be approved unless they can demonstrate sufficient cost benefit to override this major concern.
  - *Political opposition*: Overcoming political opposition may require persistence, data, and patience.
  - *Regulations prevent changes*: Practice improvement processes that violate regulations must be avoided by carefully reviewing existing regulations as part of development.

Identification of Clinical Problems Amenable to Research

Identifying **clinical problems amenable to research** is an evolving skill. Inexperienced nurses, especially those just starting out in nursing practice, are often looking to build information and skills because they lack experiential learning. They may research information about a disease or treatment that they are dealing with in order to have better skills and understanding. More experienced nurses, on the other hand, often look for information to improve patient outcomes, such as researching new procedures, treatments, or equipment for broader application. However, there is a need for both. Clinical inquiry is a program of questioning and evaluating practice through research and experience. It should include seeking a variety of data on a topic, evaluating the data, pooling results, and making determinations as to validity or applicability to the clinical practice. Clinical inquiry is also part of evidence-based practice in which data is used to support clinical decisions on an ongoing basis.

Data Definition and Collection of Data

Data definitions must be based on a solid understanding of statistical analysis and epidemiological concepts. Specific issues that must be addressed include the following:

- **3 Ss:**
  - *Sensitivity*: The data should include all positive cases, taking into account variables, decreasing the number of false negatives.
  - *Specificity*: The data should include only those cases specific to the needs of the measurement and exclude those that may be similar but are a different population, decreasing the number of false positives.
  - *Stratification*: Date should be classified according to subsets, taking variables into consideration.
- **2 Rs:**
  - *Recordability*: The tool/indicator should collect and measure the necessary data.
  - *Reliability*: Results should be reproducible.
- **UV:**
  - *Usability*: The tool or indicator should be easy to utilize and understand.
  - *Validity*: Collection should measure the target adequately, so that the results have predictive value.

Population/Sampling

Defining the **population** is critical to data collection and the criteria must be established early in the process. The population may be comprised of a particular group of individuals, objects, or events. In some cases, data is gathered on an entire population, such as all cases with a particular disease, all deaths, or all physicians in a particular discipline, usually within a specified time frame. In other cases, **sampling,** using a subset of a population, may be done to measure only part of a given population and to generalize the findings to the larger target population while accurately representing the target population. There are a number of considerations with sampling:

- The sampling must have the characteristics of the target population.
- The design of the collection must specify the size of the sample, the location, and time period.
- The sampling technique must ensure that the sampling represents the target population accurately.
- The design of the collection must ensure that the sampling will not be biased.

Types of Sampling

Depending upon the goal of data collection, different **types of sampling** or combinations of sampling may be utilized. Sampling should have a *confidence level* of 95% (.05 level), meaning that there is a 95% chance that the sample represents the population and results can be replicated. Types include non-probability and probability.

Non-Probability Sampling

This type of sampling is intentionally biased (not everyone has an equal chance of being included), and results cannot be generalized to an entire population. It utilizes qualitative judgment.

- *Convenience*: This is a type of opportunity sampling when those available are sampled, such as all those in a clinic during a certain time frame.
- *Quota*: A stratified population is divided into subgroups (such as male and female) and then a proportion is sampled, such as 5% of females over 16 with HIV. Sometimes specified numbers may be counted, such as 50 males and 50 females.
- *Purpose*: Sampling of members of a particular population, such as all women over 60 with breast implants.

Probability Sampling

Probability sampling occurs when there is an equal chance for any member of a group to be part of the sample, allowing generalization of results to the entire population. Probability sampling is usually more expensive than non-probability sampling. There are a number of sub-types:

- *Cluster*: The target population is divided into clusters or groups, and then a number of these groups are selected at random and all members of the population within the selected groups are sampled.
- *Multi-stage*: This method is similar to cluster sampling except that instead of all members of the population in selected groups being sampled, a sample of the selected groups is used, utilizing any of the methods of choosing members of a population, such as simple random sampling.
- *Simple random:* The cases in a given population are chosen randomly using a standard Table of Random Digits. This is the easiest and most commonly used method of sampling.
- *Stratified:* This is two-tier sampling method in which a group is divided into strata (mutually exclusive groups) with 2 or more homogenous characteristics. Then, a specified number of participants from each stratum are sampled. Thus, patients in outpatient surgery with intravenous solutions may be sampled by diagnosis, solution, length of stay, or complications.
- *Systematic (interval) random:* This involves random selection of the first member of the population and then other members at regular intervals. For example, if the desired sampling were 100 out of 500, then the *sampling interval* would be 5 (1 out of every 5). A random number between 1 and 5 is chosen as the *random start* and then every 5th member is sampled to a total of 100.
- *Multi-phase:* This sampling is usually done in two phases, but more can be used. In this type of sampling, certain data are obtained from an entire specified population, and then based on that data, further data are obtained from a subgroup within the original population.

Protection of Human Subjects

The Food and Drug Administration, Code of Federal Regulations, Title 21, Volume 1, regulates **protection of human subjects** and states that any researcher involving patients in research must obtain informed consent, in language understandable to the patient or the patient's agent. The elements of this informed consent must include an explanation of the research, the purpose, and the expected duration, as well as a description of any potential risks. Potential benefits and possible alternative treatments must be described. Any compensation to be provided must be outlined. The extent of confidentiality should be clarified. Contact information should be provided in the event the patient/family has questions. The patient must be informed that participation is voluntary and that he or she can discontinue participation at any time without penalty. Informed consent must be documented by a signed, written agreement.

Health and Human Services, Title 45 Code of Federal Regulations, Part 46

Protection of human subjects is covered in the **Health and Human Services, Title 45 Code of Federal Regulations, part 46.** This provides guidance for institutional review boards (IRBs) for those involved in research and outlines requirements. Institutions engaged in non-exempt research must submit an assurance of compliance (document) to the Office of Human Research Protection (OHRP) agreeing to comply with all requirements for research projects. Subjects cannot be used solely as a means to an end, but research should hold the possibility of benefit to the subject. Risks should be minimal, and selection of subjects should be equitable. Some research populations are granted additional protections because of their vulnerability and susceptibility to coercion; this includes children, prisoners, pregnant women, human fetuses and neonates, mentally disable people, and people who are economically or educationally disadvantaged. When cooperative research projects are conducted involving more than one institution, then each must safeguard the rights of subjects, ensuring informed consent and privacy.

Targeted Surveillance

Targeted surveillance is limited in scope, focusing on particular types of problems, areas in the facility, or patient population. It is less expensive than hospital-wide surveillance and may provide more meaningful data, but clusters of problems outside the survey parameters may be missed. Targeted areas are picked based on characteristics such as frequency of the disorder, mortality rates, financial costs, and the ability to use data to prevent the disorder:

- *Site-directed* targets particular sites of infection, such as bloodstream, wound, or urine.
- *Unit-directed* targets selected service areas of the hospital, such as intensive care units or neonatal units.
- *Population-directed* targets groups that are considered high-risk, such as transplantation patients and those undergoing other invasive procedures.
- *Limited periodic* involves hospital-wide surveillance of all infections for one month each quarter followed by site-directed targets for the rest of the quarter. This increases the chance of detecting clusters of infection, but those that fall outside of the hospital-wide surveillance months would still be missed.

Literature Search

Literature research requires comprehensive evaluation of current (≤5 years) and/or historical information. Most literature research begins with an Internet search of databases, which provides listings of books, journals, and other materials on specific topics. Databases vary in content, and many contain only a reference listing with or without an abstract, so once the listing is obtained, the researcher must do a further search to locate the material from a library, publisher, etc. Some databases require subscription, but access is often available through educational or healthcare institutions. To search effectively, the researcher should begin by writing a brief explanation of the research to help identify possible keywords and synonyms to use as search words.

- Truncations: "Finan*" provides all words that begin with those letters, such as "finance," "financial" and "financed."
- Wildcards: "m?n" or "m*n" provides "man" and "men."
- BOOLEAN logic (AND, OR, NOT):
    - Wound OR infect* OR ulcer

- Wound OR ulcer AND povidone-iodine
- Wound AND povidone-iodine NOT antibiotic NOT antimicrobial

Outcomes Evaluation

Outcomes evaluation is an important component of evidence-based practice, which involves both internal and external research. All treatments are subjected to review to determine if they produce positive outcomes and policies, and protocols for outcomes evaluation should be in place. Outcomes evaluation includes the following:

- *Monitoring* over the course of treatment involves careful observation and record keeping that notes progress with supporting laboratory and radiographic evidence as indicated by condition and treatment.
- *Evaluating* results includes reviewing records as well as current research to determine if outcomes are within acceptable parameters.
- *Sustaining* involves continuing treatment, but continuing to monitor and evaluate.
- *Improving* means to continue the treatment but with additions or modifications in order to improve outcomes.
- *Replacing* the treatment with a different treatment must be done if outcomes evaluation indicates that current treatment is ineffective.

Internal and External Validity, Generalizability, and Replication

Internal validity is concerned with the accuracy of the results of an experiment or study. If an experiment or study has internal validity, it demonstrates a cause and effect relationship between the variables that truly exists.

External validity is concerned with whether or not the results of an experiment or study are representative of the larger population.

Generalizability is concerned with whether or not the results of an experiment or study apply to other populations than the one studied.

Replication is concerned with whether the same results will be obtained if an experiment or study is repeated. The results of an experiment are considered to be sound if an experiment or study can be repeated and the same results are obtained.

Medical Record Review

Procedure

A systematic procedure for **medical record review** requires planning and consistency. Surveillance may involve questionnaires, medical records, or electronic review:

- *Medical record review* should be systematic and targeted as much as possible. Reporting forms should be utilized that include all necessary information in one form, paper or electronic.
- *Questionnaires* should be standardized and designed to obtain information that is quantifiable when possible. Questions should be clear, unambiguous, and non-threatening. Open-ended questions may be appropriate for some types of information gathering, especially in relation to information that may be embarrassing or indicate errors.

- *Coding* of data collection should be consistent, with specific codes for units, populations, and/or individuals to facilitate analysis. Thus, the report of a patient with a cough would have the same identification code as the laboratory work for that patient.
- *Electronic surveillance* should involve use of threshold data. Reports that are generated should be directly integrated with the data analysis system.

TYPES

There are a number of different types **medical record review** processes, and many reviews are mandated by regulations and accreditation. Types include the following:

- *Prospective*: This includes all those steps taken before an event, such as assessing need before care, checking credentials before hiring, determining ability to pay prior to doing elective procedures, and gaining preauthorization from insurance companies.
- *Concurrent*: This includes ongoing assessment while the patient is receiving care and verification of medical necessity for continued treatment as well as appropriate use of resources. Concurrent review may utilize medical records, observations of care, incidence reports, and special case studies.
- *Retrospective*: This review is done after care has been provided and provides a full picture of the continuum of care and its effectiveness. This may utilize the medical records as well as the results of prospective and concurrent review.
- *Focused*: This includes reviews done for specific pre-determined reasons, such as a specific diagnosis, procedure, or process. Criteria for case selection must be outlined.

RATES AND RATIOS

A **rate** is the number of events per a given population (a rate of 3 infections per 100 patients) or per a time period (a rate of 3 infections per 1000 device days). These figures are expressed as the **ratios** 3:100 and 3:1000. Rates and ratios are accessible. Much infection control data is expressed by these statistics. However, data should be stratified, taking risk factors into account, and different rates derived for different populations for validity. **Risk ratio** is the ratio of incidence of infection/disease among those who have been exposed compared to the incidence among those who have not been exposed. A risk ratio of 1.0 suggests that there is equal risk of infection/disease. A higher number suggests the probability that those exposed will have higher rates. Thus, a risk ratio of 1.5 shows that the exposed group is 1.5 times more likely to become infected or diseased than the group not exposed. A lower number suggests exposure brings less risk of infection/disease (immunity).

PROPORTION

Proportion is a subset of ratio in which a part of the whole is identified. That is, in the event being studied, the numerator data must be a part of the population or database used for the denominator data. This type of proportion is sometimes also referred to as a rate when looking at data over a specified period of time. Proportions are expressed as either decimals or percentages:

$$\frac{5\ people\ with\ urinary\ infections}{40\ people\ with\ Foley\ catheters} = \frac{5}{40} = \frac{1}{8} = 0.125 = 12.5\%$$

Proportion is frequently used in providing general epidemiological information about specific populations, for example, the number of smokers at different ages in a given population, such as African American teenage boys.

Incidence vs. Prevalence

Incidence and **prevalence** surveillance are both hospital-wide surveillance methods. For example, *incidence* surveillance may include ongoing surveillance of infections of all hospitalized patients, recording the number of new infections in a population of patients over a specific period of time, so incidence surveillance is both time-consuming and expensive. However, it can identify clusters of infections and allows for risk-factor analysis:

$$Incidence\ Rate = \frac{Number\ of\ new\ infections}{Total\ population\ in\ time\ period}$$

Prevalence surveillance involves both *period prevalence*, which is a specific pre-determined period of time for surveillance and *point prevalence*, which is prevalence at a specific point in time. Prevalence, then, is the number of cases of nosocomial infections that are active during the period or point of time covered by the survey:

$$Prevalence\ Rate = \frac{Number\ with\ active\ infection}{Total\ population\ in\ time\ period}$$

Prevalence surveys are less time-consuming and expensive, but results can be skewed by random infections/events, resulting in overestimation.

Risk Stratification

Risk stratification involves statistical adjustment to account for confounding issues and differences in risk factors. *Confounding issues* are those that confuse the data outcomes. For example, they involve trying to compare different populations, different ages, or different genders. For example, if there are two physicians and one has primarily high-risk patients, and the other has primarily low risk patients, the same rate of infection (by raw data) would suggest that the infection risks are equal for both physicians' patients. However, high risk patients are much more prone to infection, so in this case, risk stratification to account for this difference would show that the patients of the physician with low risk patients had a much higher risk of infection, relatively-speaking. Risk stratification is also used to predict outcomes of surgery by accounting for various risk factors (including ASO score, age, and medical conditions). Risk stratification is an important element of data analysis.

Issues Resulting in Inaccurate Data

There are a number of organizational issues that can result **in inaccurate data:**

- *Insufficient information* may be the result of incomplete medical records or lab reports at the time of survey. There may be a failure in the reporting procedure so that some data is not reported.
- *Evaluation errors* may occur even when data is available but is overlooked or the significance is not understood so that the data is not included in a survey.
- *Insufficient laboratory testing* is a frequent finding of studies. Very often indications of infection are clinically evident but cultures that would verify infection are not ordered by the physician or are not automatically triggered by established threshold rates.
- *Negligence* may relate to reluctance to verify and report infections/negative events in order to keep rates low.
- Because of *differences in efficiency of collecting data*, for example, the facility with the lowest infection rate may be the one with the least accurate data collection.

Selection and Information Bias

Selection bias occurs when the method of selecting subjects results in a cohort that is not representative of the target population because of inherent error in design. For example, if all patients who develop urinary infections are evaluated per urine culture and sensitivities for microbial resistance, but only those patients with clinically-evident infections are included, a number of patients with sub-clinical infections may be missed, skewing the results. Selection bias is only a concern when participants in studies are specifically chosen. Many surveillance studies do not involve selection of subjects.

Information bias occurs when there are errors in classification, so an estimate of association is incorrect. Non-differential misclassification occurs when there is similar misclassification of disease or exposure among both those who are diseased/exposed and those who are not. Differential misclassification occurs when there is a differing misclassification of disease or exposure among both those who are diseased/exposed and those who are not.

Incorporating Research Findings

Incorporating research findings should be central to all work of the clinical nurse specialist and should be routinely disseminated as part of practice, education, and consultation. Any time the nurse gives a presentation or provides written material, reference should be made to research findings because this provides supporting evidence and lends credence to the information the nurse is providing. Often research can provide guidance for surveillance or interventions and give valuable insights. References that are used or referred to should always be properly cited so that the work of researchers is credited. If a presentation is given orally, then the nurse should prepare a list of references. Newsletters and e-mail or Internet reports and communications should include research highlights or summaries of current studies of interest with links to online articles provided when possible to encourage people to read the research for themselves and become more knowledgeable about issues related to older adults.

Qualitative and Quantitative Data

Qualitative research involves subjective analysis. The property being studied cannot be enumerated**.** *Qualitative data* is a measure of the quality or character of the property in question. Qualitative data is classified as nominal or ordinal. Qualitative data may still be systematically analyzed. Patterns of responses are often organized into categories for analysis. Asking a person to describe his or her experience in a hospital involves collecting qualitative data.

Quantitative research measures the quantity or range of a property. This type of data is objective. *Quantitative data* can be expressed in numerical form. Quantitative data is obtained when the property in question can be measured. For example, measuring the difference in height between men and women involves collecting quantitative data.

Outcome Data

Interpretation

Outcome data provides an effective guide for performance improvement activities because it gives evidence of how well a process succeeds but not necessarily the reason; therefore, outcome data must be evaluated accordingly. There are inherent problems with outcome data that must be considered when utilizing outcomes for process improvement. First, it is almost impossible to ensure sufficient risk stratification to provide complete validity to outcome data; second, it is also difficult to accurately attribute the outcome data to any one step in a process without further study. For example, if outcome data shows a decline in deaths in an emergency department that recently changed trauma procedures but doesn't account for the fact that a gang task force has successfully decreased drive-by shootings and killings by 70%, it might be assumed that changes in the emergency department altered the outcome data when, in fact, if the data were adjusted for these external factors, the death rate may have increased.

Types

When interpreting **outcome data**, one should keep in mind that there are a number of different types of outcome data to be considered, and some data may overlap:

- *Clinical*: This includes symptoms, diagnoses, staging of disease and those indicators of patient health.
- *Physiological*: This includes measures of physical abnormalities, loss of function, and activities of daily living.
- *Psychosocial*: This includes feelings, perceptions, beliefs, functional impairment, and role performance.
- *Integrative*: This includes measures of mortality, longevity, and cost-effectiveness.
- *Perception*: This includes customer perceptions, evaluations, and satisfaction.
- *Organization-wide clinical:* This includes readmissions, adverse reactions, and deaths,

When considering outcome data, the focus may be on the process or the outcome data itself, and the team analyzing the data should clarify the purpose of reviewing the data and should understand how process and outcome data interrelate.

Triggers

Triggers are mechanisms or signals within data that indicate when further analysis (such as case review or root-cause analysis) or prioritizing needs to be done, and these triggers should be selected for each measure of performance.

Data triggers include the following:

- Sentinel events: Single clinical events that are unexpected and require assessment
- Performance rate: A pre-established level of performance in a particular measure
- Rate change: Pre-established change over a specified time period
- Difference between groups: A pattern of differences between specified groups
- Specified upper and lower control limits about a mean: Help to establish acceptable range of variation, usually set by standard deviation methods
- Control limits: Established acceptable range of variation

External triggers include the following:

- Feedback from staff, internal and external customers
- Strategic planning initiatives
- Practice guidelines
- Benchmarks

Evaluating Progress Toward Goals

Charting a patient's **progress toward goals** first requires clear delineation of what those goals are and measurable means to determine if the goals are met. Once a list of goals is developed for a patient, those responsible for noting progress should be identified as well as the time and frequency of evaluation. Often, multiple staff members are responsible for reporting on the progress of goals, so the method of reporting should communicate clearly to others on the interdisciplinary team. For example, flow charts may be used to note daily progress toward reducing the size of a pressure ulcer. Patients and/or family should understand the goals and should be actively involved in working toward those goals. Often goals are interrelated (such as reducing the size of an ulcer and increasing protein in the diet to promote healing), and these should be linked in record keeping.

Quality and Process Improvement

Practice Improvement Based on System-Level Assessment

System-level assessment is usually part of strategic planning and requires an organization to look at needs of the organization, the community, and the customers and establish goals for not only the near future (2 to 4 years) but also into the extended future (10 to 15 years) when designing practice improvement projects. Strategic planning must be based on assessments, both internal and external, to determine the present courses of action, needed changes, priorities, and methodologies to effect change. The focus of assessment and planning must be on developing services based on customer needs and then marketing those services. System-level assessment includes

- Collecting data and doing an external analysis of customer needs in relation to regulations and demographics
- Analyzing internal services and functions
- Identifying and understanding key issues, including the strengths and weaknesses of the organization, as well as potential opportunities and negative impacts
- Assessing and developing a revised mission and vision statement that identifies core values
- Establishing specific goals and objectives based on assessments

Xerox 10-Step Benchmarking Model

Benchmarking is an ongoing process of measuring practice, service, or product results against competitors or industry standards. Xerox Corporation developed the **10-step benchmarking model**. Utilizing this model requires comparing an organization's efficiency with that of others and searching for improvements. The 10-step process moves through 4 phases: planning, analysis, integration, and action. Steps include the following:

1. Identify benchmark targets.
2. Identify organizations/units/providers with which to compare data.
3. Determine and initiate methods of data collection.
4. Evaluate current performance level and deficits.
5. Project vision of future performance.
6. Communicate findings and reach group agreement.
7. Recommend changes based on benchmark data.
8. Develop specific action plans for objectives.
9. Implement actions and adjust as necessary based on monitoring of process.
10. Update benchmarks based on the latest data.

This basic benchmarking model is often modified to a 7-11 step process, depending upon the needs of the organization. Benchmarking is often used to improve cash flow as healthcare becomes more competitive and to compare infection rates.

Integration of Key Quality Concepts Within the Organization

There are a number of **key concepts** related to **quality** that must be communicated to all members of an organization through inservice, workshops, newsletters, fact sheets, and team meetings. Quality care/performance should be as follows:

- *Appropriate* to needs and in keeping with best practices.
- *Accessible* to the individual despite financial, cultural, or other barriers.
- *Competent* with practitioners well-trained and adhering to standards.
- *Coordinated* among all healthcare providers.
- *Effective* in achieving outcomes based on the current state of knowledge.
- *Efficient* in methods of achieving the desired outcomes.
- *Preventive*, allowing for early detection and prevention of problems.
- *Respectful* and caring with consideration of individual needs given primary importance.
- *Safe* so that the organization is free of hazards or dangers that may put patients or others at risk.

Resource Management

Resource management requires effective use of resources when and where they are needed in an organization or institution. Resource management in healthcare should include a focus on current, future, and emergency needs.

Resource	Issues
Human	Staffing levels: numbers, licensed vs. unlicensed, administrative vs. support, permanent vs. part-time; Assignments: permanent vs. floating, allocation, flexibility; Training: ongoing, continuing education, orientation; Supervision: hierarchy, evaluation procedures, disciplinary procedures Regulations: compliance, education, ADA
Financial	Resource leveling: balancing supply and demand with maintenance of inventories; Accounting practices: types of budgets; Costs vs. revenue: direct and indirect costs, grants, claims and payments, net vs. gross; Regulations: reporting requirements, tax implications
Information	Data collection: Responsibility, methods, frequency, duration, database design, local vs. system: Analysis: Methods, benchmarking, cost-effectiveness; Utilization: Process improvement, allocation of resources; Dissemination: Extent, method; Regulations: HIPAA, state and federal

Human and Fiscal Resource Management

The FDA maintains regulated procedures and recall information regarding contaminated equipment and supplies on a website entitled **MedWatch** (http://www.fda.gov/medwatch/index.html) to provide safety information for drugs and medical equipment. MedWatch provides electronic listing service to medical professionals and facilities for the following:

- Medical product safety alerts
- Information about drugs and devices
- Summary of safety alerts with links to detailed information

The Safe Medical Practices Act (1990) requires manufacturers and medical device user facilities to report problems with medical devices, including deaths or serious injuries (defined as requiring medical or surgical intervention), within 10 working days. Facilities must also file semiannual reports on January 1 and July1. User facilities must maintain records for 2 years and must develop written procedures for identification, evaluation and submission of medical device reports (MDR). MedWatch provides the following:

- *Reporting forms* (downloadable) for voluntary and mandatory reports
- *Recall and safety information* about recalls, market withdrawals and safety alerts, organized by months and years

Root Cause Analysis

Root cause analysis (RCA) is a retrospective attempt to determine the cause of an event, often a sentinel event such as an unexpected death, or a cluster of events. Root cause analysis involves interviews, observations, and review of medical records. Often, an extensive questionnaire is completed by the person doing the RCA, tracing essentially every step in hospitalization and care, including every treatment, every medication, and every contact. The focus of the RCA is on systems and processes rather than individuals. How did the system break down? Where did the problem arise? In some cases, there may be one root cause, but in others, the causes may be multiple. The RCA also must include a thorough review of literature to ensure that action plans based on the results of the RCA reflect current best practices. Action plans without RCA may be non-productive. If, for example, an infection was caused by contaminated air, action plans to increase disinfection of the operating room surfaces would not be effective.

Tracer Methodology

Tracer methodology is a method that looks at the continuum of care a patient receives from admission to post-discharge. A patient is selected to be "traced," and the medical record serves as a guide. Tracer methodology uses the experience of this patient to evaluate the processes in place through documents and interviews. For example, if a patient received physical therapy, surveyors may begin with the following:

- *Physical therapists*: How do they receive the orders and arrange patient transport? How is the therapy administered? How is progress noted?
- *Transport staff members*: How do they receive requests? How long does transfer take? What routes do they use? How to they transport patients? How do they clean transport equipment? What do they do if emergency arises during transport?
- *Nursing staff members*: How do they notify PT of orders? How do they prepare patients? How do they know the therapy schedule? How do they coordinate PT with the need for other treatments? How do they learn about patient progress?

Outcome Measures and Quality Improvement

An **outcome measure** is used to determine the success or failure of a process. Both short-term and long-term outcomes are important in quality improvement. Short-term outcomes are directly related to the process. Based on the outcomes, the process can be modified if necessary. Long-term outcomes, however, often relate more to general quality of care and patient satisfaction and may be used retrospectively to evaluate the process or plan for future care. Outcomes serve as an indicator that a process is effective or ineffective. Planners should focus on identifying three types of outcome measures: 1) clinical (determines if there are positive results from clinical interventions), 2) customer functioning (includes indicators of ability to perform), 3) and customer satisfaction (includes meeting expectations and needs).

Selection of Outcomes Measures

Because both process and **outcomes** are equally important in performance improvement, consideration must be given as to whether the focus is to be on the process or the outcome. Both a short term and long-term focus for outcomes should be established. Short-term outcomes show results directly related to the process, allowing for modifications/interventions of the process. Long-term outcomes, however, often relate more to general quality of care and patient satisfaction and may be used retrospectively to evaluate the process or plan for future care. Outcomes do not directly assess process, although they serve as an indicator that a process may be effective or ineffective, requiring further study or modification of process. Planners should focus on identifying **three types of outcome measures**:

- *Clinical:* Determines if there are positive results from clinical interventions
- *Customer functioning:* Includes indicators of ability to perform
- *Customer satisfaction:* Includes meeting expectations and needs

Quality Improvement

Identifying Problems/Issues and Problem Solving

Problem solving in any medical context involves developing a hypothesis and then testing the hypothesis through the assessment of data. There are steps that should be taken to prevent the recurrence of a problem:

1. *Step 1* is to define the issue. Talk with the patient or family and staff to determine the nature of the problem. For example, the problem may have arisen due to a failure in communication or due to other issues, such as culture or religion.
2. *Step 2* is the collection of data. This may involve interviewing additional staff or reviewing documentation to gain a variety of perspectives.
3. *Step 3* is the identification of important concepts. It should be determined if there are issues related to values or beliefs.
4. *Step 4* involves considering the reasons for actions. The motivation and intentions of all parties should be ascertained to determine the reason for the problem.
5. *Step 5* is making a decision. A decision on how to prevent a recurrence of a problem should be based on advocacy and moral agency.

Formulating, Testing, and Modifying Action Plans

The **development of performance improvement actions** plans usually begins with *prioritizing problems* after an initial period of monitoring and assessment. *Teams* should be assembled. Individual team members should be selected based on their knowledge of the problems and process and their commitment to improvement. There are a number of steps that should be taken. *Systematic approaches* should be taken to identify problems, conduct root cause analysis, and identify feasible changes in process. An *action plan* should be developed that outlines the expected outcomes of the change in process, chain of responsibility, time line, and methods of evaluation. A ***pilot test*** should be conducted. The *data* from the pilot test should be *analyzed. Modifications* to the change in process should be made if necessary, after the pilot test. If necessary, further pilot tests should be conducted. The plan should be adopted by individuals, departments, and leadership.

Gap Analysis in Quality Improvement

Quality improvement is an important component of managing a healthcare unit or facility well. Quality improvement methods determine where the facility is working well and providing high quality, appropriate care as well as what issues exist that need to be managed. **Gap analysis** involves assessing the gap between the current working state of the facility or unit and the goals for where it wants to be. Along with other quality improvement methods, a unit might use gap analysis to assess its current methods of documentation audits, adherence to safety protocols, or accuracy with reporting methods. It can then consider the goals that it wants to achieve in these areas. To start, gap analysis identifies the goals of the unit and what outcomes it wants to meet. It then assesses its current state to identify what areas need to be changed or updated to meet the goal outcomes. Gap analysis is important not only for identifying outcomes, but for understanding methods to achieve those outcomes.

CQI

Continuous Quality Improvement (CQI) emphasizes the organization, systems, and processes within the organization. It is not concerned with individuals. It recognizes internal customers (staff) and external customers (patients) and utilizes data to improve processes. CQI represents the concept that most processes can be improved. CQI uses the scientific method of experimentation to meet needs and improve services and utilizes various tools, such as brainstorming, multi-voting, various charts and diagrams, storyboarding, and meetings. Core concepts include the following:

- Quality and success are achieved by meeting or exceeding internal and external customers' needs and expectations.
- Problems relate to processes, and variations in process lead to variations in results.
- Change can be in small steps.

Steps to CQI include the following:

1. Forming a knowledgeable team.
2. Identifying and defining measures used to determine success.
3. Brainstorming strategies for change.
4. Plan, collect, and utilize data as part of making decisions.
5. Test changes and revise or refine as needed.

TQM

Total Quality Management (TQM) is one philosophy of quality management that espouses a commitment to meeting the needs of the customers at all levels within an organization. It promotes not only continuous improvement but also a dedication to quality in all aspects of an organization. Outcomes should include increased customer satisfaction, productivity, and increased profits through efficiency and reduction in costs. In order to provide TQM, an organization must seek the following:

- Information regarding customer's needs and opinions.
- Involvement of staff at all levels in decision making, goal setting, and problems solving.
- Commitment of management to empowering staff and being accountable through active leadership and participation.
- Institution of teamwork with incentives and rewards for accomplishments.
- The focus of TQM is on working together to identify and solve problems rather than assigning blame through an organizational culture that focuses on the needs of the customers.

PDCA

Plan-Do-Check-Act (PDCA) (Shewhart cycle) is a method of continuous quality improvement. PDCA is simple and understandable; however, it may be difficult to maintain this cycle consistently because of lack of focus and commitment. PDCA may be more suited to solving specific problems than organization-wide problems:

- *Plan*: This involves identifying, analyzing and defining the problem. The problem is clearly defined, goals are set, and a process that coordinates with leadership is established. Extensive brainstorming, including fishbone diagrams, identifies problematic processes and lists current process steps. Data is collected and analyzed and root a cause analysis completed.
- *Do*: This step involves generating solutions from which to select one or more and then implementing the solution on a trial basis.
- *Check*: This involves gathering and analyzing data to determine the effectiveness of the solution. If the solution is effective, then the next step (*ACT*) is implemented. If the solution is not effective, the previous step (*Plan*) is revisited and a different solution chosen. (*Study* may replace *Check: PDSA.)*
- *Act*: This involves identifying changes that need to be done to fully implement the solution, adopting the solution, and continuing to monitor the results while picking another improvement project.

TRACKING AND TRENDING

Tracking and trending is central to developing research-supported evidence-based practice and is part of continuous quality improvement. Once processes and outcomes measurements are selected, at least one measure should be tracked for a number of periods of time, usually in increments of 4 weeks or quarterly. This tracking can be used to present graphical representation of results that will show trends. While trends will show some normal variation, if the trend becomes erratic and measures are inconsistent, this suggests that the processes of care are not consistent or are inadequate. For example, if infections in PICC lines are tracked and the trend shows wild fluctuations with high levels of infection in one period, low in another, and vacillations in a third, then the first step is to ensure that the process is being followed correctly. If the process is stable but the variations persist, then the next course would be to modify the process by looking at best practices.

MODELS OF QUALITY IMPROVEMENT

SIX SIGMA®

Six Sigma® is a performance improvement model developed by Motorola to improve business practices and increase profits. This model has been adapted to many types of businesses, including healthcare. Six Sigma® is a data-driven performance model that aims to eliminate "defects" in processes that involve products or services. The goal is to achieve Six Sigma, meaning no more defects than 3.4 to one million opportunities. This program focuses on continuous improvement with the customer's perception as key, so that the customer defines what is critical to quality (CTQ). Two different types of improvement projects may be employed: DMAIC (define, measure, analyze, improve, control) for existing processes or products that need improvement and DMADV (define, measure, analyze, design, verify) for development of new, high quality processes or products. Both DMAIC and DMADV utilize trained personnel to execute the plans. These personnel use martial arts titles: green belts, black belts who execute programs, and master black belts who supervise programs.

FMEA

Failure mode and effects analysis (FMEA) is a team-based prospective analysis method that attempts to identify and correct failures in a process before it is implemented, to ensure positive outcomes. Steps include:

- *Definition*: Process description; Team creation.
- *Description*: Flow charts showing each step and substep in the process.
- *Brainstorming*: Each step and substep are brainstormed for potential failure modes.
- *Identification and recording* of causes of potential failures using cause and effect diagram and root cause analysis.
- Listing potential adverse outcomes.
- *Assignment of severity rating:* Potential adverse outcomes are rated on a 1 to 10 scale, 1 being slight, 10 being death.
- *Assignment of frequency/occurrence rating*: prepotential failures rated on a 1 to 10 scale with (1 remote = 1:10,000 and 10 very high) within a specified time period, usually a year.
- *Assignment of detection rating* (scale of 1 to10): Potential failures rated on a 1 to 10 scale on the likelihood that hazards, errors, or failures will be identified prior to occurrence.
- *Calculation of risk priority number* based on scales of severity, occurrence, and detection.
- Reduction of potential failures.
- Identification of performance measures.

Medical Record Review Processes

There are a number of different types **medical record review processes**, and many reviews are mandated by regulations and accreditation. Types of medical review processes include:

- *Prospective*: This category includes all those steps taken before an event, such as assessing need before care is given, checking credentials before hiring, determining ability to pay prior to doing elective procedures, and gaining preauthorization from insurance companies.
- *Concurrent*: This category includes ongoing assessment while the patient is receiving care, verification of medical necessity for continued treatment, and appropriate use of resources. Concurrent review may include medical records, observations of care, incident reports, and special case studies.
- *Retrospective*: This review is done after care has been provided and provides a full picture of the continuum of care and its effectiveness. A retrospective review may look at the medical records and the results of prospective and concurrent reviews.
- *Focused*: This category includes reviews done for specific predetermined reasons, such as a specific diagnosis, procedure, or process. Criteria for case selection must be outlined.

AHRQ Quality Indicators

The Agency for Healthcare Research and Quality (**AHRQ**) **Quality Indicators** are distributed as a software tool free of charge to healthcare organizations to help them to identify adverse events or potential adverse events that require further study. This software can prove an invaluable aid in assessing and developing the organization's patient safety culture. Discharges of patients over 18 years are assessed for the following quality indicators:

- Complications of anesthesia, death in low mortality diagnostic-related diseases (DRGs), decubitus ulcer, failure to rescue, foreign body left in during procedure, iatrogenic pneumothorax, care-related infections, post-operative hip fracture, hemorrhage or hematoma, physiologic or metabolic derangements, respiratory failure, pulmonary embolism or deep vein thrombosis, sepsis, wound dehiscence in abdominopelvic surgeries.
- Accidental puncture and laceration, transfusion reaction.
- Birth trauma.
- Obstetric trauma from vaginal delivery with and or without instrument and Caesarean section.
- The data indicators may also be used to assess safety factors at an area (such as county) level per 100,000 population.

Institute of Healthcare Improvement Bundles

The **Institute of Healthcare Improvements** is a nonprofit organization that promotes better and more cost-effective patient care with the goals of preventing needless deaths, pain and suffering, helplessness, excessive waiting, waste, or lack of care. IHI encourages such measures as the use of rapid response teams and medication reconciliation. IHI has developed **bundles**, a group of processes based on evidence-based practices that must be carried out in order to improve patient outcomes. Bundles include 3 to 5 steps, but each step is critical, and all steps should be performed as prescribed, as in the following examples:

Sepsis Resuscitation (3 hr)	Central Line
Measure Lactate Level Administer Crystalloids for hypotension or Lactate ≥4 mmol/L Obtain blood cultures before administering antibiotics Administer Broad Spectrum Antibiotics	Use of proper hand hygiene Use of barrier precautions (PPE) Skin antisepsis with chlorhexidine Selection of optimal site for catheter insertion Daily evaluation of catheter and assessment for possible removal

International Patient Safety Goals

Gerontological nurses may work in institutions accredited by the Joint Commission, but even those in other types of practices can use the **International Patient Safety Goals** as a patient-care strategy that includes adhering to goals, educating support staff, and monitoring for compliance. Nurses should adhere to the following strategies: identify patients correctly (use two identifiers for medicines, blood, or blood products); read the checklist before beginning surgery (ensure correct patient, procedure, and body part); improve effective communication (establish a procedure for taking orders and reports and read back verbal/telephone orders); remove concentrated electrolytes from patient care units, especially potassium; read the surgical checklist (ensure the proper documentation is present and the necessary equipment is in working order); mark surgical site (mark the surgical site with clear identifiable markings); comply with hand-washing standards (use Centers for Disease Control guidelines for hand washing); and assess the risk of falls (eliminate fall risks).

BENCHMARKS

External benchmarking involves analyzing data from outside an institution. It involves such actions as monitoring national rates of hospital-acquired infection and comparing them to internal rates. In order for this data to be meaningful, the same definitions must be used as well as the same populations for effective risk stratification. Using national data can be informative, but each institution is different, and relying on external benchmarking to select indicators for infection control or other processes can be misleading. Additionally, benchmarking involves the compilation of data sets that may vary considerably if analyzed individually. The problem is further compounded by anonymity that makes comparisons difficult.

Internal trending involves comparing internal rates of one area or population with another. For example, it may involve comparing infection rates in ICU with those in general surgery. This can help to pinpoint areas of concern within an institution, but making comparisons is still problematical because of inherent differences. Using a combination of external and internal data can help to identify and select indicators.

DASHBOARDS

A **dashboard** (also called a digital dashboard), like the dashboard in a car, is an easy to access and read computer program that integrates a variety of performance measures or key indicators into one display (usually with graphs or charts) to provide an overview of an organization, so it can be used for program evaluation. It might include data regarding patient satisfaction, infection rates, financial status, or any other measurement that is important to assess performance. The dashboard provides a running picture of the status of the department or organization at any point in time and may be updated as desired--daily, weekly, or monthly. An organization-wide dashboard provides numerous benefits:

- Broad involvement of all departments.
- A consistent and easy to understand visual representation of data.
- Identification of negative findings or trends so that they can be corrected.
- Availability of detailed reports.
- Effective measurements that demonstrate the degree of efficiency.
- Assistance with making informed decisions.

ACCELERATED RAPID-CYCLE CHANGE APPROACH

The accelerated rapid-cycle change approach is a response to rapid changes in healthcare delivery and radical reengineering. There are 4 areas of concern:

- *Models for rapid-cycle change:* The goal is doubling or tripling the rate of quality improvement by modifying and accelerating traditional methods. Teams focus on generating and testing solutions rather than analysis.
- *Pre-work:* Assigned personnel prepare problem statements, graphic demonstrations of data, flowcharts, and literature review. Team members are identified.
- *Team creation:* Rapid action (also sometimes called rapid acceleration or rapid achievement) teams (known as RATs) are created to facilitate rapid change.
- *Team meetings and work flow:* Meetings/work done over 6 weeks:
  - Week 1: Review information, clarification of quality improvement opportunities and identification of key customers, waste, and benchmarks.
  - Week 2: Review customer requirements and cost/benefit analysis of solutions with testing of data.

- Week 3: Complete design of solution, plan implementation and pilot tests.
- Week 4-5: Test, train, analyze, and make changes as needed.
- Week 6: Implement program.

Identifying Practice Improvement Opportunities Through Data Analysis and Monitoring

Integrating the results of **data analysis and monitoring** can help identify practice improvement processes.

- Coordinating management and leadership functions provides more efficient planning.
- Evidence-based care decisions can increase cost-effectiveness and improve outcomes.
- Duplication of effort may be reduced by sharing of information, increasing the overall efficiency of the organization.
- Staff utilization becomes more effective.
- Improved accountability allows for better performance assessment.
- Communication among departments or areas within an organization is improved.
- Using a common database facilitates tracking of patterns and trends.
- Responses can be tailored to the needs of staff, patients, and the organization as a whole.
- Organizational obstacles can be dealt with more efficiently with the supporting data.

Data Needed for Analysis to Assist with Strategic Planning

There are basically 4 **types of data** that should analyzed and summarized to assist with strategic planning:

- *Medical/clinical:* This type of information is patient-specific and includes information regarding the patient, diagnosis, treatment, laboratory findings, consultations, care plans, physician orders, and information related to informed consent and advance directives. The medical record should include records of all procedures, discharge summary, and emergency care records.
- *Knowledge-based:* This can include methods to ensure that staff is provided training, support, research, library services or other access to information, and good practice guidelines.
- *Comparisons:* This data may relate to internal comparisons or external comparisons to benchmarks or best-practice guidelines.
- *Aggregate:* This includes pharmacy transactions, required reports, demographic information, financial information, hazard and safety practices, and most things not included in the clinical record.

Risk Management Responsibilities

Risk management is an organized and formal method of decreasing liability, financial loss, and risk or harm to patients, staff, or others by doing an assessment of risk and introducing risk management strategies. Much of risk management has been driven by the insurance industry in order to minimize costs, but quality management utilizes risk management as a method to ensure quality healthcare and process improvement. An organization's risk management program usually comprises a manager and staff with a number of responsibilities:

- *Risk identification* begins with an assessment of processes to identify and prioritize those that require further study to determine risk exposure.
- *Risk analysis* requires a careful documenting of process, utilizing flow charts, with each step in the process assessed for potential risks. This may utilize root cause analysis methods.

- *Risk prevention* involves instituting corrective or preventive processes. Responsible individual or teams are identified and trained.
- *Assessment/evaluation* of corrective/preventive processes is ongoing to determine if they are effective or require modification.

Risk Management and Negligence

Risk management must attempt to determine the burden of proof for acts of **negligence**, including compliance with duty, breaches in procedures, degree of harm, and cause. Negligence indicates that *proper care* has not been provided, based on established standards. *Reasonable care* uses rationale for decision-making in relation to providing care. State regulations regarding negligence may vary but all have some statutes of limitation. There are a number of different types of negligence:

- *Negligent* conduct indicates that an individual failed to provide reasonable care or to protect/assist another based on standards and expertise.
- *Gross negligence* is willfully providing inadequate care while disregarding the safety and security of another.
- *Contributory negligence* involves the injured party contributing to his/her own harm.
- *Comparative negligence* attempts to determine what percentage amount of negligence is attributed to each individual involved.

Regulatory Compliance

HIPAA

In 1996, Congress passed the Health Insurance Portability and Accountability Act (HIPAA), which include a number of provisions that aim to improve the **portability of health information records**. The Department of Health and Human Services was charged with establishing national healthcare standards for storage and transfer of electronic health care information to improve the exchange of information from one insurance company/physician to another. Essentially, a patient's complete record would be stored and others could access these records easily. However, standardization has not yet occurred and different electronic storage systems are often incompatible. HIPAA requires that health care providers use a National Provider Identifier (NPI), which is a 10-digit number. HIPAA includes strong provisions to protect the privacy of the individual in order to prevent abuse and misuse of records.

Privacy

The **Health Insurance Portability and Accountability Act (HIPAA)** addresses the rights of the individual related to privacy of health information. The nurse must not release any information or documentation about a patient's condition or treatment without consent as the individual has the right to determine who has access to personal information. Personal information about the patient is considered protected health information (PHI) and consists of any identifying or personal information about the patient (e.g., health history, condition, or treatments in any form) and any documentation (electronic, verbal, or written). Personal information can be shared with spouse, legal guardians, those with durable power of attorney for the patient, and those involved in care of the patient (such as physicians) without a specific release, but the patient should always be consulted if personal information is to be discussed with others present to ensure there is no objection. Failure to comply with HIPAA regulations can make a nurse liable for legal action.

Americans with Disabilities Act

The 1992 **Americans with Disabilities Act** is civil rights legislation that provides the disabled, including those with mental impairment, access to employment and the community. While employers must make reasonable accommodations for the disabled, the provisions related to the community apply more directly to older Americans. The ADA covers not only obvious disabilities but also disorders such as arthritis, seizure disorders, cardiovascular disorders, and respiratory disorders. Communities must provide transportation services for the disabled, including accommodation for wheelchairs. Public facilities (schools, museums, physician's offices, post offices, restaurants) must be accessible with ramps and elevators as needed. Telecommunications must also be accessible through devices or accommodations for the deaf and blind. Compliance is not yet complete because older buildings are required to provide access that is possible without "undue hardship," but newer construction of public facilities must meet ADA regulations.

Older Americans Act/Ombudsman

The **Older Americans Act** (OAA) (Title III) of 1965 (amended in 2006) provides improved access to services for older adults and Native Americans, including community services (meals, transportation, home health care, adult day care, legal assistance, and home repair). The OAA provides funding to local area agencies on aging (AAA) or state or tribal agencies, which administer funding. These local agencies can assess community needs and contract for services. One of the programs that is commonly supported with funds from the OAA is meals-on-wheels. Low cost adult day care is also offered in some communities. The OAA includes the National Family Caregivers Support Act, which provides services for caregivers of older adults. The OAA also provides grants for programs that combat violence against older adults and others to provide computer training for older adults. Additionally, the OAA requires each state to have an ombudsman program. Ombudsmen provide services to residents of nursing homes and other facilities to ensure that care meets state standards.

EMTALA

The Emergency Medical Treatment and Active Labor Act (EMTALA) is designed to prevent patient "dumping" from emergency departments (ED) and is an issue of concern for risk management, requiring staff training for compliance:

- Transfers from the ED may be intrahospital or to another facility.
- Stabilization of the patient with emergency conditions or active labor must be done in the ED prior to transfer, and initial screening must be given prior to inquiring about insurance or ability to pay.
- Stabilization requires treatment for emergency conditions and reasonable belief that, although the emergency condition may not be completely resolved, the patient's condition will not deteriorate during transfer.
- Women in the ED in active labor should deliver both the child and placenta before transfer.
- The receiving department or facility should be capable of treating the patient and dealing with complications that might occur.
- Transfer to another facility is indicated if the patient requires specialized services not available intrahospital, such as to burn centers.

ACCREDITATION

Accreditation is a primary requirement for organization because it establishes that the organization is committed to standards based on evaluation. General accreditation is usually done by the following:

- The Joint Commission accredits more than 20,000 healthcare programs, both nationally and internationally, and is the primary accrediting agency in the United States, so accreditation by Joint Commission indicates a commitment to improving care and provides information about compliance with core measures.
- The Healthcare Facilities Accreditation Program of the American Osteopathic Association also accredits many healthcare programs, including acute care, ambulatory care, rehabilitation centers and substance abuse centers, behavioral care centers, and critical access hospitals and provides guidelines for patient safety initiatives as well as reports of common deficiencies.
- A healthcare organization may also seek to become accredited by agencies with a narrower focus to demonstrate excellence in that area, such as Intersocietal Commission for the Accreditation of Echocardiography Laboratories (ICAEL). Leadership and staff must determine what type of accreditation is most appropriate based on the programs offered and the commitment to improving standards.

COMPLIANCE WITH STANDARDS

In order to facilitate evaluation of accreditation processes, the organization must be in **compliance with standards**. Standards for accreditation are, for the most part, performance based and focus on measures of processes and outcomes and issues related to patient care and safety. Comparative performance measure data, such as core measures, are integrated into the accreditation process. Most surveyors assess compliance based on the following:

- Document review to validate compliance
- Onsite inspections and observations
- Interviews of staff
- Review of standards implementation measures
- Review of medical records
- Assessment of service and support systems of the organization
- Integration of performance measure data

The surveyors may recommend denial of accreditation if conditions exist that pose a threat to staff, public, or patients, but the organization may request the opportunity to demonstrate compliance through documentation or interviews, and in some cases, a second survey may be conducted.

PROMOTING COMPLIANCE WITH REGULATORY, ACCREDITING, AND PROFESSIONAL STANDARDS

Compliance with regulatory, accrediting, and professional standards depends on a number of factors:

- *Administrative leadership*: The importance of compliance must be stressed from the top down in all levels of leadership, because staff members who detect ambivalence or lack of direction are less likely to comply.

- *Education*: Staff members must clearly understand the purpose of standards and methods to achieve those standards. A variety of different approaches, such as one-on-one instruction, group instruction, printed materials, and computer-assisted instruction, may be used.
- *Data*: Statistical information about achieving standards must be widely disseminated to staff members, including information about statistical methods, so staff members understand goals and outcomes.
- *Personal involvement*: Staff members should be actively engaged in helping to establish methods of compliance or educating others, so they feel a part of the process. A system in which staff members are recognized or rewarded for progress toward compliance can help motivate staff.

Licensure Issues

While accreditation processes are voluntary, **licensure** is mandatory, usually through the State Department of Health Services. Organizations must be in compliance with state and federal laws and regulations in order to be licensed. Managed care organizations are usually licensed by other state departments, such as the Department of Insurance. There are a number of different types of licenses, and these may vary slightly from one state to another:

- Acute medical and psychiatric hospitals.
- Ambulatory surgical centers.
- Skilled nursing facilities and sub-acute care centers.
- Long-term care facilities.
- Home health care agencies.
- Hospice agencies.
- Assisted living programs.
- Residential programs for the behaviorally/mentally/developmentally disabled.
- Organizations that utilize beds or staffing in ways that are non-compliant risk losing their licenses. Licenses specify the number of patient beds and types of patients as well as staffing provisions, which may vary from state to state.

Organization Accreditation Standards

Magnet Recognition Program®

The American Nurses' Credentialing Center, affiliated with the ANA, developed the **Magnet Recognition Program®** to reward hospitals that meet a set of criteria for excellence in nursing and positive patient outcomes associated with high job satisfaction and low staff turnover. Hospitals must apply for magnet status and undergo extensive review for compliance. Criteria include:

- CNO with MS or doctorate in nursing; nurse managers with degrees in nursing (BS or higher).
- Evidence of innovative health care.
- Evidence of improvement in meeting the goal of nurses having professional certification by credentialing agencies.
- Patient outcome data, including falls, pressure ulcers, BSI, UTI, VAP, restraint use, pediatric IV infiltrations, and other nationally benchmarked indicators of specific specialties outperforming the mean of the selected national database.
- Patient satisfaction surveys and data on pain management, education, nursing courtesy and respect, listening, and response time.

NICHE

Nurses Improving Care for Healthsystem Elders (NICHE) is a program established in 1992 by the Hartford Institute for Geriatric Nursing at New York University College of Nursing to provide resources and material to help institutions improve geriatric care. NICHE provides models of care for older adults.

- *Geriatric Resource Nurse (GRN):* The GRNs receive training from geriatric advanced-practice nurses and then serve as a resource person for other staff on the unit to help identify risk factors and prevent injuries and complications related to the geriatric patient population.
- *Acute Care of the Elderly Medical-Surgical Unit (ACE Unit):* A special unit or section of a unit is set aside for geriatric patients and modified to meet their needs. Adaptations include flooring designed to reduce noise and glare, extra lighting, clocks and calendars on display in rooms to help keep patients oriented, and communal eating and activity areas to promote social interaction. Staff members have expertise in geriatric nursing, and interdisciplinary teams focus on preventing problems.

CARF

Commission on Accreditation of Rehabilitation Facilities (CARF) sets standards and provides accreditation for a wide range of health and human services providers. Service areas include:

- Services for the aging.
- Behavioral health, including substance abuse treatment programs.
- Business and services management networks.
- Child and youth services.
- Employment and community services, including vision rehabilitation programs.
- Medical rehabilitation, including MDEPOS.

CARFs mission is to improve the lives of people by ensuring that they are being treated with respect and receiving quality care. CARF services include developing and maintaining standards, recognizing organizations that achieve continuous improvement, conducting research, providing consultation, and providing training and resources. The accreditation process requires the organization to commit to improvement and to do a thorough review of its programs. CARF surveyors conduct on-site surveys, during which the organization must demonstrate that it meets strict standards of performance and accountability. The organization must then submit a yearly quality improvement plan (QIP).

CMS

The **Centers for Medicare and Medicaid Services (CMS)** maintains a list of approved accreditation organizations for healthcare providers. Providers and suppliers who have been accredited by one of these national accrediting agencies are exempt from state surveys to determine if they are in compliance with Medicare-mandated conditions and standards. Approved organizations include the Joint Commission, Community Health Association Program, and the Accreditation Commission for Health Care, Inc. New applicants may also apply to an approved accreditation organization, rather than waiting for state surveys, as these may be delayed because of budgetary constraints. The CMS also publishes standards for suppliers of durable medical equipment, prosthetics, orthotics, and supplies (DMEPOS). CMS has approved national accrediting agencies for DMEPOS. Prior to billing CMS, suppliers must be accredited and meet the standards of the accrediting agency.

Joint Commission

The **Joint Commission** is the primary accrediting agency for healthcare programs in the United States. The Joint Commission establishes accreditation standards for various types of healthcare programs, establishes general competencies for healthcare practitioners, and issues annual national patient safety goals. Assessment to see if facilities are compliant with Joint Commission standards is usually done by a site survey. Joint Commission survey is similar to other accreditation site surveys, in that they are performance based, comparative, and a demonstration of compliance with set standards.

Organization and System Leadership

Organizational Transparency

Organizational transparency is a fairly new concept for the health-care industry, which has been historically known for concealment of data. The public has been exerting pressure to make health-care organizations more transparent as evidence about unnecessary surgery, costs, infection rates, and other negative information has been made public. The organization must be committed to transparency of pricing and quality so that both staff and patients have realistic expectations. Information that should be available includes financial information (costs and profit information), performance measures (factors that are evaluated and measured should be clearly outlined), outcomes (both positive and negative), safety records and information about safety concerns, medical records (open to individual patients), and leadership qualities and promotion (providing a clear understanding of the basis for promotion and leadership).

Organizational Concerns

Changes in policies, procedures, or working standards are common and staff should be educated about changes related to processes. Change should be communicated to staff in an effective and timely manner.

- *Policies* are usually changed after a period of discussion and review by administration and staff, so all staff members should be made aware of policies under discussion. Preliminary information should be disseminated to staff members regarding the issue under consideration during meetings or through printed notices.
- *Procedures* may be changed to increase efficiency or improve patient safety. Changes in procedures are often instituted as a result of surveillance and outcomes data. Procedure changes are best communicated in workshops with demonstrations. Handouts should be available as well.
- *Working standards* are often changed because of regulatory or accrediting requirements. These changes may be required by regulatory agencies. Information on changes in working standards should be covered extensively so that the implications are clearly understood.

Vision Statement and Mission Statement

A **vision statement** is a description of what the organization intends to become. The vision statement outlines the commitment being made by the organization. It should include future goals rather than focusing on what has already been achieved; it is usually stated in one sentence or a short paragraph.

The **mission statement** of an organization usually reflects the current status of the organization and describes, in broad terms, the purpose of the organization and its role in the community. It should be developed in response to data and program analysis. The mission statement should be written with input from all members of the organization, and it should identify the organization or program, state its function, and outline the purpose and strategy of the program.

Motivation

Leadership must understand **motivation** because a positive perception of leadership motivates people to produce and improve performance. In order to understand what motivates staff members, the leader must set aside preconceived ideas and listen carefully, discovering the strengths of the individuals and groups within the organization or facility and providing positive reinforcement and rewards. Leadership involves expecting excellence and removing barriers to employee involvement in the process so that employees feel empowered, recognized, and acknowledged as valuable. The responses of leadership should be based on actual assessment rather than preconceived ideas or biases. Studies have shown that the 4 things that motivate employees the most include the following:

- *Autonomy*: Allowing people to use their ideas.
- *Salary*: Providing adequate compensation for work done.
- *Recognition*: Appreciating the efforts put forth by employees.
- *Respect*: Listening to ideas.

Systems Theory

Systems theory, developed by **Ludwig von Bertalanffy** in the 1940s, is an approach that considers an entire system holistically rather than focusing on component parts. Bertalanffy believed that all of the elements of a system and their interrelationships must be understood because all interact to achieve goals; a change in any one element impacts the other elements and alters outcomes. There are five elements in a system:

1. *Input*: This is what goes into a system in terms of energy or materials.
2. *Throughput*: These are the actions that take place in order to transform input.
3. *Output*: This is the result of the interrelationship between input and processes.
4. *Evaluation*: This is monitoring success or failure.
5. *Feedback*: This is information that results from the process and can be used to evaluate the end result.

To achieve desired outcomes, every part of the process must be considered. The individual parts added together do not constitute the whole because viewing the parts separately does not account for the dynamic quality of interaction that takes place.

Concepts of Systems Thinking

The promotion of organizational values and commitment requires that the organization embody systems thinking and the associated concepts. **Systems thinking** focuses on how systems interrelate with each part affecting the entire system. Concepts include the following:

- *Individual responsibility:* Individuals are encouraged to establish their own goals within the organization and to work toward a purpose.
- *Learning process:* The internalized beliefs of the staff are respected while building upon these beliefs to establish a mindset based on continuous learning and improvement.
- *Vision:* A sharing of organizational vision helps staff to understand the purpose of change and builds commitment.

- *Team process:* Teams are assisted to develop good listening and collaborative skills so that there is an increase in dialogue and an ability to reach consensus.
- *Systems thinking:* Staff members are encouraged to understand the interrelationship of all members of the organization and to appreciate how any change affects the whole.

SYSTEMS THINKING

STEPS

An approach to **systems thinking** is especially valuable in organizations in which there is lack of consensus, effective change is stalemated, and standards are inconsistent. Systems thinking is a critical thinking approach to problem solving that takes an organization-wide perspective. Steps include the following:

1. *Define the issue:* Describe the problem in detail without judgment or solutions.
2. *Describe behavior patterns:* This includes listing factors related to the problem, using graphs to outline possible trends.
3. *Establish cause-effect relationships:* This may include using the Five Whys or other root cause analysis or feedback loops.
4. *Define patterns of performance/behavior:* Determine how variables affect outcomes and the types of patterns of behavior currently taking place.
5. *Find solutions:* Discuss possible solutions and outcomes.
6. *Institute performance improvement activities:* Make changes and then monitor for changes in behavior.

BARRIERS

Barriers to system thinking can arise with the individual, the department, or the administrative level:

- *Identification with role rather than purpose*: People see themselves from the perspective of their role in the system, as nurse or physician, and are not able to step outside their preconceived ideas to view situations holistically or to accept the roles of others. They may lack the ability to look at situations as human beings first and professionals second.
- *Feelings of victimization:* People may blame the organization or the leadership for personal shortcomings or feel that there is nothing that they can do to improve or change situations. A feeling of victimization may permeate an institution to the point that meaningful communication cannot take place, and people are not open to change.
- *Relying on past experience:* New directions require new solutions, so being mired in the past or relying solely on past experience can prevent progress.
- *Autocratic views:* Some individuals feel that their perceptions and practices are the only ones that are acceptable and often have a narrow focus so that they cannot view the system as a whole but focus on short-term outcomes. They fail to see that there are many aspects to a problem, affecting many parts of the system.
- *Failure to adapt:* Change is difficult for many individuals and institutions, but the medical world is changing rapidly, and this requires adaptability. Those who fail to adapt may feel threatened by changes and unsure of their ability to relearn new concepts, principles, and procedures.
- *Weak consensus:* Groups that arrive at easy or weak consensus without delving into important issues may delude themselves into believing that they have solved problems and remain fixed rather than moving forward.

Contingency Theory

Contingency theory is a theory of organizational behavior that states that there is no one best method of organizing a company, corporation, or business but that organization is contingent on a number of factors; therefore, what works in one organization may not work in another. Some common contingency factors include the organization size, resources, technology, adaptation to the environment, operations activities, motivating forces, staff education, and managerial assumptions. Contingency theory states that the organization must be designed in such a manner as to fit into the environment. Management should utilize the best approach to achieve tasks. Fielder concluded that leadership should be appropriate for the organizational needs and different organizations require different styles of leadership depending upon contingent factors, such as staff, tasks, and other group variables. Vroom and Yetton concluded that success in decision making is contingent on a number of factors, including information available, acceptance of the decision, agreement or disagreement, and the importance of the decision.

Theory X and Theory Y

In 1960, Douglas McGregor developed 2 conflicting theories. He believed that management needs to assemble all needed components (including people) required for the company's economic benefit:

- **Theory X:** The average worker is unmotivated, dislikes work, is resistive to change, is unintelligent, and does not care about the organization. People work because they have to for money. In this case, management may become coercive, making threats to control or may be permissive, trying to placate unhappy workers so they will become more motivated.
- **Theory Y:** Work can be enjoyable, and workers can be motivated to meet goals if they result in feelings of self-fulfillment, causing workers to seek responsibility. People are basically creative and can exercise ingenuity. Management should seek to align organizational and personal goals to motivate workers, delegating, adding responsibilities, encouraging participative management, and allowing workers to set goals and evaluate their success in meeting goals.

Scientific Management Theory and Motivation Theory

Two traditional organizational behavior theories are Frederick Taylor's **scientific management theory** (1917) and Elton Mayo's **motivation theory** (1933).

- *Scientific management theory:* Management's role is to plan and control, identifying tasks and then assigning the best person to complete the tasks, utilizing both rewards and punishment as motivating forces. This theory puts the focus on the outcomes rather than on the individuals, but workers are often unmotivated with this structure.
- *Motivation theory:* This theory requires that managers take a more personal interest in the needs of workers. Mayo (in the Hawthorne experiment) found that workers responded positively to changes in the working environment when they are consulted about decisions. This theory states that workers are motivated by increased managerial interest and involvement, team work, and improved communication between management and staff.

Areas of Leadership

The clinical nurse specialist is expected to demonstrate leadership abilities in **different areas**:

- *Clinical*: The CNS serves as an advocate for patients and a leader for staff to help to facilitate change and to empower other staff members to become agents of change. The CNS provides guidance and educates others.

- *Professional organization/healthcare institution:* Professional organizations offer many different opportunities for leadership. They may develop continuing education courses and guidelines, chair committees, organize conferences, and give conference presentations. The CNS often serves as team or committee leader and often serves on institutional and administrative teams.
- *Policy*: The CNS should take an active role in helping to establish health care policies and priorities, utilizing his/her expertise and research. This may be at a local or institutional level or at a state or national level.

Leadership Styles

Leadership styles often influence the perception of leadership values and commitment: Styles include the following:

Participatory	The participatory leader presents a potential decision and then makes a final decision based on input from staff or teams. This type of leadership is time-consuming and may result in compromises that are not wholly satisfactory to management or staff, but this process is motivating to staff who feel their expertise is valued.
Democratic	The democratic leader presents a problem and asks staff or teams to arrive at a solution, although the leader usually makes the final decision. This type of leadership may delay decision-making, but staff and teams are often more committed to the solutions because of their input.
Laissez-faire	The laissez-faire leader exerts little direct control but allows employees/teams to make decisions with little interference. This may be effective leadership if the teams are highly skilled and motivated, but in many cases this type of leader-ship is the product of poor management skills and little is accomplished because of this lack of leadership.
Charismatic	The charismatic leader depends upon personal charisma to influence people and may be very persuasive, but this type leader may engage "followers" and relate to one group rather than the organization at large, limiting effectiveness.
Bureaucratic	The bureaucratic leader follows organization rules exactly and expects everyone else to do so. This is most effective in handling cash flow or managing work in dangerous work environments. This type of leadership may engender respect but may not be conducive to change.
Autocratic	The autocratic leader makes decisions independently and strictly enforces rules, but team members often feel left out of the process and may not be supportive. This type of leadership is most effective in crisis situations but may have difficulty gaining commitment of staff.
Consultative	The consultative leader presents a decision and welcomes input and questions, although decisions rarely change. This type of leadership is most effective when gaining the support of staff is critical to the success of proposed changes.

Leadership Facilitation of Leadership Values

Leadership must be consistent and succeeds by providing staff with direction and guidance that shows by example, explaining why things need to be done rather than directing how this must be achieved. A good leader fosters values by focusing on the right way to do things rather than on errors or poor performance. By engaging staff in all parts of the processes, a leader engenders a sense of commitment and collaboration on the part of the staff. This commitment cannot be achieved through rules, regulation, threats, and criticism. A good leader must demonstrate integrity, welcome diversity, be open-minded, and search for competence. While a leader must have a thorough understanding of the organization/facility and its work, he or she must be able to act holistically. The leader must motivate others by providing structure, order, and the ability to make decisions while continuing to learn and teach in order to create positive change.

Healthcare Business and Finance

Delivery of Care

The **delivery of care** in a system is impacted by numerous forces:

- *Social forces* are increasing demand for access to treatment and medical services, both traditional and complementary. As society views equitable medical care as a right, then delivery of care must be available to all.
- *Political forces* affect medical care as the federal and state governments increasingly become purchasers of medical care, imposing their guidelines and limitations on the medical system.
- *Regulatory forces* may be local, state, or federal and can have a profound effect on delivery of care and services, differing from one state or region to another.
- *Economic forces*, such as managed care or cost-containment committees, try to contain costs to insurers and facilities by controlling access to and duration of treatment and limiting products. Economic pressure is working to prevent duplication of services in a geographical area, and providers are creating networks to purchase supplies and equipment directly.

Elements of Business Plan

Elements of a **business plan** include:

- *Executive summary*: Outline all the key elements to the business proposal, including the customer, product/services, goals, risks, opportunities, costs, management, and timeline.
- *Product/Service*: Provide a detailed description, without being overly technical, including the ways in which this product or service compares to others. Note the need for patents, licenses, or any regulatory requirements.
- *Management*: Explain the hierarchy and division of duties, including an explanation of professional experience and education.
- *Market Survey*: Discuss similar products or services, target groups, and projected market volume.
- *Marketing strategies*: Explain placement, promotion, and pricing.
- *Organization*: Describe structure of business, provide flowcharts, and describe production capability, costs, quality assurance methods, and inventory, if appropriate.
- *Timeline*: Describe the timeline for implementation from the beginning to having a fully operational business.
- *Risk factors*: Describe opportunities from both gain and risk factors that may impact products or sales and methods to deal with risk factors.
- *Appendices*: Provide samples of forms and any additional information necessary.

Return on Investment, Deliverables, and Business Proposal

Return on investment is the percentage of return based on gains and costs. The formula is gains minus costs of investment divided by costs of investment ((gains – costs)/costs = ROI.) Thus, if gains are $500,000 and costs are $400,000, the calculation would be as follows:

$$ROI = \frac{500{,}000 - 400{,}000}{400{,}000} = \frac{100{,}000}{400{,}000} = 25\%$$

A deliverable is that product or service that must be delivered or supplied in accordance with an agreement or contract.

A business proposal is a request, usually submitted in writing, for a business arrangement with another entity, rather than establishment of an independent business. For example, one might submit a business proposal regarding purchase of supplies or equipment from a manufacturer. Proposals may be invited, as in response to an invitation to submit bids, or uninvited, as with a request to provide a particular service or product.

Patient Flow Management

Patient flow management is a method of tracking patients. This technique assesses the practices of the organization that influence the quality of patient care. Patient flow management assesses the way the patient flows through the system from triage to treatment. The process includes evaluating methods of routing patients through the various services. Departments are often interdependent. Organization-wide utilization management allows the evaluation and integration of information and services. For example, admissions may depend on discharges, which may depend on completion of imaging or laboratory studies, which, in turn, may depend on transmission of orders and transportation of patients. Patient flow can be improved by determining what aspects of the patient flow process are not working effectively and making changes in these areas.

Assessment of Customer Needs with Surveys

Surveys are valuable tools in assessing both progress and customer needs. However, care must be taken in the design of the survey if it is to have validity. A number of decisions must be made:

- *Target group*: Who will receive the survey? In some cases, an entire population of customers (all patients being discharged) may be targeted, but in other cases, only a percentage will be surveyed (e.g., 30% of discharges from the emergency department). Another type of sampling may also be used. Identifying the target group can be complex.
- *Type of survey:* This may be paper, telephone, or Internet. There are different investments of time and money for each.
- *Type of questions:* Questions with a yes/no decision are usually easier to quantify than open-ended questions or scales, although scales are frequently used to assess degree of satisfaction.
- *Format*: This includes font size, color, general layout, and American Disability Act compliance.
- *Follow-up:* Reminders or incentives for people to complete surveys are needed, as completion rates are often low.

Medical Costs

Even with insurance and Medicare, older adults may incur huge **medical costs.** If a patient requires nursing care at home or in a facility, the costs can range from $4,000 to more than $8,000 monthly. This quickly depletes savings. Medicare strictly limits hospital and extended care stay as well as home health care. When a patient is no longer improving, the patient's care is not paid for until he or she is eligible for hospice care. This can happen in the case of a terminal illness or Alzheimer's disease. There are also limitations on hospice care. Long-term care is not provided by Medicare or most insurance policies. There is insurance available for this purpose, but these policies are expensive. This leaves patients and families with financial burdens that they sometimes cannot pay. If savings are depleted (and the amount allowed varies from state to state), and the patient needs long-term care, state Medicaid programs may pay. However, there are few facilities willing to take Medicaid patients because the reimbursement rate is low.

Cost-Effective Drugs

Drugs are one of the most expensive aspects of medical care for patients. Even individuals with insurance drug coverage or Medicare Part D may incur considerable costs, especially when non-generic drugs are involved. Drug representatives exert great pressure on physicians to prescribe new drugs, and patients are often influenced by direct-to-consumer advertising. However, the nurse can help the patient ensure that drugs are prescribed based on need. Additionally, the benefits of the drugs must justify their cost. It is the responsibility of the nurse to act in the best interests of the patient and to educate the patient about drugs. If a less expensive drug is as effective as a more expensive or newer drug, then the nurse and patient should request that the less expensive drug be prescribed. The nurse should educate people about the use of generic drugs as a cost-saving measure. In most cases, generic drugs are as effective as name brand drugs.

Cost Allocation

One type of cost analysis involves **cost allocation.** With almost all expenditures, there are *direct* costs and *indirect* costs. A direct cost might be the salary of a team leader while indirect costs are those related to accounting and human resources. To determine cost allocation, the budget must be formatted to determine unit cost or cost per unit of service, so line item budget format is used. Direct costs must be determined as well as indirect costs. Generally, direct costs benefit just one department or service while indirect costs are shared costs, such as the cost of custodial services. Thus, a percentage of the indirect cost is allocated based upon the utilization. For a simplified example, if team leaders represent 5% of total employees, then 5% of indirect employee costs would be allocated to this line item. However, there may be many departments and services involved in indirect costs, and to arrive at a true unit cost, all of these costs must be accounted for in the calculation.

Cost-Benefit Analysis

A **cost-benefit analysis** uses the average cost of the problem (such as infection) and the cost of intervention to demonstrate savings. According to the CDC, a surgical site infection caused by *Staphylococcus aureus* results in an average of 12 additional days of hospitalization and costs $27,000. (In actuality, the cost may vary widely from one institution to another; so local data may be used.) For example, if a surgical unit were averaging 10 surgical site infections annually, the cost would be:

10 x $27,000 = $270,000 annually

If the interventions include new software ($10,000) for surveillance, an additional staff person ($65,000), benefits ($15,000), and increased staff education (including materials, $2000), the total intervention cost would be:

$10,000 + $65,000 + $15,000 + $2000 = $92,000

If the goal were to decrease infections by 50% to 5 infections per year, the savings would be calculated:

5 x $27,000 = $135,000

Subtracting the intervention cost from the savings:

$135,000 - $92,000 = $43,000 annual cost benefit

Cost-Effective Analysis, Efficacy Studies, Product Evaluation, and Incremental Cost-Effectiveness Ratio

A **cost-effective analysis** measures the effectiveness of an intervention rather than the monetary savings. Each year, about 2 million nosocomial infections result in 90,000 deaths and an estimated $6.7 billion in additional health costs. From that perspective, decreasing infections should reduce costs, but there are human savings in suffering as well, and it can be difficult to place a dollar value on that. If each infection adds about 12 days to hospitalization, then a reduction in infection by 5 would be calculated: 5 x 12 = 60 fewer patient infection days

Efficacy studies may compare a series of cost-benefit analyses to determine the intervention with the best cost-benefit. They may also be used for **process or product evaluation.** For example, a study might be done to determine the infection rates of 4 different types of catheters to determine which type resulted in the fewest infections thus, saving the most money (and infection days).

Incremental cost-effectiveness ratio is the ratio of cost change to outcome change.

Financial Management

Developing and managing a budget for a department requires an understanding of **financial management**. Management must not only include developing and assigning budget items but monitoring expenditures, analyzing, and reporting. Financial planning is a part of strategic planning in which the department demonstrates how resources will be allocated, usually for a one-year period. Financial planning should be based on the best utilization of costs in relation to revenues/outcomes. Objectives include the following:

- Developing a quantitative record of plans
- Allowing for evaluation of financial performance
- Controlling costs
- Providing information to increase cost awareness

The budget should be linked to daily operations and integrated with strategic vision, mission, goals, and objectives. Those with vested interests in the budget should participate in planning. Monitoring should be ongoing to allow for feedback and modifications as necessary.

Developing and Managing Department Budgets

Managing the budget once it is developed and established must be done on an ongoing basis to ensure that financial targets are met in relation to strategic goals. Management includes the following:

- *Accountability*: The budget team should include management/directors with an expectation of excellence.
- *Controlling expenses:* This is especially important for departments that do not produce income directly.

- *Monitoring costs in relation to best practice benchmark:* One goal of budget management should be to strive to match benchmarks.
- *Developing corrective action plans:* Any variances in the budget should be accounted for within a week and corrective actions taken.
- *Utilizing a balanced scorecard:* Various measurements, both quantitative and qualitative, should be used to manage cost containment strategies.
- *Recognizing quality:* Rewards for achieving benchmarks should be built in to the budgeting process. In some cases, this may be a bonus.

Types of Budgets

A departmental budget is part of a larger organizational budget, so an understanding of the different **types of budgets** utilized in healthcare management is helpful:

- *Operating budget:* This budget is used for daily operations and includes general expenses, such as salaries, education, insurance, maintenance, depreciation, debts, and profit. The budget has 3 elements: statistics, expenses, and revenue.
- *Capital budget:* This budget determines which capital projects (such as remodeling, repairing, purchasing of equipment or buildings) will be allocated funding for the year. These capital expenditures are usually based on cost-benefit analysis and prioritization of needs.
- *Cash balance budget:* This type of budget projects cash balances for a specific future time period, including all operating and capital budget items.
- *Master budget:* This budget combines operating, capital, and cash balance budgets as well as any specialized or area-specific budgets.

Operational Budgeting

Most **departmental budgets** will be operational, but there are a number of different approaches that can be used:

- *Fixed/forecast:* Revenue and expenses are forecast for the entire budget period and budget items are fixed.
- *Flexible*: Estimates are made regarding anticipated changes in revenue and expenses and both fixed and variable costs are identified.
- *Zero-based:* All cost centers are re-evaluated each budget period to determine if they should be funded or eliminated, partially or completely.
- *Responsibility center:* Budgeting is a cost center (department) or centers with one person holding overall responsibility.
- *Program*: Organizational programs are identified and revenues and costs for each program are budgeted.
- *Appropriations*: Government funds are requested and dispersed through this process.
- *Continuous/rolling:* Periodic updates to the budget, including revenues, costs, volume, are done prior to the next budget cycle.

Financial Costs Related to Quality

Performance improvement is not without costs, and these must be considered carefully when doing cost analysis. **Financial costs related to quality** management include the following:

- *Error-free costs* are all those costs in terms of processes, services, equipment, time, materials, and staffing that are necessary to providing a product or process that is without error from the onset. A process that is error free is relatively stable in terms of pre-established guidelines.
- *Cost of quality* (COQ) includes costs associated with identifying and correcting errors, making errors, creating defects or failures in processes, and planning as well as costs of poor quality (COPQ).
- *Conformance costs* are those costs related to preventing errors, such as monitoring and evaluation. These may include costs incurred through education, maintenance, pilot testing, and analysis.
- *Nonconformance costs* are those related to errors, failures, and defects. These may include adverse events (such as infections), poor access due to staff shortages or cancellations, lost time, duplications of service, and malpractice.

Recommending Practice, Products, and Service Modification

The CNS is in an important position to **recommend practice, products, and service modifications**, in light of fiscal situations. The CNS many times has a great amount of information regarding budget and management issues, and is also an expert in the field. The CNS can help nurses to collaborate to decide the prioritization on the purchasing of new equipment for a specific unit. As content expert, the CNS can help with the education of staff regarding the costs of supplies, equipment, and procedures. Educated staff is more likely to be on board with efforts to help with cost containment.

The CNS can also serve on committees, and encourage peers to do the same, to test new products, therefore ensuring that products that the institution purchases are high quality products, and not chose for their cost only.

FTEs

The Health Care Reform law has established a method of determining **full-time equivalency (FTE)** for employees as part of determining tax credits. Employers and accrediting agencies also use FTE when reviewing staffing levels and cost-effectiveness. FTE hours are 2080 annually, so to determine the number of FTE employees, the hours of all employees are totaled and then divided by 2080, excluding seasonal workers who work <120 days during the year, although this usually does not apply to healthcare. Note that only 2080 hours may be counted for any one employee, so hours exceeding this limit are eliminated. For example, if a single employee worked 2200 hours, 4 employees worked 2080 hours each, 4 worked 1040 hours each, and 1 worked 800 hours, the calculation is below:

- 5 x 2080 = 10,400
- 4 x 1040 = 4,160
- 1 x 800 = 800
- 10,400 + 4160 + 800 = 15,360
- 15,360/2080 = 7.38

Numbers with decimals are rounded down, not up, to the whole number, so this employer has 7 FTE employees.

Primary and Secondary Insurance

There are a number of different types of **insurance** coverage that may be available for patients. There may be exclusions for injuries/conditions not covered by the policy, such as overuse syndromes, or for pre-existing conditions. Riders may be added to a policy to override exclusions, with increased premium. Insurance includes the following:

- *Primary* insurance pays all of the costs of injury/illness to a preset dollar or percentage amount (often 80%) of what is considered usual, customary, and reasonable (UCR), usually with no deductible; however, premiums are often high, and it may require considerable paperwork to justify expenses. Some primary insurance plans include a deductible or co-payment for some types of care, such as doctor or emergency department visits. This insurance may be the patient's or may be required for an athlete by the school or organization.
- *Secondary* insurance pays remaining expenses after the primary insurance pays. Usually, there are deductibles that must be paid.

PPO, HMO, POS, and PPO

There are a number of different **models** for managed care to provide healthcare services:

- *Exclusive provider organization (EPO):* Healthcare providers provide services at discounted rates to those enrolled in a service. Some providers may be prohibited from caring for those not enrolled and enrollees are only reimbursed for care within the network.
- *Health maintenance organization (HMO):* With an HMO, there is a prepaid contract between healthcare providers, payors, and enrollees for specified services in a specified time period provided by a list of providers, usually representing a variety of specialties.
- *Point of service plans (POS):* This is a combination HMO and PPO structure so that people can receive service in the network but can opt to seek treatment outside the network in some situations.
- *Preferred provider organizations: (PPO):* This involves healthcare providers who have agreed to be part of a network providing services to an enrolled group at reduced rates of reimbursement. Care received outside of the network is usually only partially covered.

Medicare

Medicare, a federal health insurance program for those who have Social Security or those who have bought into Medicare, provides payment to private healthcare providers, such as physicians and hospitals, but limits reimbursement. Physicians receive 80% of usual customary and reasonable (UCR) fees if they accept Medicare assignment. If they do not, they can charge up to 115% of what Medicare allows. Patients are responsible for the remaining 20% or up to 115% if the physicians do not accept Medicare. Parts include the following:

- *Medicare A:* Hospital insurance covers acute hospital, limited nursing home care and/or home health care as well as hospice care for the terminally ill. There is no premium for this part.
- *Medicare B:* Medical insurance covers physicians, advance practice nurses, laboratory work and physical and occupational therapy. Patients must pay an annual deductible in addition to monthly payments.
- *Medicare D:* A prescription drug plan covers part of the costs of prescription drugs at participating pharmacies. It is administered by private insurance companies, so monthly costs and benefits vary somewhat.

Medicaid

Medicaid is a combined federal and state welfare program authorized by Title XIX of the Social Security Act to assist people with low income with payment for medical care. This program provides assistance for all ages, including children. Older adults receiving SSI are eligible as are others who meet state eligibility requirements. The Medicaid programs are administered by the individual states, which establish eligibility and reimbursement guidelines, so benefits vary considerably from one state to another. Older adults with Medicare are eligible for Medicaid as a secondary insurance. Expenses that are covered include inpatient and outpatient hospital services, physician payments, nursing home care, home health care, and laboratory and radiation services. Adults who are legal resident aliens are ineligible for Medicaid for 5 years after attaining legal resident status. Some states pay for preventive services, such as home and community-based programs aimed at reducing the need for hospitalization.

Medicare Managed Care

Medicare Managed Care is provided by a health maintenance organization (HMO), which typically receives a monthly payment per patient enrolled rather than the traditional pay-for-service Medicare payment system. The Medicare HMO programs are available in only some areas and may vary in the type of services they provide. Typically, a person must choose or is assigned a primary care physician who serves as the gatekeeper to determine what other services or physicians the patient needs, and the patient must stay within the HMO network. In general, the person must be eligible for Medicare to enroll. Further, the patient must not be in end-stage renal disease or receiving hospice care. There is an open enrollment period each year during which a patient must apply for enrollment. Many HMOs have stopped accepting Medicare patients because the costs for care were so high, so many older adults do not have access to this type of program. Some programs have been successful in lowering costs by instituting preventive health programs.

Preferred Providers and Other Plans

Medicare has made a number of modifications to allow Medicare patients to access different types of programs in addition to typical pay-for-service care and managed care through HMOs:

- *The prospective payment system* (PPS) pays a set amount for patient care, depending upon diagnosis (diagnosis-related group or DRG).
- *The preferred provider organization* (PPO) provides discounted rates for those on Medicare who choose healthcare providers from a list of those who have agreed to accept Medicare assignment.
- *Private insurance pay-for-service Medicare plans* are contracted by Medicare and may provide more benefits, but the patient may be required to work individually with the insurance company to determine benefits and may be assessed an additionally monthly fee.
- *Specialty plans* are being developed in different areas, some focusing on increased preventive care.

Certificate of Medical Necessity

In some cases, Medicare requires a **Certificate of Medical Necessity (CMN)** to indicate the need for the DME, signed by the physician or CNS. Equipment requiring the CMN includes bone growth stimulators, oxygen equipment and supplies, lymphedema pumps, patient lifts and transcutaneous electronic nerve stimulators. Medicare has established new rules for oxygen and oxygen equipment. Suppliers receive payments for 36 continuous months but then must continue to provide the oxygen and equipment for the remaining 24 months of the 5-year period. During this last period, Medicare will pay only for the oxygen contents and, if in-home, one maintenance visit every 6 months. Medicare pays 80% of the costs of durable medical equipment. If the physician or CNS feels a patient needs a motorized or power wheelchair in the home environment, the equipment may be ordered under Medicare B only after a face-to-face examination of the patient.

DRGs

Medicare's prospective payment system (PPS) pays a set amount for patient care, depending upon the **diagnosis-related group (DRG)** to which the patient is assigned. The DRG classifies patients on the basis of diagnosis, procedures, gender, age, comorbidities, complications, and condition on discharge. Medicare reimburses based on expected costs for the DRG, rather than actual cost for service. The original DRG classification included 467 potential groups, but through the years, the classification system has expanded and become more complex. A number of different DRG systems are now available, including the Medicare DRG (CMS-DRG or MS-DRG) and all-patient DRG (AP-DRG). The DRG version 27 MS-DRG listing contains 999 DRGs. The Medicare DRG releases a new version each year. For example, version 27 was released October 1, 2009, and version 31 was released October 31, 2013. Many conditions are designated as with or without major complications (MCC) and with or without complications and comorbidities (CCs). For example, the DRG listings for ventricular shunt include:

- Ventricular shunt procedures w MCC.
- Ventricular shunt procedure w CC.
- Ventricular shunt procedures w/o CC/MCC.

DME

Durable medical equipment (DME) is that equipment that can be used repeatedly (as opposed to single-use disposable items) and is used for medical purposes. Durable medical equipment (e.g., wheelchairs, walkers, hospital beds, commodes, nebulizers, and oxygen equipment) is available in hospitals and medical centers and is usually provided as part of general care. When patients return to the home environment, the costs of DME may be covered by some insurance policies. Medicare B covers the cost of DME for use in the person's dwelling (home, apartment, or residential care facility) but not for use in skilled nursing facilities, so patients covered by Medicare A who are hospitalized in skilled nursing facilities for more than the 100 days may lose DME benefits. DME not generally paid for includes exercise equipment and equipment to modify the environment, such as heaters, humidifiers, de-humidifiers, and air conditioners.

Reuse of Single-Use Devices

Single use devices (SUD), such as surgical drills, catheters, and endotracheal tubes, are manufactured for one-time use, but the reality is that for many years SUDs were reused with little regulatory oversight regarding methods of disinfecting/sterilization to determine if the SUDs were safe for use. Many hospitals reprocessed their own devices, although some sent them to third-party reprocessors. In response to concerns about this practice, the Medical User Fee and Modernization Act (MDUFMA) was issued in 2002, with requirements for reprocessing, including applications for 510(k)s and validation data demonstrating that the reprocessed SUD is essentially equivalent to the original SUD. Reprocessed devices are classified as critical (in contact with sterile tissue), semi-critical (in contact with mucous membranes), or non-critical (topical contact with skin only). The process of validation includes procedures for cleaning and sterilization, the types of materials, and product testing. Studies have shown that properly reprocessed SUDs are equivalent in safety to the original.

Tricare

Tricare is the health care program serving active military, retired military, and their spouses and dependents. Tricare provides a number of different plans, depending upon location and eligibility. For those with Medicare, Tricare becomes the secondary insurer. If patients choose to opt out of Medicare (such as those with no insurance or private insurance), Tricare pays the amount equivalent to a secondary insurer (20% of allowable), and the patient is responsible for the rest. By law, all other insurances must pay before Tricare. Patients may access care at military treatment facilities (MTF) on a space-available basis, but must enroll in Tricare Plus to receive primary care at MTFs. Those eligible for both Tricare and Veterans Affairs (VA) programs may receive care at VA medical facilities if the service is covered under Tricare and the facility is part of the Tricare network; however, the VA cannot bill Medicare, so costs not covered by Tricare must be paid by the patient even if the patient has Medicare coverage.

Long-Term Care Insurance

Yearly care in a long-term care facility can range in price from about $30,000 to $70,000 or more, depending upon the area and the type of facility. **Long-term care insurance** is provided by private insurances to cover all or part of the costs of long-term care (usually to a pre-set limit). Because these insurance plans are intended to make profit, the premiums are often high and increase (sometimes markedly) with age, so people who have paid into the system for years may be forced to cancel and end up with no benefits. Because long-term care insurance is fairly new, many current older adults do not have this coverage because if they wait until near retirement to pay for this insurance, the monthly payments are so high that there is little benefit. There is also little benefit with this type of policy for people with low income who can apply for Medicaid; however, for those with middle-to-high income, long-term care insurance may be a viable option.

Professional Development

Mentoring Overview

Mentoring occurs in many different ways. The CNS may establish one-on-one mentoring relationships; however, just as often, taking the time to assist others on a one-time basis or working with groups of staff provides an opportunity for mentoring. Mentoring is a reciprocal activity because both mentor and the mentee benefit. Mentoring is central to the role of the CNS and can be incorporated into current practice without involving extensive added responsibilities or time commitments. All interactions with other staff are essentially mentoring opportunities. The CNS should make a conscious decision to view himself/herself as a mentor and actively consider the role of mentor whenever working with other staff, especially when the CNS can identify a purpose, such as assisting others to learn new skills or providing demonstrations. The CNS can assist others to deal with issues of diversity.

Mentoring Elements

The CNS is in an ideal position to serve as a mentor, both informally and formally. There are a number of elements that enhance **mentoring**:

- *Nurturing*: Being supportive and interested in furthering the skills and education of the staff.
- *Providing clinical expertise:* Guiding the staff by demonstrating a personal commitment to excellence in provision of care.
- *Motivating others:* Encouraging others and supporting them throughout their careers.
- *Providing an example:* Teaching others by being a good example.

- *Listening*: Being non-judgmental in discussions with others and listening to determine different perspectives and needs.
- *Providing feedback:* Being honest in evaluation and assisting others to improve care, providing feedback about how their practices affect patient outcomes.
- *Role modeling:* Providing assistance to others in gaining certification and understanding the role of the CNS.

Steps to Mentoring

The most common **model for mentoring** is that of a partnership with the mentor providing the expertise and the mentee utilizing this expertise through learning, action, and reflection. There are a number of steps involved in the mentor-mentee relationship:

- *Mentor selection*: In some cases, a formal mentor program may be in effect at an institution, but in other cases the mentee may need to identify a candidate for mentor, based on mutual respect. Generally, a mentor should not be a direct supervisor as this can present conflicts. The mentor may be a peer or a nurse in advanced position.
- *Determine expectations*: Ground rules should be established, such as when and how frequently to meet.
- *Competency development*: The mentee works toward specific goals in learning with the guidance of the mentor.
- *Guidance gives way to consultation*: As the mentee gains confidence and skills, the mentor provides assistance on request, providing the mentee more independence.
- Mentorship resolves.

Coaching

Coaching is an important part of mentoring/preceptoring. Coaching can include specific training, providing career information, and confronting issues of concern. While patient safety is the primary consideration, coaching should be done in a manner that increases learner confidence and ability to self-monitor rather than in a punitive or critical manner. The CNS must develop confidence in his/her own ability to be assertive and confront issues directly in order to resolve conflicts and promote collaboration. Effective methods of coaching include the following:

- Giving positive feedback, stressing what the student is doing right
- Using questioning to help the student recognize problem areas
- Providing demonstrations and opportunities for question/answer periods
- Providing regular progress reports so the student understands areas of concern
- Assisting the student to establish personal goals for improvement
- Providing resources to help the student master material

Preceptorship

The CNS is often in the position of having many roles in clinical practice, including educating others and serving as a **preceptor** for graduate students who are studying to enter the field. While mentoring may entail a long-term relationship, preceptoring is usually a time-limited arrangement related to a term of study, such as a semester, orientation period, or a clinical rotation. The CNS must balance responsibilities and ensure that he/she is able to provide adequate clinical supervision and guidance to the student on a daily basis. This may require coordinating schedules and planning carefully to ensure all responsibilities can be met. The CNS preceptor helps the student to understand his/her impact on the spheres of influence (patient/client, nurse and nurse practice, and organization/system) by including the student in all CNS activities. The preceptor may engage in shared care as well as direct supervision in order to improve the student's skills.

Beginning Steps

The **preceptor** serves the role of teacher, supervising the clinical experience of the nursing student. In order to be successful, a relationship built on trust is critical. The preceptor trusts the student to come prepared with knowledge and skills, and the student trusts the preceptor to provide guidance and support. There are a number of steps that facilitate preceptorship:

- *Meeting the student:* If possible, this meeting should occur before preceptorship begins. Discussion should include preceptor expectations, goals, and a discussion of the student's learning style. The student should be provided with lists of materials needed and schedules.
- *Identifying learning objectives:* The preceptor helps the students to develop personal learning objectives based on essential skills and core competencies for the discipline.
- *Utilizing the nursing process:* Students should give case presentations based on the steps in the nursing process with the preceptor helping the student to see risks and benefits to actions.

CNS's Role in Nursing Orientation

The CNS's participation in the facility's **nursing orientation** program for healthcare workers is important because it signals a commitment by administration to improving performance and staff development. The CNS should clearly outline the following:

- *Area of expertise*: This should include the CNS's degree, any specialty training, and a discussion of the patient population (age, gender, specific diseases) served.
- *Experience*: The CNS should describe the type and duration of his or her experience related to the area of specialty. New graduates can explain related work history and work experience during CNS training.
- *Role in the facility*: The CNS should clearly outline responsibilities and services he or she provides to the facility and the staff, for example serving as mentor and/or resource person for staff members.
- *Availability*: Staff members need to know a schedule of when the CNS is available.
- *Methods of contact*: The CNS should provide a telephone number, pager number if appropriate, and/or an email address.

CNS's Role in Internships

The CNS's role in **internships** may vary depending on the facility and the type of nursing program. The CNS may serve as a faculty instructor or direct clinical supervisor for a nurse in a CNS program that includes an internship or for a graduate CNS nurse in a post-degree internship program. In either case, the role of the CNS as content expert is to allow the CNS intern to function in the role with as much independence as possible, while providing guidance and feedback about performance. The CNS should help provide the intern with a wide range of experiences in the three spheres of influence, seeking out learning opportunities to help the intern gain competence and confidence in providing care. The CNS may also serve as a resource person for the intern's special projects and/or presentations.

Providing Feedback

The clinical nurse specialist is often required to supervise other staff members, especially when delegating tasks, and should provide evaluation and feedback. **Feedback** may take a variety of forms. The point of feedback is to help the person to improve skills, so immediate verbal feedback is usually more useful than delayed written feedback, although the supervisory role usually requires both. Feedback should include both reference to current practice and practical advice. Although sometimes overlooked, positive feedback promotes self-esteem and is motivating and is easier than negative feedback; however, advising supervised staff members of problem areas is critical to patient safety and to helping staff members improve performance. One can begin by describing the situation and making specific observations about the person's performance. For example, a supervisor might say, without judgment, "This is what I observed." The following are examples of questioning:

- "How did you feel about the outcomes/procedure/task?"
- "What could you have done differently?"
- "How can I help you?"

If negligence requires disciplinary action, then the person should be provided with the written policy.

PRECEPTORS

The **preceptor** is responsible for evaluating the clinical expertise of the student. Basic to preceptorship is the concept that the student should provide safe and appropriate care to the patients. This requires observation and discussion as well as formal evaluation:

- *Evaluating:* Students should first engage in self-evaluation, which is then reviewed by the preceptor who provides feedback verbally and in written form. The ability of the student to look analytically and critically at his/her own performance is an important part of the learning experience. The preceptor's critiquing should be analytical rather than judgmental. Feedback should be specific and detailed and should include both positive observations as well as negative.
- *Meeting requirements:* The preceptor determines when the student has completed clinical requirements based on lists of required activities/learning experiences and evaluates the student's level of competency based on consistent accurate performance related to those activities/experiences.

EDUCATIONAL NEEDS OF HEALTHCARE WORKERS

There are a number of different methods that the CNS can use to **assess the educational needs** of health care workers:

- Review job descriptions to determine the educational qualifications/certifications for all different levels of staff to determine what, realistically, staff members should be expected to know about a particular subject.
- Review job orientation and training materials to determine what staff members have already been taught about the subject matter.
- Conduct meetings with staff members in different departments to brainstorm areas of concern and potential training needs.
- Meet with team leaders and department heads for their input about the need for education.
- Administer short quizzes to staff members asking about standard methods, such as barrier precautions and hand washing, to determine basic knowledge.
- Provide questionnaires to staff members to obtain information about their own perceptions of what they know or need to know about the subject matter.
- Make direct observations of staff members.

Educational Materials

It is impractical to believe that the CNS can produce all **educational materials,** but careful consideration must be given to a number of issues:

- *Price* ranges from free to hundreds or even thousands of dollars for educational materials, which may be handouts, videos, posters, or entire courses or series of courses available online. The CNS must first consider the budget and then look for material within those monetary constraints. Government agencies, such as the CDC, often have posters and handouts as well as PowerPoint presentations and videos available for download online at no cost.
- *Quality* varies considerably as well. The CNS should consider the goal and objectives before choosing materials, and the materials should be evaluated to determine if they cover all needed information in a clear and engaging manner.
- *Currency* must be considered as well. If material will soon be outdated because of changes in regulations, then it will have to be replaced.

Return Demonstrations

A **return demonstration** is given by learners to show mastery of a procedure. This may be done for each step during initial instruction but should eventually include a demonstration of the entire procedure:

- The nurse should ask if the learner has any questions before the demonstration.
- The learner should gather all necessary equipment, using a checklist to ensure that nothing is forgotten.
- The learner should explain the steps. The nurse can prompt: "Can you talk me through this."
- The nurse should avoid interfering if the learner makes a minor mistake, but if the learner appears confused or makes an important error (such as forgetting to apply gloves), the nurse can prompt: "Why don't you look at the checklist to make sure you've done each step."
- The nurse should provide positive feedback occasionally during the procedure: "You've placed the equipment exactly right."
- Upon completion, the nurse and learner should discuss the demonstration and determine if an additional return demonstration is needed.

Audience Size

There are a number of issues related to **audience size** that must be considered when planning presentations.

- Class participation is more difficult in a large class because there may not be time for all participants to speak individually. Breaking the class into small groups or pairs for discussion for part of the class time can increase participation, but there must be a focused purpose to the discussion so that people stay on task.
- In small groups, placing chairs in a circle or sitting around a table allows people to look at each other and have more active discussions than if they are sitting in rows.
- Online "virtual" classes can vary considerably in size, depending upon the type of presentation and whether or not scores and replies are automated or posted by the instructor. If a large group is taking an online course, setting up a "chat room" can facilitate exchange of ideas.

Steps to Program Improvement Training

Development of organizational **performance improvement training** for quality requires a number of steps:

1. Assess training needs in order to provide needs-based training and to determine the type and extent of training needs. Assessment must be done while keeping in mind the organizational outcomes to be achieved. Assessing current level of knowledge for targeted information can be helpful.
2. Use strategic goals to establish specific learning goals and objectives tied to the mission and vision of the organization.
3. Determine methods of outcomes measurement.
4. Assess appropriate learning styles and teaching techniques in developing teaching strategies.
5. Develop course materials.
6. Train instructors or assistants as necessary.
7. Pilot test training materials and program with small group and utilize feedback to make modifications if necessary,
8. Implement training program.
9. Conduct measurements to determine outcomes.

Continuing Education

Continuing education is the education and training that are required to remain current in the nursing profession. Continuing education is an obligation of all nurses. Employers may require continuing education for continued employment. In some cases, employers may require that nurses take specific courses or types of courses. Continuing education requirements for renewal of an RN license (regardless of the type of program) are established by individual states and vary widely. Some states require no continuing education. Other states require a minimum number of units (one contact hour per unit). This often comes out to 20 to 30 units for each licensing period, which is typically every two years. Some states specify certain courses that must be taken for license renewal (end-of-life or human immunodeficiency virus/acquired immune deficiency syndrome [HIV/AIDS], for example). State boards of nursing must approve all providers of continuing education courses. This is to ensure that the courses meet minimum standards. Continuing education courses may be delivered in a traditional classroom setting, via the Internet, or through self-study materials.

CNS Practice Test

1. Which adventitious lung sound is most often associated with congestive heart failure?

a. Rales.
b. Wheezing.
c. Stridor.
d. There are no abnormal breath sounds associated with CHF.

2. An 82-year-old male has been diagnosed with ischemic heart disease and it is believed that a coronary artery bypass graft (CABG) could help him. Which of the following would NOT be a contraindication to him undergoing this procedure?

a. Severe COPD.
b. Severe CHF.
c. His age.
d. Current chemotherapy therapy for prostate cancer.

3. On exam, a patient is found to have a systolic ejection murmur that is heard best at the right second intercostal space and radiating to the neck. Imaging shows a calcified, bicuspid aortic valve. Which of the following would be appropriate at this time?

a. Valve replacement surgery.
b. Cardiac catheterization.
c. Echocardiogram.
d. Temporary valvuloplasty.

4. For a patient diagnosed with schizophrenia, which of the following is usually an indicator of a better outcome with this disease?

a. Age of onset at 20-years-old or older.
b. Insidious onset of symptoms.
c. Slow rate of progression of the illness.
d. Low socioeconomic status.

5. A 72-year-old male with glaucoma is seen for an exacerbation of COPD with low-grade fever. His current medications include lisinopril, simvastatin, timolol eye drops, albuterol inhaler, and Advair inhaler. One of the medications he should not receive for this exacerbation is:

a. albuterol via nebulizer.
b. Levaquin.
c. Tessalon Perles.
d. prednisone.

6. Which heart murmur would most likely be associated with aortic stenosis?

a. A pansystolic murmur heard best over the left sternal border at the 4th-5th intercostal space.
b. A mid-systolic murmur heard best over the right sternal border at the 1st-2nd intercostal space.
c. A mid-systolic click with a crescendo-decrescendo murmur at the apex.
d. A low-pitched and rumbling pandiastolic murmur heard best at the apex.

7. A 74-year-old female is seen for weakness and shortness of breath that started this morning. An EKG is completed and shows ST elevation and Q waves in leads II, III, and aVF. The most likely diagnosis is:

a. anterior wall infarction.
b. inferior wall infarction.
c. lateral wall infarction.
d. posterior wall infarction.

8. An anterior wall infarction is caused by occlusion of the:

a. left anterior descending coronary artery.
b. right coronary artery.
c. left circumflex coronary artery.
d. left marginal coronary artery.

9. A 76-year-old female with mild dementia is brought in by her daughter for a routine appointment. Her daughter expresses interest in having her mother try one of the medications to "cure her dementia." It is important she understand that:

a. the medications are very expensive and may not be covered by her insurance.
b. frequent monitoring of blood tests is necessary if one of these medications is started.
c. there is no known cure for dementia and the medication will only temporarily improve the symptoms.
d. these medications are reserved for use in those patients with severe dementia.

10. The medication with a mechanism of action of decreasing insulin resistance and increasing glucose utilization is:

a. glipizide (Glucotrol).
b. metformin (Glucophage).
c. acarbose (Precose).
d. pioglitazone (Actos).

11. In the patient who comes in with complaints of a depression in the center of their fingernails and the edges curling up, the first test that should be done is:

a. a CBC.
b. renal function tests.
c. a liver panel.
d. a biopsy of the nail material.

12. A patient is seen for complaints of low back pain that radiates into the thighs. An x-ray is completed and shows blurriness over the sacroiliac joints. Labs are completed and the HLA-B27 is positive. The demographic of this patient is most likely:

a. 62-year-old black female.
b. 42-year-old white female.
c. 17-year-old black male.
d. 21-year-old white male.

13. A patient is in the critical care unit being treated for sepsis. On his second day of treatment, he develops hypokalemia that is not responding to potassium administration. Which other electrolyte abnormality should be looked for?

a. Hyperglycemia.
b. Hypernatremia.
c. Hypocalcemia.
d. Hypomagnesemia.

14. According to the U.S. Preventive Services Task Force, the latest recommendation for routine PSA screening is:

a. it should be done annually on men >50-years-old.
b. it is not recommended.
c. it should be done annually on men >60-years-old.
d. it should be done every 5 years on men >40-years-old.

15. A 59-year-old female is seen for complaints of weakness and dyspnea for 2 days. Vital signs show a pulse of 42 bpm and BP of 162/50 mm Hg. EKG shows irregularly spaced P waves with wide, slow QRS complexes. The most appropriate intervention for this patient at this time is:

a. IV atropine.
b. IV fluid bolus.
c. synchronized cardioversion.
d. temporary pacemaker.

16. Which of the following is true regarding the murmur heard with mitral valve prolapse?

a. It is best heard over the right sternal border.
b. It is louder when the patient is standing and decreases with squatting.
c. It is heard best during the diastolic phase.
d. It is associated with a loud carotid bruit.

17. A patient presents with complaints of general malaise and a throbbing headache over her left temple which has last lasted all day. On exam, the left temporal artery reveals a bounding palpable pulse and scalp tenderness. The most appropriate test to do at this time to confirm the diagnosis is:

a. ultrasound of the temporal artery.
b. erythrocyte sedimentation rate.
c. temporal artery biopsy.
d. rheumatoid factor.

18. Changes that may be seen on a CBC in a patient with Grave's disease include:

a. elevated white blood cell count and decreased red blood cell count.
b. increased red blood cell count and increased hemoglobin.
c. decreased white blood cell count and decreased red blood cell count.
d. elevated white blood cell count and elevated red blood cell count.

19. Which recommendation from the U.S. Preventive Services Task Force regarding cervical cancer screening is true?

a. A Pap smear is recommended annually for all women age 30 to 75.
b. A Pap smear and HPV testing is recommended every 3 years for all women age 30 to 75.
c. A Pap smear is not recommended for women under the age of 21.
d. HPV testing should be done on all women, regardless of age, every 3 years.

20. The best option for treatment of osteoarthritis in the knees is:

a. acetaminophen (Tylenol).
b. naproxen (Naprosyn).
c. capsaicin cream.
d. hydrocodone (Vicodin).

21. If a patient is blind in his right eye, which of the following would be true?

a. A light shined in the opposite eye will cause both pupils to constrict.
b. A light shined in the blind eye will cause both pupils to dilate.
c. A light shined in the opposite eye will cause only that pupil to constrict.
d. A light shined in the blind eye will cause only the opposite pupil to dilate.

22. The gold standard for diagnosing polymyositis is:

a. serum antinuclear antibodies.
b. electromyography.
c. muscle biopsy.
d. serum aldolase level.

23. A teenage girl is newly diagnosed with polycystic ovarian syndrome, or PCOS. She is asking why she has been having increasing facial hair and acne with this. The best explanation is:

a. she has more estrogen than normal because of the disease.
b. she has more progesterone than normal because of the disease.
c. her blood sugar levels are high which causes these changes.
d. she has a higher than normal testosterone level.

24. What is the difference between palliative care and hospice care?

a. Palliative care is for inpatient end of life care and hospice care is performed in the home.
b. Palliative care can be started at the time of diagnosis during treatment and hospice care is started when the patient is not going to survive the illness and the end of life is nearing.
c. Palliative care can be provided by a patient's primary care provider and hospice care is provided by a certified hospice care agency.
d. Palliative care specializes in only the different forms of therapy that a patient needs and hospice care specializes in end of life comfort care.

25. An adult with asthma is using his levalbuterol (Xopenex) inhaler daily. He also is woken up with wheezing a few times a month. Which of the following should be started at this time?

a. Inhaled long-acting beta agonist.
b. Inhaled steroid plus a long-acting beta agonist.
c. Nebulized short-acting beta agonist.
d. Oral steroid on a tapering dose.

26. During a routine assessment, the AGCNS notices a patient has some dryness of his conjunctivae with white patches present there. This is indicative of a deficiency in which vitamin?

a. A.
b. B_{12}.
c. D.
d. Niacin.

27. A 54-year-old female is taking levothyroxine 0.125 mg daily. Her most recent labs show TSH increased at 8.1 and T4 decreased at 4.2. What is the most appropriate step to take next?

a. Continue the levothyroxine at the current dosage and recheck labs at her next follow-up.
b. Decrease the levothyroxine dosage to 0.1 mg daily and recheck labs in 6-8 weeks.
c. Increase the levothyroxine dosage to 0.137 mg daily and recheck labs in 6-8 weeks.
d. Increase the levothyroxine dosage to 0.3 mg daily and recheck labs in 6-8 weeks.

28. Of the following, the illness that requires airborne precautions be followed is:

a. influenza.
b. rubella (German measles).
c. varicella (chickenpox).
d. pertussis (whooping cough).

29. In order for a patient with congestive heart failure to qualify for Hospice care, which of the following requirements must be met?

a. One or more hospitalizations for a CHF-related flare-up within the past year.
b. Symptoms are well-controlled with medications, but the patient is noncompliant and suffers frequent exacerbations because of the disease.
c. Along with CHF, there is a concomitant diagnosis of coronary artery disease or COPD.
d. The patient's ejection fraction is measured at <20% and there are symptoms at rest despite maximum medical treatment.

30. A 65-year-old male with a history of coronary artery disease and hypertension presents with altered mental status for the past 2 hours. On exam, his BP is 220/120 mm Hg and papilledema is seen on funduscopic exam. Which of the following should be started immediately?

a. Enalapril.
b. Hydralazine.
c. Labetalol.
d. Nitroglycerin.

31. A 75-year-old man is seen with complaints of dyspnea on exertion and bilateral ankle swelling. He has a history of hypertension and COPD, both of which have been well-controlled. On exam, he has 2 cm of JVD and 2+ pitting edema at the ankles. Which abnormal sound would the AGCNS expect to hear during his cardiac exam?

a. An ejection click.
b. A thrill.
c. S_3.
d. S_4.

32. Which of the following is indicative of right-sided heart failure?

a. Elevated jugular venous pressure.
b. Hypotension.
c. Interstitial edema on chest x-ray.
d. Significant orthopnea.

33. An AGCNS is seeing a gentleman who underwent a total hip replacement 2 weeks ago. He has complaints of shortness of breath and pain in the lower leg in which he had the hip surgery. Which of the following studies is the best for confirming the suspected diagnosis?

a. D-dimer serum test.
b. P/V scintigraphy.
c. Pulmonary angiogram.
d. Spiral CT of the chest.

34. An AGCNS sees a patient who would like to have a skin lesion removed. The lesion is on her upper arm, is 4 mm round with well-defined margins. She had noticed that it was black, but she thinks it has developed some purple discoloration recently. The best way to assess this would be:

a. excisional biopsy.
b. KOH prep.
c. punch biopsy.
d. Wood's lamp assessment.

35. A 65-year-old female has a long history of untreated hypercalcemia. The finding that the AGCNS would also be expect to find is:

a. a DEXA score of 2.0.
b. decreased thirst.
c. shortness of breath.
d. nephrolithiasis.

36. A 59-year-old male is seen for complaints of a tremor in his right hand when he is at rest. On exam, he has a resting tremor, no arm movement when walking, and cog wheeling in the shoulders. The most likely diagnosis is:

a. multiple sclerosis.
b. Huntington's disease.
c. amyotrophic lateral sclerosis.
d. Parkinson's disease.

37. Which of the following is more likely to occur in COPD due to emphysema as opposed to COPD due to bronchitis?

a. Dyspnea on exertion.
b. Peripheral edema.
c. Productive cough.
d. Weight loss.

38. In the patient with complaints of decreased hearing in the left ear due to impacted cerumen, what finding would one expect to see on a Weber test?

a. Sound is heard longer through the air than through bone in the left ear.
b. Sound is heard longer through bone than through the air in the left ear.
c. Sound would lateralize to the left ear.
d. Sound would lateralize to the right ear.

39. A 52-year-old male has started to play golf after several years of not playing. He has developed pain over the medial side of the right elbow. What would the AGCNS expect to find on physical exam?

a. Bulging of the biceps muscle.
b. Pain with a valgus stress of the elbow.
c. Pain with resisted wrist extension.
d. Pain with resisted wrist flexion.

40. The rash that can be seen with Stevens-Johnson Syndrome can be described as:

a. a pale pink, papular rash on the extremities.
b. target-like lesions with the center being a vesicle, purpuric, or necrotic, surrounded by erythema.
c. a widely scattered vesicular rash that crusts over after the lesions rupture.
d. a lacy-type rash scattered all over the body.

41. Which of the following patients would be most likely to show impairment on the Mini Mental Status Exam?

a. A 54-year-old female attorney with mild short-term memory impairment.
b. A 62-year-old male college professor with moderate short-term memory impairment.
c. A 57-year-old male engineer with very mild short-term memory impairment.
d. A 67-year-old male, educated through grade 6, with moderate short-term memory impairment.

42. Which of the following patients would be a candidate for a left ventricular assist device (LVAD)?

a. A 73-year-old male with chronic atrial fibrillation.
b. A 55-year-old female with worsening mitral valve prolapse.
c. A 62-year-old male with coronary artery disease who had 3 cardiac stents placed within the past year.
d. A 57-year-old male with end-stage congestive heart failure undergoing evaluation for a heart transplant.

43. Which of the following is not normally examined when assessing a patient's functional status?

a. Learned activities of daily living.
b. Basic activities of daily living.
c. Intermediate activities of daily living.
d. Advanced activities of daily living.

44. One of the first signs of a urinary tract infection in an 86-year-old female patient is:

a. dysuria.
b. confusion.
c. urinary frequency.
d. polydipsia.

45. Which of the following patients is at most risk for developing an abdominal aortic aneurysm?

a. A 75-year-old female smoker with hypertension, well-controlled with medication.
b. A 51-year-old male, non-smoker, with elevated LDL cholesterol.
c. A 79-year-old male smoker with hypertension, hypercholesterolemia, and COPD.
d. A 62-year-old male smoker with no chronic medical problems.

46. A 65-year-old man has had chest pain that was diagnosed as angina. When taking his history, he tells his AGCNS that he is a heavy smoker, drinks alcohol daily, has a very poor diet, drinks a lot of caffeine every day, and does not exercise. What is the most important lifestyle change he should make?

a. Quit drinking alcohol.
b. Quit smoking.
c. Improve his diet.
d. Start a regular exercise routine.

47. A definitive diagnosis of Parkinson's disease is made with:

a. the presence of neurofibrillary tangles on brain MRI.
b. the development of hallucinations and dementia-type symptoms.
c. frequent falls due to shuffling gait.
d. the presence of at least two of the four main symptoms of Parkinson's disease.

48. A 52-year-old male is seen in the office for complaints of left great toe pain. He woke up this morning with the pain and rates his pain level as a 10/10. He denies any trauma. On exam, the left great toe is erythematous and edematous with significant pain with movement or palpation. The lab test that would be most appropriate at this time is:

a. a uric acid level.
b. a chemistry panel.
c. a CBC.
d. no lab tests are available to diagnose this condition.

49. All of the following are early signs/symptoms of temporal arteritis EXCEPT:

a. headache.
b. jaw pain.
c. loss of vision.
d. tenderness of the scalp.

50. The EKG changes that are seen with severe hyperkalemia include:

a. absent P waves, a prolonged PR segment, ST depression, and inverted T waves.
b. prolonged QRS, a bundle branch block, sinus bradycardia, and a sine wave.
c. sinus tachycardia rhythm with ST segment elevation.
d. irregularly irregular rhythm with rate usually >120 and inverted T waves.

51. An elderly female patient has a nasogastric drain. The results of her arterial blood gases are as follows: pH 7.5, HCO_3 31, pCO_2 37. Based on these values, which acid-base disorder has this patient developed?

a. Respiratory alkalosis.
b. Respiratory acidosis.
c. Metabolic alkalosis.
d. Metabolic acidosis.

52. The T-score the AGCNS would expect to see on the DEXA scan of an osteopenic female is:

a. -1.0 to -2.5.
b. less than -2.5.
c. -1.0 to 1.0.
d. 1.0 to 2.0.

53. An AGCNS would expect the results of a pulmonary function test (PFT) in an asthmatic patient to be:

a. FEV_1 90%, FVC 92%, FEV_1/FVC 97%.
b. FEV_1 70%, FVC 83%, FEV_1/FVC 84%.
c. FEV_1 94%, FVC 90%, FEV_1/FVC 100%.
d. FEV_1 89%, FVC 84%, FEV_1/FVC 104%.

54. The diagnostic test of choice in a patient with coffee grounds emesis and dark tarry stools is:

a. abdominal CT scan.
b. colonoscopy.
c. upper endoscopy.
d. upper GI series.

55. The modifiable risk factors used to calculate cardiac risk are:

a. age, HDL cholesterol, LDL cholesterol, and smoking history.
b. gender, total cholesterol, blood pressure, and smoking history.
c. smoking history, HDL cholesterol, total cholesterol, and systolic blood pressure.
d. age, gender, LDL cholesterol, and HDL cholesterol.

56. A decubitus ulcer that has exposed adipose tissue and eschar present would be classified as:

a. stage III.
b. stage II.
c. stage I.
d. an unstageable ulcer.

57. Which of the following is true regarding an asymptomatic patient with a positive PPD test?

a. The patient has latent tuberculosis.
b. The patient is contagious.
c. Pharmacotherapy is not needed.
d. The patient should be in respiratory isolation.

58. What is the rationale for initiating beta blocker therapy in a patient with congestive heart failure?

a. Beta blockers are contraindicated in patients with CHF.
b. Beta blockers will reduce catecholamine stimulation in patients with CHF.
c. Beta blockers will stimulate serotonin release to improve mood and decrease anxiety.
d. Beta blockers can help improve renal function.

59. During an annual physical of a 35-year-old female, small granulomatous nodules are seen in the bilateral conjunctivae. Based on that finding, further work-up should be done for:

a. systemic lupus erythematosus.
b. multiple sclerosis.
c. rheumatoid arthritis.
d. sarcoidosis.

60. Most patients with plaque psoriasis are eligible candidates for treatment with a biologic if the disease is considered severe. All of the following are considered severe characteristics of psoriasis EXCEPT:

a. thickened plaques that do not respond to topical treatments.
b. lesions covering more than 5-10% of the body.
c. significant psoriatic arthritis.
d. severe impact on quality of life.

61. The recommended treatment for chronic lymphocytic leukemia after initial diagnosis, is usually:

a. chemotherapy.
b. radiation.
c. combination of chemotherapy and radiation.
d. continue to monitor for progression of the disease.

62. One of the differences in symptom presentation with Crohn's disease versus ulcerative colitis is:

a. Crohn's disease is more likely to cause rectal bleeding.
b. Crohn's disease is less likely to cause rectal bleeding.
c. Crohn's disease is more likely to cause occasional abdominal pain versus chronic pain with ulcerative colitis.
d. Crohn's disease is less likely to cause perianal symptoms such as fistulas and skin breakdown.

63. The mineral that is often very low after the administration of intravenous Lasix is:

a. calcium.
b. magnesium.
c. iron.
d. fluoride.

64. The form of macular degeneration associated with deterioration of the central retina is:

a. wet macular degeneration.
b. congenital macular degeneration.
c. dry macular degeneration.
d. acquired macular degeneration.

65. What is the most common cause of ARDS, or acute respiratory distress syndrome?

a. Congestive heart failure.
b. Sepsis.
c. COPD.
d. Malignant hypertension.

66. The most common cause of a small bowel obstruction in an elderly patient is:

a. use of multiple pain medications.
b. frequent laxative use.
c. history of past abdominal surgery.
d. uncontrolled diabetes mellitus.

67. Of the following, the food that is most likely to cause a flare-up of gout is:

a. broccoli.
b. oranges.
c. trout.
d. peanut butter.

68. The most common cause of petechiae is:

a. excessive straining.
b. endocarditis.
c. warfarin therapy.
d. thrombocytopenia.

69. A 48-year-old male has abdominal obesity with a waist circumference of 45 inches. He is also being treated for hypertension and blood pressure is 142/90. The third finding that would confirm a diagnosis of metabolic syndrome is:

a. fasting glucose of 98 mg/dL.
b. HDL cholesterol 45 mg/dL.
c. LDL cholesterol 120 mg/dL.
d. triglycerides 200 mg/dL.

70. In the patient with COPD, a long-acting bronchodilator should be used:

a. after prednisone has been given for at least 3 months and is not controlling the symptoms.
b. as a first-line treatment.
c. in nebulizer form only.
d. when a short-acting inhaler is not adequate in controlling symptoms throughout the day.

71. A geriatric patient with anemia is receiving a blood transfusion. The AGCNS would be alerted to a possible transfusion reaction if the patient develops:

a. dysuria.
b. the hiccups.
c. ear pain.
d. tenderness at the IV site.

72. Current recommendations for screening mammography in women 75-years-old and older state:

a. annual mammography screening should be performed until it is deemed unnecessary due to other medical co-morbidities.
b. screening mammography should be performed in this age group every 2 years.
c. screening mammography is not recommended for women in this age group.
d. annual mammography screening should be performed for all women until death or end-of-life issues are present.

73. When teaching tracheostomy care at home, it is important the caregivers understand:

a. cleaning and changing the trach tube must be done under sterile conditions.
b. the trach tube can be reused after it has been cleaned properly.
c. the trach tube can only be changed by a Respiratory Therapist who will come to the home.
d. a new, sterile trach tube must be used each day.

74. The diet that would be most appropriate for the geriatric patient hospitalized with liver disease is:

a. low sodium, high carbohydrate.
b. high protein.
c. low carbohydrate, high protein.
d. non-dairy, high protein.

75. The level of care received by the patient who sees a Cardiologist and is then admitted to the hospital for coronary artery bypass grafting is:

a. primary care.
b. secondary care.
c. tertiary care.
d. terminal care.

76. The recommendations for colorectal cancer screening apply to those adults:

a. age 40-80.
b. age 45-75.
c. age 55-80.
d. age 50-75.

77. One of the benefits of adopting a patient- and family-centered plan of care is:

a. relieving the burden on patients in making healthcare decisions and transferring that responsibility to the family instead.
b. increasing and improving communication between the staff and patients and families.
c. to decrease the amount of money spent on improving facilities.
d. to increase the length of hospital stays to ensure that all members of the healthcare team are collaborating on a patient's care.

78. The purpose of using a clinical pathway when caring for a patient with a specific problem is:

a. to allow each member of the healthcare team to individualize their plan of care for the patient.
b. to explore new, or more experimental, treatments for a patient.
c. to provide a template for standardized care for a patient while helping to control medical costs.
d. to more easily enroll the patient into a clinical trial to treat their condition.

79. An AGCNS has seen a patient and prescribed an antibiotic for an ear infection. The pharmacy calls shortly after they leave to say the medication is not covered by insurance and it is very expensive. The most appropriate response is:

a. unfortunately, there is no other option than to treat the infection with that particular medication.
b. the patient should try to contact the pharmaceutical company to see if he can get approved for their patient assistance program.
c. call in a less expensive antibiotic to the pharmacy.
d. the insurance should be contacted to see if a prior authorization or another process can be completed to get drug coverage.

80. An 82-year-old male is seen for a laceration on his left hand. He builds sculptures out of scrap metal as a hobby and occasionally suffers a laceration. He is unsure when he last received a tetanus shot. The best medical advice that could be provided would be:

a. tetanus shots are no longer necessary after the age of 75.
b. tetanus has been eradicated in the U.S. and shots are no longer necessary.
c. only major trauma or surgery require a tetanus shot.
d. he should receive a tetanus shot today to reduce his risk of developing the disease.

81. When preparing a treatment plan for a patient, it is imperative that it include:

a. a very specific, refined goal that is to be reached.
b. multiple goals that will need to be reached.
c. measurable objectives for the identified goal.
d. one measurable objective per identified goal.

82. A 17-year-old girl is prescribed Cipro for treatment of a UTI. She and her mother should be told that:

a. there is a chance that this antibiotic could permanently stain her teeth.
b. she will need to return for blood work after she has finished the antibiotic to check her liver function tests.
c. avoid taking any ibuprofen while taking Cipro.
d. she should not drink any milk or milk products 2 hours before and 4 hours after taking the antibiotic.

83. The AGCNS have ordered a dopamine infusion for a patient in the ICU. Once it is completed, the effects from the medication should be gone:

a. within 10 minutes.
b. within 1 hour.
c. within 4 hours.
d. within 12 hours.

84. A normally healthy male presents to the ER with complaints of productive cough and fever for the past three days. Chest x-rays reveals a small infiltrate in the right lower lobe. The most appropriate antibiotic therapy for this patient is:

a. azithromycin 500 mg PO on day one, then 250 mg PO once daily for 4 days.
b. ceftriaxone 1 g IM today, followed by doxycycline 100 mg PO twice daily for 10 days.
c. amoxicillin 875 mg PO twice daily for 10 days.
d. no antibiotic therapy is necessary because the cause of these findings is most likely viral.

85. A pre-menopausal woman who has been treated for breast cancer is taking tamoxifen. She asks her AGCNS how long she will need to take this medication. The most appropriate answer is:

a. two years following treatment of the cancer.
b. five years following treatment of the cancer.
c. seven years following treatment of the cancer.
d. ten years following treatment of the cancer.

86. A contraindication for using gentamicin ear drops to treat otitis externa is:

a. renal failure.
b. a perforated ear drum.
c. liver failure.
d. hearing loss.

87. Appropriate dosing of valacyclovir for treatment of a herpes zoster infection in a patient with normal kidney function is:

a. 1 g PO three times daily for 7 days.
b. 500 mg PO twice daily for 10 days.
c. 1 g PO twice daily for 10 days.
d. 500 mg PO three times daily for 7 days.

88. A 69-year-old male is taking Plavix for a history of coronary artery disease. His cardiac condition has been stable, but he requires treatment for GERD symptoms. The medication that is most appropriate to treat these symptoms is:

a. Nexium.
b. Prilosec.
c. Pepcid.
d. Dexilant.

89. A 64-year-old male has type 2 diabetes that has not been well-controlled with metformin alone. His past medical history is significant for hypertension, hypercholesterolemia, congestive heart failure, and coronary artery disease. Which of the following medications would be contraindicated in this patient?

a. Byetta.
b. Glipizide.
c. Actos.
d. Lantus insulin.

90. A 52-year-old obese male is seen for a routine medical checkup after several years without medical care. After review of screening labs, he is started on atorvastatin for hyperlipidemia and metformin for type 2 diabetes mellitus. His blood pressure was 188/100 in the office and he says it has been close to that when his wife has checked it at home. The most appropriate antihypertensive medication to start him on at this time would be:

a. metoprolol.
b. lisinopril.
c. hydrochlorothiazide.
d. carvedilol.

91. Which of the following antibiotics may cause an allergic response cross-reaction in a patient with a penicillin allergy?

a. Cefdinir.
b. Azithromycin.
c. Ciprofloxacin.
d. Sulfamethoxazole.

92. Why are albuterol and ipratropium (Duoneb) given together?

a. Adding ipratropium to the albuterol decreases the tremors that are often associated with albuterol.
b. The albuterol requires ipratropium be present to aid in absorption of the drug in the airway.
c. These two drugs are not available on their own, only as a combination medication.
d. They work together by causing dilation of the airway (ipratropium) along with relaxation of the bronchial smooth muscle (albuterol).

93. The medication that will require a dosage adjustment in the patient with renal failure is:

a. lisinopril.
b. hydrochlorothiazide.
c. vitamin D.
d. ranitidine (Zantac).

94. A 67-year-old male presents to the clinic with complaints of vision changes causing some yellowish discoloration in his visual field. He has a past medical history of hypertension, coronary artery disease, and congestive heart failure. He is currently taking lisinopril, metoprolol, digoxin, and Plavix. Which of these medications is most likely causing his symptoms?

a. Plavix.
b. Metoprolol.
c. Digoxin.
d. Lisinopril.

95. Which of the following drugs would be least likely to help with the bradykinesia associated with Parkinson's disease?

a. Amantadine.
b. Anticholinergics.
c. Levodopa.
d. MAOIs.

96. A 72-year-old male with type 2 diabetes mellitus is seen for irritation inside his mouth. On exam, he has white, cheesy-like lesions in his mouth that can easily be scraped off with a tongue depressor. The most appropriate therapy for this is:

a. acyclovir.
b. fluconazole.
c. penicillin.
d. prednisone.

97. A patient has had GERD-type symptoms for a couple of months and tests positive for *Helicobacter pylori* infection. The treatment regimen consists of:

a. amoxicillin, bismuth subsalicylate, and a proton pump inhibitor.
b. amoxicillin, clarithromycin, and a proton pump inhibitor.
c. clarithromycin, tetracycline, and bismuth subsalicylate.
d. a proton pump inhibitor alone.

98. A 52-year-old male is diagnosed with an uncomplicated UTI. The antibiotic that would be the least effective for this patient is:

a. ciprofloxacin.
b. levofloxacin.
c. nitrofurantoin.
d. trimethoprim-sulfamethoxazole.

99. A 42-year-old male with rheumatoid arthritis is beginning to develop increased symptoms with joint pain and deformity. His past medical history is significant for Hodgkin's' lymphoma as a teenager and he has been in remission for 27 years. He is also being treated for hypertension and hypercholesterolemia, both well-controlled with medications. Based on his history, which factor is a contraindication for treatment with a biologic agent for his RA symptoms?

a. Age.
b. History of lymphoma.
c. Hypertension.
d. Hypercholesterolemia.

100. A 63-year-old female is seen for a dental abscess because she cannot get in with her Dentist for another week. Her past medical history is significant for a cardiac stent one year ago, hypothyroidism, hypertension, and hyperlipidemia. She is taking Plavix, levothyroxine, lisinopril, and atorvastatin. Based on her history, which antibiotic would be contraindicated?

a. Amoxicillin.
b. Clarithromycin.
c. Amoxicillin-clavulanate.
d. Trimethoprim-sulfamethoxazole.

101. The pain reliever that would be the safest for treating arthritis knee pain in an elderly patient is:

a. acetaminophen.
b. naproxen.
c. ibuprofen.
d. diclofenac.

102. The purpose of nursing informatics is to:

a. streamline the communication process among health care providers.
b. form a database that can be used by nurses at all professional levels to promote networking.
c. utilize input from all levels of nursing care to formulate information technology resources to provide better care to patients.
d. integrate nursing science with analytics to communicate data and information.

103. The criteria set forth for utilizing the electronic health record in order to provide coordinated care and improve patient quality and safety is:

a. meaningful use.
b. health measures.
c. quality management.
d. clinical analytics.

104. Which of the following is true regarding provider-patient boundaries?

a. It is acceptable for a provider's involvement with a patient to extend into personal or business relationships.
b. It is reasonable to believe that the CNS, as the patient's provider, are the only one who really understands the patient or who can help the patient.
c. It is appropriate to divert personal questions the patient has about the CNS or CNS's family back to the patient to focus the attention on the patient's problems.
d. It is appropriate to meet with a patient somewhere outside of work to discuss any problems they are having.

105. When communicating with a non-English speaking patient and her family, it is best to:

a. have another family member serve as an interpreter, if possible.
b. improvise using pictures and video to teach the patient about their medical care.
c. hold most of the conversation through an online translating program.
d. arrange to have an interpreter familiar with medical terminology present.

106. One of the main advantages to using the Teach-Back system for educating patients and their families is:

a. improving education documentation in the patient's medical record.
b. to ensure that information that is taught is fully understood.
c. to limit the number of people involved in the patient's care.
d. to meet staff continuing medical education credit requirements.

107. The goal of the Quality and Safety Education for Nurses initiative is to:

a. provide extensive education for nurses so they can go on to assist in meeting quality measures and meaningful use goals.
b. prepare nurses so they can go forth and improve the quality and safety of the health care system in which they work.
c. establish specific protocols within a healthcare setting that can be used to improve patient safety.
d. ensure the nursing staff within a healthcare setting has completed annual continuing education course requirements.

108. The purpose of quality improvement is to:

a. improve employee satisfaction.
b. monitor the leadership skills of the administration of a healthcare facility.
c. implement specific changes in healthcare which have a measurable improvement for a group of patients.
d. provide specific training and education opportunities to employees to ensure the quality of the care provided is reaching high standards.

109. The measure in place to protect patients from unsafe or incompetent practice is the:

a. Nurse Practice Act.
b. Nurse Competency Act.
c. Nurse Oversight Committee Act.
d. Medical Peer Review Act.

110. The AGCNS receives a phone call from a local cardiologist's office requesting the discharge summary on a patient who was recently hospitalized whom the CNS cared for. The best response is:

a. they must first fax over a release of information form signed by the patient.
b. it will be faxed right over to them.
c. they must ask the patient to obtain this for them.
d. the information must be mailed and cannot be faxed.

111. What is informatics as it pertains to healthcare?

a. The study of the legalities of patient confidentiality.
b. A healthcare information program that enables students of the medical sciences to easily access core medical knowledge.
c. A model of communication used by healthcare corporations to inform employees of changes in policy.
d. The combination of computer science with healthcare.

112. Which of the following is the responsibility of the referring provider in a consultation?

a. Explain to the patient the purpose for a consultation and the name of the consulting provider.
b. Contact the patient's insurance carrier to request a peer-to-peer review for any future treatments.
c. Inform the patient that they will need to seek the services of a provider within a certain specialty on their own.
d. Wait for a request for records and any diagnostic testing that has been completed.

113. The Thomas-Kilmann Instrument is used for:

a. hip replacement surgery.
b. assessing a patient's respiratory status.
c. conflict resolution.
d. creating ergonomic work environments.

114. What is the definition of cultural encounter?

a. A negative interaction between a healthcare provider and someone who is of a different cultural background.
b. Encouraging medical professionals to interact with those of a different cultural background from their own.
c. A coordinated effort between two cultural groups to gather and work through their differences.
d. The egocentric behaviors of a set of individuals who are intolerant of those from a different culture.

115. Which of the following situations would require the services of a content expert?

a. A hospital launching a new electronic health record program.
b. A private medical practice changing their policy regarding pharmaceutical representative visits.
c. A change in the hospital employee parking area while renovations are being made at the facility.
d. The decision of a hospital advisory board expanding their members to include a Clinical Nurse Specialist.

116. A poster presentation should:

a. explain in detail the purpose of the presentation.
b. be made up of illustrations with very little language content.
c. provide a summary of the work with features that will engage viewers so that they will want to learn more.
d. contain more information than the paper it represents.

117. The difference between a preceptor and a mentor is:

a. a mentor is performing job evaluations and identifying training needs while a preceptor carries out the training needs.
b. a preceptor provides hands-on training or orienting in a new position while a mentor provides encouragement and feedback when a problem is encountered.
c. a mentor is a general co-worker and a preceptor is a supervising or charge nurse responsible for disciplinary action on the job.
d. a preceptor provides guidance when requested and a mentor is in charge of peer review proceedings.

118. The nursing model that promotes group accountability and responsibility in decision making using basic values and belief systems is:

a. evidence-based nursing practice.
b. professional practice model.
c. shared governance.
d. relationship-based care.

119. The core principles of the humanistic learning theory encourage:

a. following a strict doctrine when teaching without variation.
b. promoting pro-life opinions.
c. simplifying information to ensure different people will understand it.
d. emotional, mental, and physical health.

120. A role model in nursing is different than a preceptor or mentor in that the role model:

a. is looked up to for their professionalism and clinical skills without holding a formal responsibility to educate others.
b. has a more hands-on approach to providing training to nursing students.
c. has more responsibility in regards to making hiring decisions.
d. is responsible for providing all of the professional constructive criticism to new nurses.

121. The certification exams available for the clinical nurse specialist including all of the following EXCEPT:

a. Critical Care.
b. Adult/Gerontology.
c. Pediatrics.
d. Neonatal.

122. An acquaintance that an AGCNS is friends with on Facebook is seen for a UTI. Two days after her appointment, she messages the CNS requesting the results of her urine culture. The most appropriate response is to:

a. reply with the urine culture and susceptibility results, but make sure it is sent as a private message that no others can view.
b. post on her Facebook account that, based on the culture results, she was prescribed the appropriate antibiotic and she should be feeling well soon.
c. send her a text message on her phone with the urine culture results.
d. reply to the message that they are not able to share any personal medical information through social media and she would need to contact the office for those results.

123. The clinical nurse specialist nurse functions as a patient advocate by:

a. reporting any medication errors that occur involving the patient.
b. following the Clinical Pathway for the patient's diagnosis.
c. not sharing any personal information the patient has shared.
d. protecting the health, safety, and rights of the patient.

124. In order to obtain the certification to be an Adult-Gerontology Clinical Nurse Specialist, the provider must have completed:

a. an LPN program, RN program, and an accredited masters level nursing program.
b. an RN program and an accredited master's degree program.
c. an accredited master's degree program only.
d. an LPN program and an RN program.

125. Regarding the legal authority to prescribe medications, the clinical nurse specialist:

a. has full prescriptive authority in all states for all categories of medications.
b. has full prescriptive authority in all states for non-controlled medications, but cannot prescribe any controlled substances.
c. has variable prescriptive rights depending on the state laws in which they practice.
d. is not allowed to prescribe any medications in the United States.

126. Capacity as it refers to medical issues is defined as:

a. the assessment of a person's ability to understand and interpret information in order to make decisions, as determined by a medical evaluation.
b. a legal term that defines whether a person has the mental competence to make legal decisions.
c. the amount of information a person can interpret at one time to be an informed decision maker in their health care.
d. the approved amount of medical services a person can receive within a given time period as determined by their insurance carrier.

127. An elderly Orthodox Jewish man has died after suffering multiple strokes. The AGCNS knows that before his body is transported from the hospital:

a. all of the family members must come in his room one by one to pay their respects.
b. any machines should be disconnected, but no tubes or probes should be removed from his body.
c. the body should be stripped and washed thoroughly.
d. he should be dressed in his regular clothes rather than a hospital gown.

128. One of the goals of the Healthy People 2020 program is to:

a. acknowledge those individuals who have excelled at promoting health and wellness in their communities.
b. set up a program that rewards those who have lost the most weight by the year 2020.
c. establish surroundings that encourage healthy living.
d. decrease the number of fast food establishments in communities by the year 2020.

129. The medical service that is covered under Medicare Part A is:

a. durable medical equipment.
b. appointments with a primary care provider.
c. appointments with a specialist.
d. prescription drug coverage.

130. The practice by which the clinical nurse specialist has an ongoing commitment to apply the knowledge and skills necessary to practice safely and effectively is known as:

a. quality control.
b. professional role playing.
c. shared governance.
d. continued competence.

131. Which of the following is a certifying body for the clinical nurse specialist?

a. American Medical Association.
b. Certification of clinical nurse specialists is optional and performed at the state level.
c. American Nurses Credentialing Center.
d. There is no certification requirement to be a clinical nurse specialist.

132. The rate of reimbursement under Medicare for the clinical nurse specialist is:

a. 100%, equal to that of the physician's reimbursement.
b. 80% of the physician's reimbursement.
c. 75% of the physician's reimbursement.
d. 50% of the physician's reimbursement.

133. An example of a third-party payer is:

a. the patient.
b. the patient's employer.
c. a health insurance company.
d. a worker's compensation coverage company.

134. What is benchmarking as it relates to nursing?

a. When an organization reaches record levels of success in a particular field.
b. When an organization undergoes a review process for a particular level of care provided.
c. When an organization is identified for being a leader within a particular field of medicine.
d. When an organization compares its processes to other organizations.

135. The information that is used to determine the benefits of health care to be provided is called:

a. a cost-benefit analysis.
b. an analytics outcome report.
c. a quality measure review.
d. a risk-benefit outcome.

136. The purpose of quality improvement is to:

a. improve employee satisfaction.
b. monitor the leadership skills of the administration of a healthcare facility.
c. implement specific changes in healthcare which have a measurable improvement for a group of patients.
d. provide specific training and education opportunities to employees to ensure the quality of the care provided is reaching high standards.

137. The organization responsible for providing accreditation to thousands of health care organizations in the United States is:

a. The National Hospital Review Board.
b. The Commission on Accreditation and Review.
c. The U.S. Food and Drug Administration.
d. The Joint Commission.

138. The theory that provides a way of describing, analyzing, understanding, and improving systems is called:

a. feedback theory.
b. organizational theory.
c. distributed benefit theory.
d. quality control theory.

139. The most relevant comprehensive list of diseases and their billing codes established by the World Health Organization is:

a. the ICD-10.
b. the ICD-9.5.
c. the ICD-9.
d. the CPT.

140. The basic principle behind the transformational style of leadership in healthcare is:

a. a pyramid-type structure of managerial leadership with one person leading and the rest following.
b. having multiple leaders who come to a consensus regarding managerial decisions.
c. leadership raising the motivation and morality among those under them to empower them.
d. the method of rotating managers, or leaders, to allow for different perspectives in the leadership role.

141. Clinical pathways have been criticized as being potentially harmful to the patient because:

a. they increase the out of pocket medical expenses.
b. a patient may be discharged from the hospital earlier than they should be.
c. they do not allow for flexibility and individualizing a plan of care for the patient.
d. they may result in more medication errors.

142. The ACO health care delivery model:

a. is available under only certain health insurance plans.
b. was a failed attempt at streamlining patient care across the healthcare spectrum by organizing all aspects of care into one location.
c. focuses on the whole patient and requires all specialties and treatment modalities coordinate their treatment of the patient.
d. uses a traditional transaction-based reimbursement plan.

143. Which of the following can be a sign of excessive stress in the work environment?

a. Good working relationships with co-workers.
b. Insomnia.
c. Having an alcoholic drink twice a month during a social outing.
d. Using all of one's allotted vacation days each year.

144. A set of orders pre-written for a specific diagnosis is called a(n):

a. medication administration record (MAR).
b. Pyxis.
c. care plan.
d. order set.

145. The concept that emphasizes learning and accountability rather than blame and punishment when reporting medical errors is called:

a. just culture.
b. risk stratification.
c. self-reporting.
d. quality improvement.

146. What is an evidence-based clinical practice guideline?

a. A comprehensive listing of research data gathered on a specific subject.
b. An algorithm created for the nursing and support staff to follow when caring for a patient.
c. The standards that all hospital staff are held to according to the institution's employee handbook.
d. A set of recommendations for the care that should be provided to a patient with a specific condition.

147. The method for examining a process for potential failures, and the potential impact of these failures, is called:

a. a quality improvement analysis.
b. a failure modes and effects analysis.
c. a root cause analysis.
d. a gap analysis.

148. What is a root cause analysis?

a. The process of identifying who is at fault for a medical error that has occurred.
b. An evaluation performed to determine why hospital profits are decreasing.
c. A method of problem solving used to identify the root cause of a problem that has occurred.
d. Identifying an individual or department within an organization that has improved a process.

149. The comparison between actual performance and desired performance within an organization is called:

a. gap analysis.
b. quality analysis.
c. actual goal analysis.
d. outcome performance analysis.

150. Which of the following is a resource used for process improvement?

a. Joint Commission accreditation standards.
b. Practice inquiry and innovation.
c. Cost/benefit analysis.
d. National Patient Safety Goals.

151. What is a care bundle?

a. Materials sent home with a patient following hospitalization to help them perform self-care.
b. An evaluation of a hospital process to help improve the quality of care.
c. Specific evidence-based practices that help to improve patient outcomes.
d. A multi-specialty team of healthcare providers brought together to evaluate a patient.

152. What are nursing quality indicators?

a. Evaluation gathered from employee reviews regarding nursing performance.
b. Information released quarterly and annually regarding the quality of nursing care at the unit level.
c. A reward system utilized by organizations to recognize those nurses who have high evaluation scores.
d. A tool used for evaluating potential employees to ensure they have received good reviews in the past.

153. All of the following are types of nursing indicators EXCEPT:

a. quality indicators.
b. structural indicators.
c. process indicators.
d. outcome indicators.

154. A nursing home patient is admitted to a local hospital for pneumonia. After one week of a complicated course, it is noted that he has developed a stage 2 pressure ulcer on his right buttock. This would be an example of a(n):

a. structural indicator.
b. process indicator.
c. outcome indicator.
d. sentinel event.

155. A sentinel event is:

a. a sudden decline in patient satisfaction scores.
b. a local national disaster that requires implementation of the hospital's emergency management plan.
c. a situation within a healthcare facility that places the employees and patients in a position of danger.
d. an unplanned incident within a healthcare facility that results in death or psychological damage to a patient.

156. All of the following are examples of a sentinel event EXCEPT:

a. an infant abduction from the newborn nursery.
b. the suicide of a patient one week after discharge from an acute-care setting.
c. surgery on the wrong patient or wrong body part.
d. blood transfusion reaction due to blood group incompatibilities.

157. A patient who has been diagnosed with Lewy body dementia has reached a point at which his wife can no longer care for him at home. She is working on having financial assets placed in her name, but to do so, her attorney has told her that she will need to file the legal documents that say her husband does not have:

a. the capacity to make financial decisions on his own.
b. the legal right to make financial decisions on his own.
c. the competency to make financial decisions on his own.
d. children who can manage his finances for him.

158. In order to accurately code a patient's diagnosis using the ICD-10 coding system, the provider must include:

a. qualifiers.
b. CPT codes.
c. the equivalent ICD-9 code.
d. the differential diagnoses.

159. Delays in the check-in process at a busy Cardiology office have increased patient complaints about being seen much later than their appointment time. This has also led to increased frustration levels with the staff and providers who take these complaints. What could be done to evaluate the cause of the delay to determine how this process could be made more efficient?

a. Gap analysis.
b. Root cause analysis.
c. Quality improvement review.
d. Quality data evaluation.

160. Using standardized instructions and controlling any extraneous variables will improve what aspect of a research study?

a. Control variables.
b. Power analysis.
c. Internal validity.
d. External validity.

161. Which of the following interventions would the AGCNS expect to see on an order set for a patient on a ventilator?

a. Advance to a normal diet as soon as possible.
b. Ambulating the patient daily.
c. Prophylactic antibiotic therapy.
d. DVT prophylaxis.

162. A major academic-based teaching hospital is rolling out an initiative to have patients enroll in an online service which will enable them to access their medical record. They will be able to view lab results, orders for diagnostic studies, and schedule their own appointments. Before this program is instituted, the best way to plan for any potential problems is to perform a:

a. failure modes and effects analysis.
b. gap analysis.
c. root cause analysis.
d. power analysis.

163. A busy Urgent Care is reviewing their patient satisfaction scores regarding wait time to see a provider. They have set a goal of having patients wait no more than 30 minutes to be seen during a busy flu season. The actual wait time has been 40-45 minutes. This evaluation is known as a:

a. clinical practice guideline.
b. sensitivity level.
c. specificity level.
d. gap analysis.

164. When conducting a research study, the element to analyze to determine whether the results will be consistent if the variables are applied to the full population rather than just the study subject sample is:

a. the organizational theory.
b. the level of significance.
c. continuous quality improvement measures.
d. the process improvement analysis.

165. The governmental organization that ensures the safety and protection of humans participating in research studies is the:

a. Drug Enforcement Agency.
b. National Institutes of Health.
c. Office for Human Research Protections.
d. World Health Organization.

166. For an in-office influenza test to be at its most accurate level in diagnosing, it should have:

a. a low sensitivity and a low specificity.
b. a low sensitivity and a high specificity.
c. a high sensitivity and a low specificity.
d. a high sensitivity and a high specificity.

167. Which of the following is an example of how a quality improvement registry can be used to assist in providing appropriate evidence-based care?

a. A registry of diabetic patients that tracks when diabetic eye screening exams should be performed.
b. An automatic computer program that schedules routine chart and file back up for a medical office.
c. An analysis of the flow of check in and registration through discharge during a patient's appointment.
d. Obtaining patient feedback following every encounter with a specific medical office.

168. What process should be completed to compare the actual number of patients being identified for referral for screening colonoscopies, versus the patients who should be referred for these studies based on evidence-based clinical guidelines?

a. An examination of the gap analysis.
b. A comparison of internal and external validity.
c. A healthcare audit.
d. An actual goal analysis.

169. A urine pregnancy test is performed on a 38-year-old female. The result is positive, but a serum pregnancy test is negative with normal hCG levels. The urine test would be considered:

a. a type II error.
b. a type I error.
c. a syntax error.
d. a quality data error.

170. The power of statistical tests is influenced by all of the following EXCEPT:

a. the results of the test.
b. the level of statistical significance.
c. the size of the treatment effect.
d. the sample size.

171. Due to sub-optimal level of sensitivity, the rapid flu tests performed via nasopharyngeal swab have almost a 30% probability of:

a. a type I error.
b. a false positive result.
c. a syntax error.
d. a false negative result.

172. The Hospital Inpatient Quality Reporting Program was started by:

a. Joint Commission.
b. Medicare and Medicaid.
c. Social Security.
d. National Institutes of Health.

173. What is the leading cause of accidental death in the United States?

a. Motor vehicle accidents.
b. Drug overdose.
c. Suicide.
d. Other accidents in the home.

174. Which of the following would not be considered a restraint for a very restless patient who continues to try to remove IVs, oxygen, and other necessary medical equipment?

a. Mittens.
b. Padded wrist bracelets that attach to the bed rail.
c. A prn dose of a benzodiazepine.
d. A Posey vest.

175. Which of the following is an example of an iatrogenic condition?

a. A femur fracture following a motorcycle accident.
b. A self-inflicted gunshot wound.
c. Joint deformities due to rheumatoid arthritis.
d. Hair loss following chemotherapy.

Answer Key and Explanations

1. A: Rales develop with congestive heart failure due to fluid-filled alveoli in the lungs. Wheezing is normally seen with COPD due to airway constriction. Stridor is present with croup.

2. C: Age alone is not a contraindication to undergoing a surgical procedure for ischemic heart disease. Given his other co-morbidities, however, this patient would not be a good surgical candidate. Severe COPD, severe CHF and current chemotherapy treatment for prostate cancer make him vulnerable to complications due to overall weakness of the heart and lungs, and the immunosuppressive effects of chemotherapy.

3. B: Before any plans can be made for possible heart valve replacement surgery, further workup needs to be done to include a cardiac catheterization. Valve replacement surgery is performed only for symptomatic patients who are having shortness of breath, heart failure, or syncopal episodes due to the faulty valve. A valvuloplasty is less effective and has had high restenosis rates.

4. A: A diagnosis at 20-years-old or older is associated with a better outcome. An insidious onset in disease symptoms with a slow rate of progression of the disease are considered to be poorer outcomes. Being from a lower socioeconomic class is also associated with a poor outcome.

5. D: In patients with glaucoma, prednisone orally and any steroid via eye drop should be avoided. These can cause an increase in intraocular pressure, which can worsen glaucoma symptoms. Patients receiving the steroid via an eye drop are going to be more likely to develop the increase in pressure.

6. B: The murmur associated with aortic stenosis is best described as a mid-systolic ejection murmur. It is heard best over the righter, upper sternal border. An early peaking murmur is usually heard with a milder form of the disease while a late peaking murmur is usually heard when the aortic stenosis is more advanced.

7. B: EKG changes consistent with an infarct in the inferior wall are evident in leads II, III, and AVF. An anterior wall infarct is evident in leads I, AVL, and V2-V6. A lateral wall infarct is evident by ST depression, as opposed to ST elevation, in leads I, AVL, and V5-V6. Posterior wall infarcts also show ST depression except in leads V1-V3 where ST elevation is present.

8. A: The left anterior descending artery supplies blood to the anterior wall of the left ventricle and the anterior two-thirds of the interventricular septum. The right coronary artery supplies the posterior heart and the AV node. The left circumflex artery supplies the posterolateral surface of the heart and the left marginal artery supplies the left lateral wall of the heart.

9. C: The daughter must understand that there is no known cure for dementia. Cholinesterase inhibitors have been proven to have some success with controlling some of the symptoms of dementia and in slowing down the progression of the disease. Unfortunately, the symptoms do continue to worsen with time. It is important that patients and families have proper understanding and expectations of treatment measures for dementia.

10. D: Pioglitazone works by decreasing insulin resistance and increasing glucose utilization. Glipizide increases insulin secretion. Metformin lowers blood sugar levels by decreasing glucose production in the liver and increasing glucose utilization. Acarbose works be delaying the absorption of glucose.

11. A: Koilonychia, or "spooning," is most often associated with iron-deficiency anemia. The nails are very thin and may break or chip easily. This usually occurs when the anemia has been present for a lengthy amount of time. Therefore, a CBC is the most appropriate test to conduct first in diagnosing and treating the cause of this condition.

12. D: The symptoms, x-rays, and lab findings are most consistent with a diagnosis of ankylosing spondylitis. This disease is more common in males than females and it effects whites more often than blacks. The age of onset is usually in the late teens or early 20s.

13. D: Magnesium is necessary for potassium uptake and maintenance. If hypokalemia will not improve despite administration of potassium, this may be due to low levels of magnesium preventing the potassium from being used.

14. B: It is no longer recommended that routine, annual PSA screening be performed. It has been found that this often leads to unnecessary prostate biopsy procedures and an increased risk of adverse outcomes from the biopsy. A digital rectal exam is still felt to be a helpful screening tool for prostate lesions.

15. D: Her symptoms and EKG findings are consistent with a 3rd-degree heart block and a temporary pacemaker is necessary until a permanent unit can be surgically implanted. AV block will not respond to atropine. Cardioversion will not be helpful either because she has a functioning sinus node, but her ventricles are not responding appropriately. Atropine is indicated in symptomatic sinus bradycardia.

16. B: The murmur associated with mitral valve stenosis is heard best over the apex of the heart while a patient is standing or performing a Valsalva maneuver. During those activities, the volume within the left ventricle is decreased, which makes the murmur worse. If the patient is squatting, there is an increase in venous return and diastolic filling which will hold the valve shut and decrease the murmur.

17. C: The gold standard for diagnosing temporal arteritis is by temporal artery biopsy. This needs to be performed as soon as possible once the diagnosis is suspected and steroids should be started immediately to begin treatment. The rheumatoid factor is not relevant for this diagnosis and a sedimentation rate is too nonspecific to confirm diagnosis. An ultrasound will also not provide a definitive diagnosis of this condition.

18. C: With Grave's disease, it is not uncommon to see decreased white blood cells and decreased red blood cells on a CBC. It is important to have a baseline CBC before medical treatment is started for the disease because the medication can also cause a slight decrease in neutrophils.

19. C: The current recommendations regarding cervical cancer screening state that Pap smears should be done every 3 years for women age 21 to 65. This can be lengthened to every 5 years with a Pap smear and HPV testing for women age 30 to 65. Screening is not recommended for women under the age of 21 or over the age of 65 if they have never had an abnormal Pap smear in the past.

20. B: NSAIDs such as naproxen have been proven to relieve pain due to osteoarthritis more efficiently than other medications. The anti-inflammatory action of this class of drugs helps to relieve the pain due to degenerative joint disease. While narcotics, such as hydrocodone, are effective at relieving pain, they are not the ideal choice for treating chronic arthritis pain.

21. A: As long as there is still sympathetic and parasympathetic nerve innervation, a light shined into the opposite eye will cause both pupils to constrict. If a light is shined into the blind eye, neither pupil will change.

22. C: Polymyositis is a type of inflammatory myopathy in which only a biopsy of the involved muscle can be used to definitively diagnose the disease. It causes progressive proximal muscle weakness and the facial muscles are spared. The other test choices can be ordered, but their results will not definitively diagnose the condition.

23. D: Polycystic ovarian syndrome can cause the pancreas to secrete more insulin than is necessary. Higher levels of insulin can stimulate the ovaries to make more testosterone than is normal. This increase in testosterone can cause increased facial hair growth and acne.

24. B: Palliative care is often utilized to offer a patient the extra care or therapy they need when faced with a chronic illness. Some palliative care patients will "graduate" from this and others may need to transition to hospice care as their chronic disease progresses.

25. B: Based on his symptoms, this patient has moderate to persistent asthma and would benefit from a combination of an inhaled steroid along with a long-acting beta agonist. An oral steroid tapering dose is usually reserved for acute exacerbations of asthma symptoms.

26. A: A deficiency in vitamin A can cause xerosis, or dry conjunctivae, and the white patches are called Bitot's spots. The patient will often have problems with decreased vision at night. Vitamin A is found in foods rich in beta carotene, such as carrots.

27. C: An increased TSH level and decreased T4 level would indicate mild hypothyroidism and her medication dosage should be increased. It is recommended that levothyroxine be increased in increments of 0.0125 to 0.025 mg and then have labs rechecked before adjusting the medication again.

28. C: An illness that requires airborne precautions be followed means that the virus or bacteria will suspend in the air to be breathed in by another person. Varicella is one of these illnesses, along with SARS, anthrax, and tuberculosis.

29. D: In order for a CHF patient to qualify for hospice care, they must be suffering from chronic, debilitating symptoms of the disease despite being on maximum medical treatment. In addition to this, the ejection fraction should be less than or equal to 20%. Once these conditions are met, the patient is considered a candidate for hospice care.

30. C: Labetalol functions as a beta and alpha-blocker and is the most effective at lowering blood pressure quickly. Enalapril and hydralazine will lower blood pressure, but not as quickly or effectively as the labetalol in this situation. Nitroglycerin is used for patients with chest pain.

31. C: An S3 is present when there is increased resistance in the ventricle as the atria are emptying. It is present with congestive heart failure. An S4 is the extra heart sound heard when there is increased resistance in the ventricle as the atria are contracting. An ejection click is heard with mitral valve prolapse or aortic stenosis. A thrill is felt when a harsh murmur is present.

32. A: Of these symptoms, only the elevated jugular venous pressure is seen in right-sided heart failure. All of the other symptoms listed are present with left-sided heart failure.

33. D: A spiral CT of the chest is the most accurate, non-invasive assessment for a pulmonary embolism. The pulmonary angiogram is considered the gold standard to definitively diagnose, but it is invasive and has its risks. If there is a low probability of a pulmonary embolism, a D-dimer can be performed, and if it is negative, it will rule out the presence of an embolus.

34. A: With the discoloration present in this skin lesion, there is some concern for malignant melanoma. Excisional biopsy with clean margins is the preferred method for removing this lesion for it to be fully assessed. Though the ABCDs are always assessed with skin lesions, not all of the factors need to have negative findings in order for the skin lesion to be concerning.

35. D: Hypercalcemia is due to hyperparathyroidism and can cause kidney stones. Most patients are asymptomatic, but some may have polyuria and polydipsia due to diabetes insipidus. With the elevated serum calcium level, there is decreased calcium in the bones which will affect the DEXA scan score, but this is usually less than -0.1.

36. D: These are the typical symptoms seen with Parkinson's disease. Multiple sclerosis presents with weakness, numbness and paresis that is intermittent. Huntington's disease is genetically acquired and presents with flowing chorea movements and dementia. ALS begins with numbness and weakness in the lower extremities and speech difficulties.

37. D: Weight loss is seen more commonly with emphysema. Dyspnea on exertion can be seen with either emphysema or bronchitis, but it is generally worse with bronchitis. Peripheral edema is more common with bronchitis. A productive cough is common with bronchitis while a dry cough is seen with emphysema.

38. C: Cerumen impaction will cause a conductive hearing loss. This would cause a Weber test to reveal lateralization of the sound to the left ear. With sensorineural hearing loss, air conduction is stronger than bone conduction in the affected test, which is called a Rinne's test.

39. D: His symptoms are consistent with medial epicondylitis. Pain can be reproduced with resisted wrist flexion. Pain on resisted wrist extension is seen with lateral epicondylitis. A biceps muscle bulge would be expected if the biceps muscle had ruptured. A posterior elbow impingement would be most likely to cause pain with a valgus stress of the elbow.

40. B: Stevens-Johnson Syndrome is a reaction that is usually due to a medication exposure or acute illness. It starts with flu-like symptoms of fever, chills, headache, and general malaise. The rash develops with target-like lesions that are initially macular, but then develop into vesicular, purpuric, or necrotic lesions centrally surrounded by a ring of erythema.

41. D: The MMSE is used as a preliminary screening tool for determining whether a patient has some cognitive impairment, however, it does have its limitations. Patients over the age of 60 and those with a low education level have been shown to score lower on the test than others. Further testing and work up is indicated in order to make the diagnosis of dementia and this should not be relied upon alone.

42. D: The LVAD was designed to function as a pump to assist the left ventricle with muscle contraction and increase cardiac output. It is used for patients waiting for a heart transplant and for those who are not a candidate for transplantation, but who will require the device long-term.

43. A: Basic ADLs are those activities which are necessary for basic care. These include bathing, dressing, personal hygiene, and feeding oneself. Intermediate ADLs are more advanced activities, such as cooking, cleaning, driving, and managing medications. Advanced ADLs are the most advanced activities such as performing work duties, fulfilling family responsibilities, and participating in community activities. Learned ADLs are not examined when assessing a patient's functional status.

44. B: A urinary tract infection will usually cause dysuria, urinary frequency, and urinary urgency. These classic symptoms are usually not very pronounced, though, in the elderly population, especially those with underlying dementia, confusion is very common, along with other behavior changes.

45. C: The 79-year-old male smoker with hypertension, hypercholesterolemia, and COPD is at highest risk for developing an abdominal aortic aneurysm. Being of older age and male are the two biggest risk factors to developing an abdominal aortic aneurysm. Other risk factors include hypertension, COPD, smoking, and peripheral arterial disease.

46. B: All of the choices are modifications that should be made to improve his general overall health, but smoking is the leading cause of cardiovascular death. He should work on all of these habits, but the smoking should go first.

47. D: The four main symptoms of Parkinson's disease are a tremor, bradykinesia, stiffness of the extremities or trunk, and postural instability causing frequent falls. At least two of these symptoms must be present in order to make a diagnosis of Parkinson's disease. There is not one, definitive test for Parkinson's disease. Rather, the diagnosis is made based on these clinical findings.

48. A: Acute gout occurs when the body does not excrete enough uric acid and it accumulates within a joint space. A serum uric acid level is usually elevated with this condition. One way to prevent gout flare-ups is to eat a low-purine diet.

49. C: Temporal arteritis is the inflammation of the temporal artery. This inflammation initially causes headaches, pain in the jaw, tenderness of the scalp and changes in vision. If left untreated, a late onset symptom of temporal arteritis is vision loss, therefore it is important to identify and treat this condition based on the early signs and symptoms noted.

50. B: Severe hyperkalemia is classified as a serum potassium level >7 mEq/L. When the potassium level is slightly elevated, tall and peaked T waves can be seen on EKG. As this worsens, the PR segment becomes longer and the P waves eventually disappear. Once severe, the changes listed (prolonged QRS, a bundle branch block, sinus bradycardia, and a sine wave) are present on EKG. If this continues to worsen, it will result in cardiac arrest.

51. C: Metabolic alkalosis will cause the arterial blood pH and bicarbonate levels to increase (normal bicarbonate range is 22-30 mEq/L). Conversely, metabolic acidosis will cause arterial pH and bicarbonate levels to decrease. Respiratory acidosis will increase the arterial carbon dioxide level while decreasing the pH, and respiratory alkalosis will have the opposite results with a decrease in CO2 level and an increased pH.

52. A: The T-score is the measure used with bone densitometry, or DEXA, scans to determine whether someone has adequate bone density, if they are osteopenic, or if they have osteoporosis. A T-score -1.0 or higher is considered normal. A T-score of -1.0 through -2.5 indicates osteopenia is present. A T-score of -2.5 or greater indicates osteoporosis.

53. B: FEV_1 70%, FVC 83%, and FEV_1/FVC 84% indicates asthma. The FEV_1 is the amount of air that can be exhaled within the first second after inhaling the maximum amount of air a person can inhale (the FVC). The normal range for the FEV_1 and the FVC is 80-120%. The FEV_1/FVC ratio is calculated and should be about 85%. A decrease in FEV_1 and the FEV_1/FVC ratio indicates asthma as a diagnosis.

54. C: His symptoms sound more like the source of bleeding could be from the upper portion of the GI tract. Because of this, an upper endoscopy procedure would be best to visualize the esophagus, stomach, and duodenum. A colonoscopy is indicated when the lower GI tract needs further evaluation.

55. C: These are the modifiable risk factors used to calculate a patient's cardiac risk, which identifies whether they have an increased risk of a cardiovascular event occurring. Age and gender are not modifiable risk factors. Identifying those patients with an increased cardiac risk can help to implement a treatment plan to try to prevent the complications of cardiovascular disease.

56. A: Stage I decubitus ulcers exhibit erythematous skin with no breakdown present. Stage II decubitus ulcers have a partial thickness skin loss with the dermis being visible. Stage III decubitus ulcers have a full thickness skin loss with exposed adipose tissue and sometimes eschar present.

57. A: A positive PPD test indicates that the patient has been exposed to someone with tuberculosis, not that they have an active infection themselves. It is recommended that they be further evaluated with a chest x-ray and be treated with medications to prevent activation of the infection.

58. B: Beta blockers have been shown to decrease catecholamine stimulation in patients with CHF. Catecholamine has been found to impair heart function by affecting ejection fraction, ventricular hypertrophy, and even contributing to cardiac muscle cell death. By decreasing the amount of catecholamine present, the heart is not subjected to the potential injury that can occur.

59. D: Sarcoidosis can cause chronic inflammation in the eyes that can cause granulomatous growths in the conjunctiva. Uveitis is another common ocular finding with this disease. Routine eye exams are necessary for patients with this disorder.

60. A: Thickened plaques are not considered a severe characteristic of psoriasis. With severe psoriasis, topical treatments frequently are not strong enough to effectively decrease the lesions. For third party payment purposes, the failure of methotrexate to effectively control the symptoms of psoriasis is usually required for approval for treatment with a biologic drug.

61. D: Upon initial diagnosis, CLL is usually not treated with chemotherapy or radiation. The symptoms are monitored and treatment is reserved for later in the course of the disease. Early treatment has not been shown to prolong life or decrease the progression of the disease.

62. B: Crohn's disease is less likely to cause rectal bleeding, whereas rectal bleeding is more common with ulcerative colitis. This may be due, in part, to the location of the diseases within the GI tract. Crohn's disease can affect any portion of the GI tract from the mouth to the anus. Ulcerative colitis is confined to the colon.

63. A: Calcium excretion is increased when a person receives Lasix. In the geriatric patient, this can affect bone density if it becomes severe. Calcium levels should be monitored and supplementation administered if necessary.

64. C: There are two main types of macular degeneration: wet and dry. Wet macular degeneration involves formation of leaky blood vessels behind the retina. Dry macular degeneration occurs when there is wearing away of the center of the retina. Both forms can result in permanent blindness.

65. B: Sepsis is the most common cause of ARDS. Severe infection causes vascular instability within the lungs which leads to leakage of blood from the blood vessels to the lung tissue. This prevents adequate oxygenation of the blood and results in hypoxemia and multi-system organ failure due to poor perfusion.

66. C: Past abdominal surgeries can cause adhesions within the abdominal cavity. This has been found to be the most common cause of a small bowel obstruction due to the scar tissue affecting the motility of the small intestine. Frequent use of pain medications may also slow down GI motility, leading to constipation and small bowel obstruction, but this is not seen as often as adhesions as a cause for this condition.

67. C: A gout flare-up can be triggered by eating any foods which are high in purines. This includes meat, some seafood (such as trout), and any type of alcohol. Aged cheeses, shellfish, and processed foods are also known to be high in purines.

68. A: Prolonged straining that occurs with coughing, excessive vomiting, or weight lifting can cause the tiny surface capillaries to rupture, leading to the small, bruised-appearing lesions on the skin. These are especially evident on the face, neck, and chest.

69. D: Metabolic syndrome consists of central obesity (>40 inches in men, >35 inches in women), HDL <40 mg/dL in men and <50 mg/dL in women, and triglycerides >150 mg/dL. A diagnosis of metabolic syndrome means a patient is at greater risk for diabetes, heart disease, and stroke.

70. D: Long-acting bronchodilators can be very effective at controlling the symptoms of COPD. When a patient is having to use their short-acting bronchodilator several times during the day, a long-acting medication should be considered to better control the symptoms and decrease the risk of exacerbations of the disease.

71. D: One of the first signs that an acute intravascular hemolytic reaction is occurring is pain at the IV site. Other early signs include fever, chills, elevated heart rate, nausea, and dyspnea. This potentially life-threatening reaction usually occurs within 10 minutes of the beginning of the infusion of blood or blood products.

72. C: According to the U. S. Preventive Services Task Force, routine screening mammography is not recommended in women 75-years-old and older. It is felt that this age group may be more adversely affected by complications from over-diagnosing breast cancer. This population of patients are also at much greater risk of dying from other medical conditions rather than from any breast cancer that is detected.

73. B: Tracheostomy care can be taught to caregivers so this can be performed at home without having a Respiratory Therapist come to the home each day. The trach tube can be reused at home once it has been cleaned with soap and water and mucus inside the tube has been cleaned out. In the hospital setting, trach care is done using aseptic technique to prevent contamination, but it is done under "clean" conditions at home.

74. A: Generally, patients dealing with liver disease need to decrease their sodium intake to help prevent swelling. Though some protein is needed in the diet, the majority of calories should come from carbohydrates, followed by fats, and then protein, which should be low.

75. B: Primary care is the care received by the primary care physician and is usually the first care a patient receives. Secondary care involves the care from specialists and the care may involve services provided in a hospital. Tertiary care is the management and recovery from an acute or chronic illness that requires more intensive therapies. An example would be the services a patient receives at a skilled nurse facility following a total hip replacement.

76. D: According to the U.S. Preventive Services Task Force, it is recommended that adults age 50 through 75 undergo colorectal screening. It is recommended that a fecal occult blood test be performed every year with sigmoidoscopy every 5 years and colonoscopy every 10 years. These guidelines are for those patients who have not had a personal history of colorectal cancer.

77. B: The patient- and family-centered care model was designed to open communication between patients, their family members who are helping to provide care, and the nursing and medical providers delivering care. It involves developing more effective communication with everyone involved in the patient's care with a common goal to improve the patient's outcome.

78. C: The purpose of a clinical pathway is to provide a plan that can be followed for a specific clinical diagnosis. These have been proven to improve the patient's prognosis while helping to control the medical costs of treating the illness. Clinical pathways were first used in the 1980s and have been proven to assist with providing organized and efficient care for the patient.

79. C: There are many different antibiotics available on the market, many of them generic, which are lower priced. If this was a long-term medication, it would be worthwhile to contact the pharmaceutical company to inquire about any programs that could help with the cost of the medication. For a short antibiotic prescription, it is more appropriate to call in a less expensive option to the pharmacy.

80. D: Tetanus is caused by the *Clostridium tetani* spores that enter an open wound and mature into bacteria. This has a detrimental effect on the motor neurons which leads to severe muscle spasms. The spasms can be severe enough to break the underlying bones. A tetanus shot should be given every 10 years to prevent the disease from occurring. When the patient does not recall the last time he/she received the tetanus shot, the shot should be administered as a precaution.

81. C: The first step in implementing a treatment plan for a patient is to identify the main goal that is to be achieved. This should be broad and describe what is to be achieved with the program put into place. Once the goal is identified, measurable objectives should be listed to describe how the end goal is to be achieved. There are usually several objectives for each goal identified.

82. D: Milk and milk products can bind with Cipro and other drugs in this classification, which prevents the antibiotic from being absorbed. Milk should be avoided 2 hours before and 4 hours after taking the antibiotic.

83. A: The half-life of dopamine is less than 2 minutes, so the total time in which the effects from the medication are seen is around 10 minutes. Dopamine is used to improve heart function, increase blood pressure, and increase renal perfusion.

84. A: The type of pneumonia that is most common in a person who is normally healthy is community-acquired pneumonia. Without any other co-morbidities present, the most appropriate treatment is with azithromycin. Azithromycin is the appropriate choice. Clarithromycin and doxycycline are also options for treatment if there is an allergy to azithromycin.

85. D: The ATLAS trial evaluated the benefits of long-term tamoxifen treatment in thousands of women worldwide who had been treated for breast cancer. It was found that completing a ten-year treatment with tamoxifen provided longer survival rates and a lower repeat incidence of breast cancer.

86. B: Gentamicin ear drops should not be used if a perforated ear drum is present. This may cause systemic absorption of the medication which can increase the risk of ototoxicity and hearing loss. If indicated, oral medications should be used.

87. A: Valacyclovir (Valtrex) should be dosed at 1 g PO three times daily for 7 days for an acute outbreak of herpes zoster. This dose should be adjusted as appropriate for the patient suffering from renal insufficiency. Two other medications that can be used to treat this condition are Famvir and Zovirax.

88. D: Certain medications categorized as proton pump inhibitors (Nexium, Prilosec, Prevacid), can decrease the effectiveness of Plavix, which may cause an increased risk of cardiac events. They prevent full absorption of the medication. Dexilant is a PPI, but has been found to be safe when taken with Plavix.

89. C: Actos has a black box warning for its risk of increasing the incidence of congestive heart failure. With there being multiple medications on the market to treat type 2 diabetes, it should be avoided with those patients who are known to have congestive heart failure.

90. B: While all of these choices are adequate at lowering blood pressure, lisinopril would be the best choice because of its renal protection qualities. He has been diagnosed with type 2 diabetes and an ACE inhibitor is recommended for diabetics to help provide some protection from diabetes-associated renal insufficiency.

91. A: There is a 1% chance that a patient with a penicillin allergy may develop an allergic response to cefdinir, or other drugs in the cephalosporin class. The benefit of the cephalosporin with certain illnesses often outweighs the risk of developing a reaction. Unless there is no other choice, cephalosporins are avoided if the patient has had an anaphylactic reaction to medications in the penicillin class.

92. D: Ipratropium and albuterol can be given independent of each other, but they work well together to help with bronchospasm. The ipratropium works as an anticholinergic to dilate the airway while albuterol helps to relax the bronchial smooth muscle to prevent bronchospasm. They are both considered short-acting medications.

93. D: Zantac is the only medication of these that will require a dosage adjustment in those patients with renal failure. Once the creatinine clearance becomes less than 50 mL/min., the dosage of Zantac needs to be decreased.

94. C: One of the earliest signs of digoxin toxicity is a yellowish discoloration in vision, especially while looking at light. This is called xanthopsia. A digoxin level should be drawn and the normal range is 0.5-2 ng/mL.

95. B: Anticholinergic drugs can help with some of the rigidity seen with Parkinson's, but they do little to help with the bradykinesia. The side effects seen with this class of drugs can be more severe in elderly populations. The other medications listed are helpful with all of the symptoms of Parkinson's disease.

96. B: This patient is presenting with symptoms of thrush. Oral thrush lesions respond well to the antifungal fluconazole. Another option is to use nystatin in liquid form to use as a mouthwash.

97. B: Amoxicillin, clarithromycin, and a proton pump inhibitor is the combination therapy necessary to treat *H. pylori* peptic ulcer disease. Metronidazole can be substituted for amoxicillin if the patient is allergic to amoxicillin. The patient may need to continue with the proton pump inhibitor after the treatment regimen is completed.

98. C: Though it has been effective at treating urinary tract infections in females, nitrofurantoin has been shown to not be as effective in men due to low tissue concentrations of the drug. Nitrofurantoin has also been shown to not be effective at treating underlying prostatitis. Medications from the fluoroquinolone class and sulfa drugs are usually the best antibiotics to use, pending urine culture results.

99. B: The biologic agents used for treatment of rheumatoid arthritis pose an increased risk of lymphoma. Therefore, any patients with lymphoma or a history of lymphoma, cannot receive medications from this class. The CBC is routinely monitored in those patients who are taking a biologic agent.

100. B: Clarithromycin can interfere with the efficacy of Plavix by decreasing its effectiveness. This could lead to an increased risk of blood clots. A different antibiotic should be chosen, when possible, for those patients who are taking Plavix for anticoagulation.

101. A: Acetaminophen would be the safest due to its tolerability. The other medications listed are NSAIDs which pose the threat of GI bleed and increased risk of cardiovascular events. NSAIDs can be used in low doses for limited periods of time in this class of patients, but this should be monitored.

102. D: Nursing Informatics uses the data information and knowledge gathered to better inform those involved in patient care. The goal is to better inform not just those who make up the healthcare team, but to help to use the data gathered to provide better care for patients and to better inform patients of their care. Nursing Informatics is a growing field that has become more popular in recent years with the changing face of healthcare.

103. A: Meaningful use was established to provide an incentive through Medicare and Medicaid by utilizing the electronic health record to its fullest potential. It sets forth specific objectives and goals to improve the quality of patient care, patient safety, and result in better patient outcomes. It has been released in three separate stages. The American Recovery and Reinvestment Act of 2009 authorized Medicare and Medicaid to offer these incentives to those healthcare professionals who meet the criteria for meaningful use.

104. C: It is appropriate to divert personal questions the patient has about the CNS or CNS's family back to the patient to focus the attention on the patient's problems. Providers must be very cognizant of the relationships they establish with patients and their families. It is easy to become attached to patients, but it is unprofessional and harmful to place oneself in a position in which the relationship has lost the boundary between provider and patient. Always be wary of the relationships established with patients and continue to re-evaluate those boundaries so that the best care possible can be provided to the patient.

105. D: Whenever possible, have an interpreter present in these types of situations, ideally one who has undergone some training in medical terminology. Using a family member is not ideal because it is not known that any medical training or terms will be correctly translated. Online software may not be accurate and there is no way to verify that the terms and concepts are being interpreted appropriately.

106. B: The Teach-Back system is a method used to improve patient and family understanding of the plan of care. After teaching a patient and/or family about an illness or treatment, they are then asked to repeat or demonstrate what was reviewed. This ensures that there is full understanding of the treatment plan which improves patient compliance and decreases potential complications.

107. B: The Quality and Safety Education for Nurses initiative was started in 2005 with the objective to prepare future nurses for the challenge of improving the healthcare settings in which they work. It provides these nurses with the knowledge, skills, and attitudes (KSAs) needed to accomplish this goal.

108. C: Quality improvement is instrumental in improving the way healthcare services are provided, while continually measuring the effect those changes have on the health status of the patients served. This is often measured through patient satisfaction information.

109. A: In 1902, the United States government outlined the Nurse Practice Act and gave the authority of regulating nursing practice to each individual state. This was established to ensure that certain standards of care are upheld in nursing practice in order to keep patients safe. The specific scope of practice for nursing is also established by each state legislature and falls under this statute.

110. B: According to HIPAA, information regarding the care of a patient can be shared with other members of the healthcare team without permission from the patient or patient representative. This information can be faxed over to the cardiologist's office.

111. D: Informatics is the combination of computer-based information with healthcare. Early informatics started with the development of the electronic health record in the 1970s. Since then, the computer-based resource available to healthcare professionals in order to gather patient information has grown exponentially. This access to information helps with the coordination of care for patients, as well as aide in providing timely and efficient care.

112. A: The referring provider should be open with the patient regarding the need for a specialty consultation. The reason for the consultation, along with the names of appropriate provider should be discussed. Once the patient is in agreement to be referred, all pertinent records should be sent to the consultant so that he or she is adequately informed of the patient's history.

113. C: The Thomas-Kilmann Conflict Mode Instrument (TKI) is used to measure the behavior of a person who is in a conflict situation. It assesses whether a person's behavior is assertive in order to reach their own goal or whether they are cooperative in order for the other person within the conflict to attain their goals. The TKI is used in all types of conflict situations and is not specialized to use only within the healthcare work environment.

114. B: Cultural encounter is the process of encouraging medical staff to interact with those patients who are from a different cultural background. It has been found that the more a person interacts with those from different cultures, the more their beliefs and practice can be understood. Communities have become very diverse and the medical professional needs to be prepared to address the individual needs and practices of those from different cultures.

115. A: A content expert is a person who has undergone extensive training in a particular subject matter so they are capable to then go forth and train others on that subject. An example of this would be an IT specialist who specializes in a particular computer program. When a hospital has a change to a new electronic health records system, there is extensive training that is coordinated with all employees before the change is made in order for everyone to be prepared. Content experts are responsible for coordinating this effort and ensuring as much training as possible is completed in order to make this a smooth transition.

116. C: The purpose of a poster presentation is to gain the attention of a reader with a brief summary that draws them in. There can be many poster presentations at conferences and meetings, so the poster presentation needs to gain the attention of the attendee passing by. The poster presentation should also contain a summary of the purpose, methods, and findings of a more formal paper.

117. B: The preceptor is the person who will work with a new nurse or a nurse new to a department to ensure the protocols and specific skills are understood. A mentor is someone who provides advice and guidance when asked, but in a much more informal way than a preceptor.

118. C: The shared governance model of nursing practice has been utilized to promote job satisfaction and nurse retention. It enables the nurses to function as a group, making shared decisions, and implementing plans for the betterment of the patient.

119. D: The humanistic learning theory fosters emotional and mental health, in addition to physical health. Its purpose is to help patients grow by learning in a healthy and creative way. This theory also takes in consideration that the patient is unique and an individual with individual needs in learning. This helps to create a learning plan based on these needs.

120. A: The role model in nursing is someone that is looked up to because of their day-to-day interactions with patients and the way in which they perform their job responsibilities. The role model is the nursing professional that other nurses, or nursing students, strive to emulate. This is not necessarily a formal position with set responsibilities in educating others, though others can learn how to provide compassionate care from this person.

121. A: Practice laws for clinical nurse specialists vary from state to state, but generally there are three areas of practice in which the clinical nurse specialist can specialize: Adult/Gerontology, Pediatrics, and Neonatal. The certification that is chosen by the clinical nurse specialist indicates what population of patients they will be evaluating, diagnosing, and treating for a variety of conditions.

122. D: With social media being used by most people, it is frequently misinterpreted as a means of communication for all aspects of our lives. It is important to note, however, that only secure methods should be used for discussing healthcare issues with a patient in order to prevent the violation of privacy laws. In this case, the patient should be informed that her lab results cannot be discussed through social media and she will need to contact the office.

123. D: The clinical nurse specialist functions as a patient advocate through many different actions, but the overall goal is to keep the patient safe and ensure they are receiving the highest quality of care possible. This can involve providing necessary education about a disease state or coordinating efforts with many providers for the patient to receive all of the necessary care they need.

124. B: In order to qualify to obtain the certification to be an Adult-Gerontology Clinical Nurse Specialist, the provider must be an RN that has completed an accredited masters level nursing program that enables them to sit for the clinical nurse specialist national certification exam.

125. C: Like most mid-level providers, the clinical nurse specialist must adhere to the state laws in which they practice. Some states will allow full prescriptive authority, to include controlled substances with appropriate DEA licensure, while others limit the medications that can be prescribed. It is important that the clinical nurse specialist is fully aware of the prescribing laws within their practicing state to remain compliant.

126. A: Capacity is often mistaken to mean the same thing as competency. Capacity is determined by a physician, often a psychiatrist, after a series of mental status tests are performed. Once the evaluation is completed, the physician can make a determination whether a person has the capacity to make important legal decisions.

127. B: Any tubes, including IV tubing, should be cut with the end still inserted in the body. It is Jewish tradition that the body be buried in its entirety, with as much of the blood and tissue left intact as possible. The funeral home will remove any devices or tubing while following Jewish law.

128. C: The Healthy People 2020 program was established to promote overall health and wellness throughout the nation. This includes promoting environments that help to promote good health, such as community recreation centers, walking trails, and recreational parks.

129. A: Medicare Part A covers the services available outside of a physician's office. This includes hospitalization, skilled nursing home care for the first 100 days after a 3-day hospital stay, hospice care, home care, and durable medical equipment. Medicare Part B covers the care provided within the physician's office.

130. D: Continued competence is an ongoing process for all healthcare professionals in order to provide safe care for the patient. It is a commitment that is made when one goes into the healthcare field so that the responsibilities of this role can be fulfilled. This continued competence can chance as the healthcare provider's role changes, also, so that the most effective and knowledgeable care available can be offered.

131. C: The American Nurses Credentialing Center is one of the certifying bodies that offers certification to those who hold a current RN license and have completed an accredited master's degree program that qualifies them to be a clinical nurse specialist. The ANCC is a subsidiary of the American Nurses Association and offers certification in many sub-specialties of nursing practice.

132. B: The reimbursement rate for nurse practitioners seeing Medicare patients is 80% of the physician's reimbursement rate. Supervising physicians do not need to be on site for the nurse practitioner to receive reimbursement. There is also no restriction on the type of patient that is seen, whether they are an "old" or "new" patient.

133. C: A third party payer is an organization that pays for the medical expenses of a person. This is usually a health insurance company such as Medicare, Medicaid, or private health insurance. The patient is the first party payer who purchases the health insurance policy.

134. D: Benchmarking is when health care organizations are compared to other organizations to assess their proficiency in a particular area of health care. This is utilized as a means of identifying their strengths and weaknesses to help with improving the level of care offered. An organization will usually compare themselves to another organization that is known to be a leader within a particular field.

135. A: A cost-benefit analysis examines the amount of expenditures relative to the possible medical benefits. This is especially helpful when there are limited resources and priorities need to be established as to which choices should be made first. By doing this, it determines which health care services are going to be provided.

136. C: Quality improvement is instrumental in improving the way healthcare services are provided, while continually measuring the effect those changes have on the health status of the patients served. This is often measured through patient satisfaction information.

137. D: The Joint Commission was established in 1951 with the primary goal of ensuring that health care organizations are providing the safest and highest quality of care available. Organizations must undergo on-site reviews and analysis of policies and procedures that are used to ensure this care is being provided effectively. The on-site surveys are performed every three years, or more frequently if necessary.

138. B: Organizational theories assist managers in achieving the missions and goals of a healthcare system. This process can help to fully analyze how a system functions, and helps managers to diagnose and fix organization and process problems. This can help to prevent major problems within an organization and lead to successful outcomes.

139. A: The International Statistical Classification of Diseases and Related Health Problems (ICD) is now in its 10th revision. This is created by the World Health Organization and work on the 10th version started in 1983 and was finished in 1992. The United States started to use this version in 2015. The ICD-10 contains over 14,000 disease states and symptoms for which there is a diagnosis code.

140. C: The transformation leadership theory involves having a leader that motivates their followers to participate in making organizational decisions. This encourages them to develop ideas and problem solving skills to help make the healthcare setting more productive. This empowers everyone to take responsibility for organizational problems and create productive solutions for the betterment of the organization.

141. C: A clinical pathway is a structured plan of care for a specific diagnosis. The intent of this is to outline the steps to follow when caring for a patient, from admission to discharge. One criticism of this tool is that it does not allow for personalization of the patient's care and may result in negative outcomes if the appropriate care for the patient is delayed.

142. C: The ACO, or Accountable Care Organization model, coordinates the efforts of all specialties and treatment modalities for the patient. The reimbursement plan varies, but there is extra incentive to address wellness and disease prevention.

143. B: Stress in a person's work environment is normal to a certain degree. When the stress is excessive, though, it begins to affect our everyday lives and is exhibited by being short-tempered, not sleeping well, withdrawing, feeling overwhelmed, or self-medicating with alcohol or drugs. It is important to recognize these signs of stress so that they can be addressed when they occur and steps can be taken to decrease stress within the work environment. Prolonged stress can increase the risk for hypertension, heart disease, and diabetes.

144. D: Order sets are created to ensure the orders specific to particular diagnosis or post-op procedure are complete and accurate. These should be current, using the best evidence-based practice protocols, and complete to address all potential issues associated with a particular diagnosis. These can be altered to meet the individual needs of a specific patient.

145. A: The Just Culture concept focuses on finding a system improvement that could prevent a medical error from happening again, rather than focusing on the individual who performed erroneously. It accepts the fact that errors can occur, but avoids the blame and punishment being placed on one individual. It is an effective tool to improve the process leading up to the error rather than ignoring the problems with that process and focusing on the individual.

146. D: Clinical Practice Guidelines were formulated by the Institute of Medicine to serve as a template for appropriate care to be provided to a patient based upon a specific diagnosis. This helps to improve patient care by outlining the specific elements of care that should be provided to patients in order to optimize their treatment plan.

147. B: The failure modes and effects analysis (FMEA) is used to identify potential failure in a process that is going to be used. By identifying the area of potential failure, the impact of this failure, if it occurs, can be better analyzed for the effect it will have on the process as a whole. This analysis also helps to formulate solutions to potential failures before they occur.

148. C: A root cause analysis is an in-depth evaluation of a system process to identify what has caused a problem within the process. It provides a very thorough examination into a full process system so that errors and problems can be evaluated and corrected to improve the process. This is not specific to healthcare and can be used for any failure that has been identified within an established process.

149. A: A gap analysis identifies the difference between what is actually being accomplished versus what is the desired performance outcome. This analysis identifies specific items which may need to be approached in a different manner in order to achieve the desired outcome. It can also be beneficial in identifying those goals which may not be attainable using the current process in place.

150. D: National Patient Safety Goals are established by Joint Commission and have been used in practice since 2003. They are used for process improvement by identifying specific areas of concern in regard to patient safety. They involve specific actions that should be taken by organizations who undergo accreditation in order to prevent medical errors.

151. C: A care bundle, or Institute of Healthcare Improvement (IHI) bundle, is a set of evidence-based practices that can improve the overall outcome for a patient. This is usually a set of three to five practices that have been proven to provide the optimal level of care associated with the highest outcomes possible.

152. B: Nursing quality indicators are part of a national database that is updated quarterly and annually. This reports the structure, process, and outcome indicators used to evaluate nursing care. These are measures that are considered nursing-sensitive because they are dependent upon the quality of nursing care. Nursing job satisfaction is also considered to be an indicator.

153. A: Structural indicators, process indicators, and outcome indicators are all categories of indicators evaluated in the National Database of Nursing Quality Indicators. Structural indicators evaluate the skill level and education level of the nursing staff. Process indicators measure the methods used for patient assessment. Outcome indicators evaluate patient outcomes that are determined to be nursing-sensitive because they are dependent upon the quality of nursing care received.

154. C: Developing a pressure ulcer during a hospital stay is evaluated as an outcome indicator. These reflect patient outcomes that are determined by be dependent upon the quality and quantity of nursing care the patient receives during their hospitalization. It is reasoned that, if the patient had been checked more frequently and repositioned in bed while avoiding excessive resting on pressure points, the pressure ulcer may not have developed.

155. D: A sentinel event is defined by The Joint Commission as any event that occurs in a healthcare setting that results in the death or significant psychological damage of a patient. A root cause analysis is performed when a sentinel event takes place to identify the cause of the incident, as well as put forth measures to help prevent this from happening again.

156. B: The suicide of a patient within 72 hours of discharge from an acute-care setting would be considered a sentinel event, but not one week after discharge. All of the other options are considered sentinel events. Other examples of a sentinel event include rape or suicide of a patient while they are within an acute-care setting, unexpected death of a full-term infant, and radiation therapy to the wrong body part or at a dose 25% higher than what was planned.

157. C: Competency is the legal term used to mean a person does not have the mental ability to make decisions for themselves, such as managing finances. It is often confused with capacity, which is determined by a physician, often a psychiatrist, after a series of mental status tests are performed. The legal system is responsible for deeming someone incompetent to make their own decisions.

158. A: The ICD-10 diagnosis coding system was established by the World Health Organization. It contains over 14,000 disease states and symptoms for which there is a diagnosis code. Along with these codes, there are additional qualifiers that must be added to indicate specific information regarding the patient's condition, which makes this more specific. For example, instead of only using a code for type 2 diabetes mellitus, qualifiers are added on to indicate whether this controlled or uncontrolled, whether there is associated retinal disease or kidney disease, and whether they are controlling this with insulin or oral medications.

159. B: In order to evaluate the cause of a delay of service, and to determine how the process could be more efficient, a root cause analysis is the most appropriate tool to utilize. It provides a very thorough examination into a full process system so that errors and problems can be evaluated and corrected to improve the process. In this case, every step of the check-in process can be evaluated to determine what system improvements could be made to prevent the delays.

160. C: Internal validity examines whether the research in a study was performed correctly. It identifies the validity of the independent variable in the study and evaluates whether there is more than one independent variable that could be acting at the same time. The less chance of having more than one independent variable will lend a higher internal validity to a study.

161. D: DVT prophylaxis should be included on an order sets or bundles for patients on ventilators because they non-ambulatory. The risk of DVT increases with decreased activity and being sedentary, so compression stockings and passive range of motion exercises should be performed regularly if tolerated by the patient. Including DVT prophylaxis in an order set helps to address a potential issue associated with a particular diagnosis.

162. A: The failure modes and effects analysis (FMEA) is used to identify potential failure in a process that is going to be used. By identifying the area of potential failure, the impact of this failure, if it occurs, can be better analyzed for the effect it will have on the process as a whole. This analysis also helps to formulate solutions to potential failures before they occur.

163. D: This review is focused on comparing actual wait times with the clinic's goal for patient wait times; therefore, they are utilizing a gap analysis in this instance. A gap analysis examines the difference between what is actually being accomplished versus the desired outcome. It identifies specific items which may need to be approached differently in order to achieve the set goal. It can also be helpful in identifying those goals which may not be attainable using the current process in place.

164. B: Statistical power is a measure of the likelihood that a researcher will find statistical significance in a sample if the effect exists in the full population. Power is a function of three primary: sample size, effect size, and significance level. The most common reason to conduct a power analysis is to determine the sample size needed for a particular study. However, power analysis may also be used after a study has been completed to determine if the reason an effect was not significant was insufficient power.

165. C: The Office for Human Research Protections, or OHRP, provides education, clarification, and guidance, as well as advice on ethical and regulatory issues in biomedical and behavioral research. It is a division of the U.S. Department of Health and Human Services.

166. D: The more sensitive a diagnostic test is, the more likely it is to accurately indicate a positive result in the presence of the disease for which it is testing. The higher the specificity, the more likely it is to accurately indicate a specific variable in the testing. For example, in-office influenza tests should be high in sensitivity to detect the presence of influenza virus in the testing specimen, but should also have a high level of specificity to determine if the infective organism is from type A or type B influenza virus.

167. A: Quality improvement registries track specific data to improve the quality of care. This is frequently done through the electronic health record to identify specific health maintenance recommendations, such as diabetic eye screening exams, so that the provider can be alerted to the clinical practice guideline requirements for a patient. This is based on evidence-based clinical practice guidelines put in place to ensure the highest level of care for a specific condition or disease state.

168. C: A healthcare audit reviews the care being provided and compares it against current recommendations in healthcare to improve the quality of care. For example, an audit of the data of a specific patient population can identify those who are actually being referred for a routine screening colonoscopy versus the full set of patients who should be referred for screening colonoscopies.

169. B: A type I error, or a false positive, occurs when something is said to be positive, when in reality it is actually negative. This can apply to any clinical situations in which something is believed to be true when it is not. This differs from a type II error, which is a false negative reading.

170. A: The power of any test of statistical significance is defined as the probability that it will reject a false null hypothesis. Statistical power is affected mainly by the size of the effect and the size of the sample used to detect it, and lesser so by the level of statistical significance.

171. D: A decreased sensitivity level of nasopharyngeal swab flu tests may produce up to a 30% incidence of false negative results. This is also called a type II error. This differs from a type I error, which is also called a false positive result.

172. B: The Hospital Inpatient Quality Reporting Program was established by the Departments of Medicare and Medicaid Services. This program has implemented a system in which hospitals report specific quality measures in order to receive a higher annual update to their payment rates. This was placed in effect to provide a measurable way in which to improve patient care.

173. B: According to the American Society of Addiction Medicine, drug overdose is the leading cause of accidental death in the U.S. Of the more than 52,000 drug overdose-related deaths in 2015, over 20,000 were due to overdose of prescription pain relievers.

174. A: Mittens are not considered a restraint because they do not immobilize the hands or fingers. If they are tight and constrict movement, they would be considered a restraint. Mittens are used to prevent patients from picking, scratching, or grasping IV and oxygen lines and removing them.

175. D: An iatrogenic condition is caused as a result of any medication, treatment, procedure, or a combination thereof. This includes expected or adverse negative effects from a medication that is necessary to treat an illness. This is not necessarily a negative outcome, though, such as weight loss with some diabetic medications.

How to Overcome Test Anxiety

Just the thought of taking a test is enough to make most people a little nervous. A test is an important event that can have a long-term impact on your future, so it's important to take it seriously and it's natural to feel anxious about performing well. But just because anxiety is normal, that doesn't mean that it's helpful in test taking, or that you should simply accept it as part of your life. Anxiety can have a variety of effects. These effects can be mild, like making you feel slightly nervous, or severe, like blocking your ability to focus or remember even a simple detail.

If you experience test anxiety—whether severe or mild—it's important to know how to beat it. To discover this, first you need to understand what causes test anxiety.

Causes of Test Anxiety

While we often think of anxiety as an uncontrollable emotional state, it can actually be caused by simple, practical things. One of the most common causes of test anxiety is that a person does not feel adequately prepared for their test. This feeling can be the result of many different issues such as poor study habits or lack of organization, but the most common culprit is time management. Starting to study too late, failing to organize your study time to cover all of the material, or being distracted while you study will mean that you're not well prepared for the test. This may lead to cramming the night before, which will cause you to be physically and mentally exhausted for the test. Poor time management also contributes to feelings of stress, fear, and hopelessness as you realize you are not well prepared but don't know what to do about it.

Other times, test anxiety is not related to your preparation for the test but comes from unresolved fear. This may be a past failure on a test, or poor performance on tests in general. It may come from comparing yourself to others who seem to be performing better or from the stress of living up to expectations. Anxiety may be driven by fears of the future—how failure on this test would affect your educational and career goals. These fears are often completely irrational, but they can still negatively impact your test performance.

Review Video: 3 Reasons You Have Test Anxiety
Visit mometrix.com/academy and enter code: 428468

Elements of Test Anxiety

As mentioned earlier, test anxiety is considered to be an emotional state, but it has physical and mental components as well. Sometimes you may not even realize that you are suffering from test anxiety until you notice the physical symptoms. These can include trembling hands, rapid heartbeat, sweating, nausea, and tense muscles. Extreme anxiety may lead to fainting or vomiting. Obviously, any of these symptoms can have a negative impact on testing. It is important to recognize them as soon as they begin to occur so that you can address the problem before it damages your performance.

Review Video: 3 Ways to Tell You Have Test Anxiety
Visit mometrix.com/academy and enter code: 927847

The mental components of test anxiety include trouble focusing and inability to remember learned information. During a test, your mind is on high alert, which can help you recall information and stay focused for an extended period of time. However, anxiety interferes with your mind's natural processes, causing you to blank out, even on the questions you know well. The strain of testing during anxiety makes it difficult to stay focused, especially on a test that may take several hours. Extreme anxiety can take a huge mental toll, making it difficult not only to recall test information but even to understand the test questions or pull your thoughts together.

Review Video: How Test Anxiety Affects Memory
Visit mometrix.com/academy and enter code: 609003

Effects of Test Anxiety

Test anxiety is like a disease—if left untreated, it will get progressively worse. Anxiety leads to poor performance, and this reinforces the feelings of fear and failure, which in turn lead to poor performances on subsequent tests. It can grow from a mild nervousness to a crippling condition. If allowed to progress, test anxiety can have a big impact on your schooling, and consequently on your future.

Test anxiety can spread to other parts of your life. Anxiety on tests can become anxiety in any stressful situation, and blanking on a test can turn into panicking in a job situation. But fortunately, you don't have to let anxiety rule your testing and determine your grades. There are a number of relatively simple steps you can take to move past anxiety and function normally on a test and in the rest of life.

Review Video: How Test Anxiety Impacts Your Grades
Visit mometrix.com/academy and enter code: 939819

Physical Steps for Beating Test Anxiety

While test anxiety is a serious problem, the good news is that it can be overcome. It doesn't have to control your ability to think and remember information. While it may take time, you can begin taking steps today to beat anxiety.

Just as your first hint that you may be struggling with anxiety comes from the physical symptoms, the first step to treating it is also physical. Rest is crucial for having a clear, strong mind. If you are tired, it is much easier to give in to anxiety. But if you establish good sleep habits, your body and mind will be ready to perform optimally, without the strain of exhaustion. Additionally, sleeping well helps you to retain information better, so you're more likely to recall the answers when you see the test questions.

Getting good sleep means more than going to bed on time. It's important to allow your brain time to relax. Take study breaks from time to time so it doesn't get overworked, and don't study right before bed. Take time to rest your mind before trying to rest your body, or you may find it difficult to fall asleep.

Review Video: The Importance of Sleep for Your Brain
Visit mometrix.com/academy and enter code: 319338

Along with sleep, other aspects of physical health are important in preparing for a test. Good nutrition is vital for good brain function. Sugary foods and drinks may give a burst of energy but this burst is followed by a crash, both physically and emotionally. Instead, fuel your body with protein and vitamin-rich foods.

Also, drink plenty of water. Dehydration can lead to headaches and exhaustion, especially if your brain is already under stress from the rigors of the test. Particularly if your test is a long one, drink water during the breaks. And if possible, take an energy-boosting snack to eat between sections.

Review Video: How Diet Can Affect your Mood
Visit mometrix.com/academy and enter code: 624317

Along with sleep and diet, a third important part of physical health is exercise. Maintaining a steady workout schedule is helpful, but even taking 5-minute study breaks to walk can help get your blood pumping faster and clear your head. Exercise also releases endorphins, which contribute to a positive feeling and can help combat test anxiety.

When you nurture your physical health, you are also contributing to your mental health. If your body is healthy, your mind is much more likely to be healthy as well. So take time to rest, nourish your body with healthy food and water, and get moving as much as possible. Taking these physical steps will make you stronger and more able to take the mental steps necessary to overcome test anxiety.

Review Video: How to Stay Healthy and Prevent Test Anxiety
Visit mometrix.com/academy and enter code: 877894

Mental Steps for Beating Test Anxiety

Working on the mental side of test anxiety can be more challenging, but as with the physical side, there are clear steps you can take to overcome it. As mentioned earlier, test anxiety often stems from lack of preparation, so the obvious solution is to prepare for the test. Effective studying may be the most important weapon you have for beating test anxiety, but you can and should employ several other mental tools to combat fear.

First, boost your confidence by reminding yourself of past success—tests or projects that you aced. If you're putting as much effort into preparing for this test as you did for those, there's no reason you should expect to fail here. Work hard to prepare; then trust your preparation.

Second, surround yourself with encouraging people. It can be helpful to find a study group, but be sure that the people you're around will encourage a positive attitude. If you spend time with others who are anxious or cynical, this will only contribute to your own anxiety. Look for others who are motivated to study hard from a desire to succeed, not from a fear of failure.

Third, reward yourself. A test is physically and mentally tiring, even without anxiety, and it can be helpful to have something to look forward to. Plan an activity following the test, regardless of the outcome, such as going to a movie or getting ice cream.

When you are taking the test, if you find yourself beginning to feel anxious, remind yourself that you know the material. Visualize successfully completing the test. Then take a few deep, relaxing breaths and return to it. Work through the questions carefully but with confidence, knowing that you are capable of succeeding.

Developing a healthy mental approach to test taking will also aid in other areas of life. Test anxiety affects more than just the actual test—it can be damaging to your mental health and even contribute to depression. It's important to beat test anxiety before it becomes a problem for more than testing.

Review Video: Test Anxiety and Depression
Visit mometrix.com/academy and enter code: 904704

Study Strategy

Being prepared for the test is necessary to combat anxiety, but what does being prepared look like? You may study for hours on end and still not feel prepared. What you need is a strategy for test prep. The next few pages outline our recommended steps to help you plan out and conquer the challenge of preparation.

Step 1: Scope Out the Test

Learn everything you can about the format (multiple choice, essay, etc.) and what will be on the test. Gather any study materials, course outlines, or sample exams that may be available. Not only will this help you to prepare, but knowing what to expect can help to alleviate test anxiety.

Step 2: Map Out the Material

Look through the textbook or study guide and make note of how many chapters or sections it has. Then divide these over the time you have. For example, if a book has 15 chapters and you have five days to study, you need to cover three chapters each day. Even better, if you have the time, leave an extra day at the end for overall review after you have gone through the material in depth.

If time is limited, you may need to prioritize the material. Look through it and make note of which sections you think you already have a good grasp on, and which need review. While you are studying, skim quickly through the familiar sections and take more time on the challenging parts. Write out your plan so you don't get lost as you go. Having a written plan also helps you feel more in control of the study, so anxiety is less likely to arise from feeling overwhelmed at the amount to cover.

Step 3: Gather Your Tools

Decide what study method works best for you. Do you prefer to highlight in the book as you study and then go back over the highlighted portions? Or do you type out notes of the important information? Or is it helpful to make flashcards that you can carry with you? Assemble the pens, index cards, highlighters, post-it notes, and any other materials you may need so you won't be distracted by getting up to find things while you study.

If you're having a hard time retaining the information or organizing your notes, experiment with different methods. For example, try color-coding by subject with colored pens, highlighters, or post-it notes. If you learn better by hearing, try recording yourself reading your notes so you can listen while in the car, working out, or simply sitting at your desk. Ask a friend to quiz you from your flashcards, or try teaching someone the material to solidify it in your mind.

Step 4: Create Your Environment

It's important to avoid distractions while you study. This includes both the obvious distractions like visitors and the subtle distractions like an uncomfortable chair (or a too-comfortable couch that makes you want to fall asleep). Set up the best study environment possible: good lighting and a comfortable work area. If background music helps you focus, you may want to turn it on, but otherwise keep the room quiet. If you are using a computer to take notes, be sure you don't have any other windows open, especially applications like social media, games, or anything else that could distract you. Silence your phone and turn off notifications. Be sure to keep water close by so you stay hydrated while you study (but avoid unhealthy drinks and snacks).

Also, take into account the best time of day to study. Are you freshest first thing in the morning? Try to set aside some time then to work through the material. Is your mind clearer in the afternoon or evening? Schedule your study session then. Another method is to study at the same time of day that you will take the test, so that your brain gets used to working on the material at that time and will be ready to focus at test time.

Step 5: Study!

Once you have done all the study preparation, it's time to settle into the actual studying. Sit down, take a few moments to settle your mind so you can focus, and begin to follow your study plan. Don't give in to distractions or let yourself procrastinate. This is your time to prepare so you'll be ready to fearlessly approach the test. Make the most of the time and stay focused.

Of course, you don't want to burn out. If you study too long you may find that you're not retaining the information very well. Take regular study breaks. For example, taking five minutes out of every hour to walk briskly, breathing deeply and swinging your arms, can help your mind stay fresh.

As you get to the end of each chapter or section, it's a good idea to do a quick review. Remind yourself of what you learned and work on any difficult parts. When you feel that you've mastered the material, move on to the next part. At the end of your study session, briefly skim through your notes again.

But while review is helpful, cramming last minute is NOT. If at all possible, work ahead so that you won't need to fit all your study into the last day. Cramming overloads your brain with more information than it can process and retain, and your tired mind may struggle to recall even previously learned information when it is overwhelmed with last-minute study. Also, the urgent nature of cramming and the stress placed on your brain contribute to anxiety. You'll be more likely to go to the test feeling unprepared and having trouble thinking clearly.

So don't cram, and don't stay up late before the test, even just to review your notes at a leisurely pace. Your brain needs rest more than it needs to go over the information again. In fact, plan to finish your studies by noon or early afternoon the day before the test. Give your brain the rest of the day to relax or focus on other things, and get a good night's sleep. Then you will be fresh for the test and better able to recall what you've studied.

Step 6: Take a practice test

Many courses offer sample tests, either online or in the study materials. This is an excellent resource to check whether you have mastered the material, as well as to prepare for the test format and environment.

Check the test format ahead of time: the number of questions, the type (multiple choice, free response, etc.), and the time limit. Then create a plan for working through them. For example, if you have 30 minutes to take a 60-question test, your limit is 30 seconds per question. Spend less time on the questions you know well so that you can take more time on the difficult ones.

If you have time to take several practice tests, take the first one open book, with no time limit. Work through the questions at your own pace and make sure you fully understand them. Gradually work up to taking a test under test conditions: sit at a desk with all study materials put away and set a timer. Pace yourself to make sure you finish the test with time to spare and go back to check your answers if you have time.

After each test, check your answers. On the questions you missed, be sure you understand why you missed them. Did you misread the question (tests can use tricky wording)? Did you forget the information? Or was it something you hadn't learned? Go back and study any shaky areas that the practice tests reveal.

Taking these tests not only helps with your grade, but also aids in combating test anxiety. If you're already used to the test conditions, you're less likely to worry about it, and working through tests until you're scoring well gives you a confidence boost. Go through the practice tests until you feel comfortable, and then you can go into the test knowing that you're ready for it.

Test Tips

On test day, you should be confident, knowing that you've prepared well and are ready to answer the questions. But aside from preparation, there are several test day strategies you can employ to maximize your performance.

First, as stated before, get a good night's sleep the night before the test (and for several nights before that, if possible). Go into the test with a fresh, alert mind rather than staying up late to study.

Try not to change too much about your normal routine on the day of the test. It's important to eat a nutritious breakfast, but if you normally don't eat breakfast at all, consider eating just a protein bar. If you're a coffee drinker, go ahead and have your normal coffee. Just make sure you time it so that the caffeine doesn't wear off right in the middle of your test. Avoid sugary beverages, and drink enough water to stay hydrated but not so much that you need a restroom break 10 minutes into the test. If your test isn't first thing in the morning, consider going for a walk or doing a light workout before the test to get your blood flowing.

Allow yourself enough time to get ready, and leave for the test with plenty of time to spare so you won't have the anxiety of scrambling to arrive in time. Another reason to be early is to select a good seat. It's helpful to sit away from doors and windows, which can be distracting. Find a good seat, get out your supplies, and settle your mind before the test begins.

When the test begins, start by going over the instructions carefully, even if you already know what to expect. Make sure you avoid any careless mistakes by following the directions.

Then begin working through the questions, pacing yourself as you've practiced. If you're not sure on an answer, don't spend too much time on it, and don't let it shake your confidence. Either skip it and come back later, or eliminate as many wrong answers as possible and guess among the remaining ones. Don't dwell on these questions as you continue—put them out of your mind and focus on what lies ahead.

Be sure to read all of the answer choices, even if you're sure the first one is the right answer. Sometimes you'll find a better one if you keep reading. But don't second-guess yourself if you do immediately know the answer. Your gut instinct is usually right. Don't let test anxiety rob you of the information you know.

If you have time at the end of the test (and if the test format allows), go back and review your answers. Be cautious about changing any, since your first instinct tends to be correct, but make sure you didn't misread any of the questions or accidentally mark the wrong answer choice. Look over any you skipped and make an educated guess.

At the end, leave the test feeling confident. You've done your best, so don't waste time worrying about your performance or wishing you could change anything. Instead, celebrate the successful completion of this test. And finally, use this test to learn how to deal with anxiety even better next time.

Review Video: 5 Tips to Beat Test Anxiety
Visit mometrix.com/academy and enter code: 570656

Important Qualification

Not all anxiety is created equal. If your test anxiety is causing major issues in your life beyond the classroom or testing center, or if you are experiencing troubling physical symptoms related to your anxiety, it may be a sign of a serious physiological or psychological condition. If this sounds like your situation, we strongly encourage you to seek professional help.

Tell Us Your Story

We at Mometrix would like to extend our heartfelt thanks to you for letting us be a part of your journey. It is an honor to serve people from all walks of life, people like you, who are committed to building the best future they can for themselves.

We know that each person's situation is unique. But we also know that, whether you are a young student or a mother of four, you care about working to make your own life and the lives of those around you better.

That's why we want to hear your story.

We want to know why you're taking this test. We want to know about the trials you've gone through to get here. And we want to know about the successes you've experienced after taking and passing your test.

In addition to your story, which can be an inspiration both to us and to others, we value your feedback. We want to know both what you loved about our book and what you think we can improve on.

The team at Mometrix would be absolutely thrilled to hear from you! So please, send us an email at tellusyourstory@mometrix.com or visit us at mometrix.com/tellusyourstory.php and let's stay in touch.

Additional Bonus Material

Due to our efforts to try to keep this book to a manageable length, we've created a link that will give you access to all of your additional bonus material.

Please visit https://www.mometrix.com/bonus948/cnsadultgeron to access the information.